Clinical Manual of Psychosomatic Medicine

A Guide to Consultation-Liaison Psychiatry

Second Edition

Clinical Manual of Psychosomatic Medicine

A Guide to Consultation-Liaison Psychiatry

Second Edition

by

Kemuel L. Philbrick, M.D.
Assistant Professor of Psychiatry, College of Medicine at Mayo Clinic,
Rochester, Minnesota

James R. Rundell, M.D.
Professor of Psychiatry, College of Medicine at Mayo Clinic,
and Consultant in Psychiatry at Mayo Clinic, Jacksonville, Florida

Pamela J. Netzel, M.D.
Assistant Professor of Psychiatry, College of Medicine at Mayo Clinic,
Rochester, Minnesota

James L. Levenson, M.D.
Professor of Psychiatry, Medicine, and Surgery,
Virginia Commonwealth University School of Medicine, Richmond, Virginia

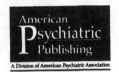

American Psychiatric Publishing
A Division of American Psychiatric Association

Washington, DC
London, England

Copyright © 2012 American Psychiatric Association
ALL RIGHTS RESERVED

15 14 13 12 11   5 4 3 2 1
First Edition

Typeset in AGaramond and Fomata Regular.

American Psychiatric Publishing, a Division of American Psychiatric Association
1000 Wilson Boulevard
Arlington, VA 22209-3901
www.appi.org

Library of Congress Cataloging-in-Publication Data
Clinical manual of psychosomatic medicine : a guide to consultation-liaison psychiatry / by Kemuel L. Philbrick ... [et al.]. — 2nd ed.
    p. ; cm.
    Rev. ed. of: Clinical manual of psychosomatic medicine / Michael G. Wise, James R. Rundell. 1st ed. c2005.
    Includes bibliographical references and index.
    ISBN 978-1-58562-393-8 (pbk. : alk. paper) 1. Consultation-liaison psychiatry. 2. Medicine, Psychosomatic. I. Philbrick, Kemuel L., 1956– II. Wise, Michael G., 1944– Clinical manual of psychosomatic medicine.
    [DNLM: 1. Psychophysiologic Disorders—diagnosis. 2. Psychophysiologic Disorders—therapy. 3. Mental Disorders—diagnosis. 4. Mental Disorders—therapy. 5. Psychotherapy—methods. 6. Referral and Consultation.   WM 90]
    RC455.2.C65W568 2012
    616.89¢14—dc23

                                                                            2011026355

British Library Cataloguing in Publication Data
A CIP record is available from the British Library.

Contents

PART I
General Considerations

PART II
Syndromes

PART III
Treatments

PART IV
Unique Issues in
Psychosomatic Medicine Settings

List of Tables and Figures

Preface

"Doctors learn at two levels: 1) the scientific, when the variables can be properly controlled, and 2) experiential, frequently without understanding, when the variables are uncontrolled." So wrote Eugene Stead, M.D., longtime Chair (1947–1967) of the Department of Medicine at Duke University. Although an internist, he also mused, "Many nervous systems are capable of doing things that you think your nervous system wouldn't think possible." Capturing the intersection of art and science, Dr. Stead summarized, "All disease sits in the substrate of a person: the soil in which things grow."

(Wagner et al. 1981, pp. 14, 16, 77)

The physician who finds the collision—or collusion—of medical, surgical, and psychiatric difficulties fascinating, fun, and challenging will find a friend in this volume. Internists, family physicians, psychiatry residents, and psychiatric consultants alike commonly encounter patients in whom the interface of medicine and psychiatry complicate disease and suffering. The authors intend the 28 chapters of this book to provide rich but practical and concise resources for the busy clinician in four sections:

1. *General Considerations,* such as medicolegal issues, mental status, personality, and suicidal issues in the medically ill;
2. *Syndromes* that occur frequently, such as anxiety, delirium, mood disorders, somatoform disorders, and substance abuse problems;
3. *Treatments,* including biological and psychopharmacological as well as psychosocial strategies; and

4. *Unique Issues in Psychosomatic Settings,* which include 13 areas such as cardiology, disaster and terrorism, fatigue and fibromyalgia, gastroenterology, oncology, and transplantation.

We believe it is essential for the informed physician who has trained as a psychiatrist to maintain 1) expertise in the administration and interpretation of the mental status examination, 2) knowledge about medical conditions and treatments, 3) expertise in identifying toxic and medical causes of psychiatric signs and symptoms, 4) skill in both psychopharmacology and psychotherapy, 5) dexterity in forming comprehensive biopsychosocial differential diagnoses, and 6) the ability to work comfortably and communicate clearly with medical-surgical colleagues.

We dedicate this second edition of the *Clinical Manual of Psychosomatic Medicine* to Michael G. Wise, M.D. In 1987, Dr. Wise coauthored the first edition of the *Concise Guide to Consultation Psychiatry.* He also coauthored the second and third editions of that text, published in 1994 and 2000, respectively. The Concise Guide was the predecessor to the first edition of the *Clinical Manual of Psychosomatic Medicine,* published in 2005, a work also coauthored by Dr. Wise. He further coauthored the first comprehensive textbook of Psychosomatic Medicine, *The American Psychiatric Publishing Textbook of Consultation-Liaison Psychiatry,* the first edition of which was published in 1996 and the second edition in 2002. These important textbooks blazed the trail for the current flagship textbook of our subspecialty, *The American Psychiatric Publishing Textbook of Psychosomatic Medicine,* and were accompanied by study guides and condensed versions. Dr. Wise, through his ground-breaking writing and through his loving mentorship of literally hundreds of general psychiatrists and psychosomatic medicine psychiatrists, has made an enduring impact on our subspecialty. In fact, he trained and mentored two of the authors of this book. For all of his contributions to our field, we owe Michael Wise an enormous debt of gratitude, and we are honored to dedicate this work to him.

Special thanks are due John McDuffie and Rebecca Richters of American Psychiatric Publishing (APP). Mr. McDuffie, Editorial Director at APP, orchestrated the conception and development of the project. Once a manuscript emerged, Ms. Richters, Senior Editor, Books, at APP choreographed the transformation of 500 pages of raw text into the book you are now reading. The finished product would simply never have seen the light of day but for their patient perspicacity and good humor.

Kemuel L Philbrick, M.D.
James R. Rundell, M.D.
Pamela J. Netzel, M.D.
James L. Levenson, M.D.

Reference

Wagner GS, Cebe B, Rozear MP, eds: To care for the person who has the illness, and, Most medical problems are not curable, in E.A. Stead, Jr.: What this patient needs is a doctor. Edited by Wagner GS, Cebe B, Rozear MP. Durham, NC, Duke Hospital, 1981, pp 14, 16, 77

Disclosure of Competing Interests

The authors had no competing interests during the year preceding manuscript submission.

PART I

General Considerations

Effective Psychiatric Consultation

History of Psychiatric Consultation

1920s–1930s

Psychosomatic medicine (PM) and consultation-liaison (CL) psychiatry began in the 1920s and 1930s with the development of general hospital psychiatry units and the PM movement (Lipowski and Wise 2002).

1930s–1950s

Rockefeller Foundation grants in 1934 and 1935 aided development of consultation psychiatry by establishing closer collaboration between psychiatrists and other physicians. A number of psychoanalysts contributed specific psychosomatic theories to the field during the 1930s through 1950s.

1960s–1970s

During the 1960s and 1970s, the number of CL psychiatry services grew, and a subspecialty scientific literature developed. In 1974, under the leadership of James Eaton, the Psychiatry Education Branch of the National Institute of

Mental Health (NIMH) supported the development and expansion of CL services throughout the United States, in part by providing grants for CL fellowships (Eaton et al. 1977). By 1980, NIMH supported 130 programs and materially contributed to the training of more than 300 CL psychiatry fellows (Lipowski and Wise 2002).

1980s–1990s

Federal budget cuts in the 1980s dramatically decreased the number of stipends for the "Eaton fellowships." Nevertheless, CL psychiatry continued to grow and develop during the 1980s and 1990s (Lipowski and Wise 2002), especially in academic and larger medical centers.

Since 2000

In 2003, the American Board of Medical Specialties (ABMS) approved PM as a subspecialty, and the American Board of Psychiatry and Neurology (ABPN) established a certifying examination. These actions have resulted in an expansion of PM fellowships and a move toward standardization of training requirements by the Accreditation Council for Graduate Medical Education (ACGME). The scope of the subspecialty, as defined by a list of competencies developed by the Academy of Psychosomatic Medicine (APM), the American Psychiatric Association (APA), and the ABPN, has become firmly established in both outpatient and inpatient consultative settings (Rundell et al. 2008; Worley et al. 2009). The emphasis on multidisciplinary, integrated care delivery is increasing in both primary care and specialty care settings (Kathol et al. 2009).

Trends Affecting Psychosomatic Medicine Practice

Limited Reimbursements

Direct reimbursement for psychiatric consultations, especially inpatient consultations, is limited. Medicare recently abolished consultation billing codes. PM psychiatrists must educate institutional physician and administration leaders about the value of consultation psychiatry in cost offset and quality of care outcomes. Payers often "carve out" psychiatric and other mental health payment structures from medical and surgical ones, increasing the difficulty of receiving reimbursements for psychiatric services to medical-surgical patients.

Outpatient Consultation

The scope of practice of PM in the outpatient setting is distinct from that of general outpatient psychiatry (Rundell et al. 2008). The most frequent conditions seen in the outpatient PM setting are depression and/or anxiety in patients who are medically ill, and unexplained medical symptoms. The enriched case mix, when added to the most frequent cases seen in inpatient CL work (delirium, depression, capacity determination, dementia), is an asset for fellowship and residency training.

Integrated Care

Psychiatric care provided in settings other than mental health sites has always been part of PM practice. Concepts of liaison psychiatry have evolved to the current models of integrated care. Integrated care involves the provision, by multidisciplinary team members, of individualized but evidence-based care based on either a clinical condition (e.g., obesity, infertility) or treatment setting (e.g., primary care, transplantation) (Kathol et al. 2009). Data support the efficacy of integrated care in terms of clinical outcomes, financial performance, and patient and provider satisfaction (Hunkeler et al. 2006; Kathol et al. 2009).

Subspecialty Certification

Since 2003, PM has been a recognized subspecialty of the ABMS. Although this status has not necessarily translated into improved financial viability of PM or CL services, it has resulted in standardization across training programs and academic departments. Consensus core competencies that define the subspecialty have been adopted and serve as benchmarks for skill development and affirmation (Worley et al. 2009).

Business of Consultation Practice

Make the Case to Payors That Psychiatric Disorders Are Frequent and Add to the Cost of Health Care

- *Psychiatric disorders are frequent.* From 30% to 60% of general hospital inpatients have diagnosable psychiatric disorders (Hall et al. 2002).

- *Psychiatric disorders increase health care costs.* Depression, anxiety, and cognitive dysfunction each has been shown to predict longer hospital stays and greater hospitalization costs, even after accounting for demographics, degree of physical impairment, type of hospital unit, medical diagnosis, and circumstances of admission (Levenson et al. 1990; Saravay and Lavin 1994).
- *Comorbidity increases health care costs.* Medical-psychiatric comorbidity predicts poorer outcomes and increased health care use and cost (Druss and Rosenheck 1999).
- *Psychiatric consultation is cost-effective.* Psychiatric consultation for general hospital patients and medical-surgical outpatients may reduce mortality, morbidity, length of stay, and hospital costs (Hall et al. 2002).

Make the Case That Maintaining the Financial Viability of Psychosomatic Medicine Services Is Essential to Overall Institutional Financial Performance

Psychiatric consultation services need to make the case that maintaining the financial viability of these services is essential to overall institutional financial performance. To help in proving this point, consultant services can do the following:

1. *Become involved in billing processes.* Because centralized billing departments often place a lower priority on psychiatric billing than on more lucrative surgical and procedure-based reimbursements, a psychiatric consultation service must have direct input into its inpatient and outpatient billing processes.
2. *List all diagnoses.* For each consult, a consultant should list all appropriate medical and psychiatric diagnoses and document specific diagnostic criteria for each major psychiatric diagnosis made.
3. *Rate complexity.* The consultant should keep in mind that the complexity of the case, number of diagnoses, amount of time spent, and amount of information included in the note may significantly alter the level of billing submitted for an initial consult or specialty evaluation.
4. *Work with administration.* The PM service chief should work closely with hospital administration to define and document sources of cost savings produced by the consultation service.

Characteristics of Effective Psychiatric Consultants

1. *Respond promptly to consultation requests.* Do today's work today.
2. *Establish the level of urgency:* emergent, urgent, or routine.
3. *Determine the center of gravity of the case.* Having time to address comprehensively all biopsychosocial issues a patient may have, especially in inpatient settings, is rare.
4. *Be flexible.* Perform consultations in both inpatient and outpatient settings.
5. *Respect patients' rights to know that the identified "customer" is the consulting physician.*
6. *Review medical data and spend time collecting essential information.* Helpful information sources include the medical record, physicians, nurses, family, friends, and caregivers.
7. *Use the biopsychosocial model.* Consider patients' predispositions, precipitants, and strengths.
8. *Make a well-reasoned differential diagnosis.* Consider medical, neurological, and psychiatric syndromes.
9. *Avoid not otherwise specified (NOS) diagnoses.* They usually do not convey helpful or specific information.
10. *Make specific recommendations* that are brief, goal oriented, and free of psychiatric jargon.
11. *Discuss findings and recommendations* with consultee physicians in person whenever possible.
12. *Follow up with a patient in the hospital until the goals of the consultation have been met, and arrange outpatient care when indicated.*
13. *Respect boundaries.* Do not take over aspects of the patient's medical care unless asked to do so.
14. *Read medical journals, and remain part of the medical community.*
15. *Educate medical administrators about cost-offset advantages of psychiatric consultation.*
16. *Work with the business office and staff to optimize reimbursement.*

Approach to Consultation

Consultation Style

Structured Versus Unstructured Interview Styles

Structured versus unstructured interview styles are not mutually exclusive, and both are necessary to obtain valuable longitudinal and cross-sectional information. The relative merits of an open-ended interview versus a structured clinical examination are debated (Shakin Kunkel et al. 2002).

Structured examination is necessary for some historical data and for parts of the mental status examination.

Value of Listening and Observing

Simply listening and observing provide much information needed to make a diagnosis and a biopsychosocial formulation. Use open-ended questions, such as the following:

- "What brings you into the clinic?"
- "How has this illness affected your life?"
- "Why do you think your doctor asked the psychiatrist to see you?"

Patient Confidentiality

Psychiatric consultation is a new experience for many patients. Many patients have never seen a psychiatrist before, did not request the consultation, and in the inpatient setting, may not have been informed about the consultation. The patients need to be made aware of confidentiality issues.

Confidentiality Limits

Confidentiality has limits in the consultation setting. Maintaining absolute doctor-patient confidentiality is not possible for a psychiatric consultant (Simon and Walker 2002), because the physician requesting the consult is the identified "customer" and expects an answer to the consultation. The best approach is to explain this dual relationship to the patient from the start.

Sharing of Medical Records

Medical records are read by others. The outpatient or inpatient medical record is a relatively public document. Notes regarding consultation visits are available not only to the referring physician but also to other providers in the health care system.

The Health Insurance Portability and Accountability Act (HIPAA) increased document protection requirements in health care settings. Particular care should be taken to satisfy these requirements when considering transmitting patient information via fax or electronic means (Office for Civil Rights 2002).

Patient Follow-Up

Patients should be followed up until the goals of consultation are met. Psychiatric consultants generally should follow up patients until they are discharged from the hospital or clinic or until the goals of the consultation are achieved. This is necessary for three reasons:

- *Urges to "sign off" on patients are sometimes related more to negative reactions* toward patients than to resolution of the presenting symptoms.
- *Symptoms can evolve and recur.* Premature sign-off creates a potential loss of credibility and may lead to reconsultation.
- *Follow-up enhances credibility.* Follow-up instills confidence that the consulting psychiatrist is available and willing to help.

The frequency and duration of psychiatric follow-up will vary depending on patient needs and financial circumstances (Simon and Walker 2002):

- *Focused consultation.* Many patients benefit from a single consultation visit, consisting of management recommendations to the consulting physician.
- *Brief intervention period.* Some patients need a brief intervention or follow-up, followed by referral back to the referring specialty or primary care physician.
- *Transfer to a specialty mental health setting.* Other patients need transfer to specialty mental health care clinics or units, for ongoing follow-up.
- *Shared follow-up or team management.* In many situations, a period of shared follow-up with an outpatient physician or team allows for continued involvement and learning.

Outpatient Psychosomatic Medicine Consultation Models

Traditional Outpatient Consultation

An outpatient primary care physician or specialist may ask a psychiatric consultant to see a patient regarding one or more specific questions. The consultant may see the patient once or for one or two follow-up visits to help "right the ship," with the expectation that the referring physician will resume overall care of the patient after the consultation or brief intervention. Occasional patients will need ongoing follow-up in an outpatient general psychiatry or PM practice.

Collaborative Consultation

Teams of PM psychiatrists, health psychologists, psychiatric nurses, and mental health allied health providers can provide collaborative team care for patients referred for consultation (Rundell et al. 2008). These teams work out of a mental health clinic, can discuss cases, see patients together or see patients consecutively, and conduct brief interventions. Having nurses and allied health providers collect basic historical information can increase efficiency and improve financial performance without detracting from patient or consultee satisfaction (Rundell and Seime 2008).

Integrated Care

Primary Care Settings

Teams of case managers, primary care physicians, and PM psychiatrists work together in primary care systems to detect and manage depression and other psychiatric disorders. Education, behavioral activation, antidepressants, and brief focused psychotherapy (problem-solving treatment) are used to manage the disorders before patients need specialty mental health treatment settings or programs. These programs deliver long-term benefits, better function, and enhanced quality of life for patients (Hunkeler et al. 2006).

Specialty Care Settings

PM psychiatrists often participate in integrated teams in specialty care outpatient settings and programs (Rundell et al. 2008). These specialty and subspecialty teams are becoming more common in major medical centers. Financial arrangements, which have to be negotiated with sponsoring clinical services, are often favorable when compared to fee-for-service consultation reimbursements. Examples of specialty care integrated teams include transplantation, bariatric surgery, oncology, women's health, infertility, dermatology, movement disorder, dementia, and rehabilitation services.

References

Druss BG, Rosenheck RA: Patterns of health care costs associated with depression and substance abuse in a national sample. Psychiatr Serv 50:214–218, 1999

Eaton JS Jr, Goldberg R, Rosinski E, et al: The educational challenge of consultation-liaison psychiatry. Am J Psychiatry 134 (March suppl):20–23, 1977

Hall RCW, Rundell JR, Popkin MK: Cost-effectiveness of the consultation-liaison service, in The American Psychiatric Publishing Textbook of Consultation-Liaison Psychiatry: Psychiatry in the Medically Ill, 2nd Edition. Edited by Wise MG, Rundell JR. Washington, DC, American Psychiatric Publishing, 2002, pp 25–32

Hunkeler EM, Katon W, Tang L, et al: Long term outcomes from the IMPACT randomised trial for depressed elderly patients in primary care. Br Med J 332:259–263, 2006

Kathol RG, Kunkel EJ, Weiner JS, et al: Psychiatrists for medically complex patients: bringing value at the physical health and mental health/substance-use disorder interface. Psychosomatics 50:93–107, 2009

Levenson JL, Hamer RM, Rossiter LD: Relation of psychopathology in general medical inpatients to use and cost of services. Am J Psychiatry 47:1498–1503, 1990

Lipowski ZJ, Wise TN: History of consultation-liaison psychiatry, in The American Psychiatric Publishing Textbook of Consultation-Liaison Psychiatry: Psychiatry in the Medically Ill, 2nd Edition. Edited by Wise MG, Rundell JR. Washington, DC, American Psychiatric Publishing, 2002, pp 3–11

Office for Civil Rights, Department of Health and Human Services: Standards for privacy of individually identifiable health information: final rule. Fed Regist 67:53182–53273, 2002

Rundell JR, Seime R: Comparison of an integrated, multidisciplinary outpatient psychosomatic medicine assessment model with traditional outpatient consultation. Poster presented at the annual meeting of the Academy of Psychosomatic Medicine, Miami, FL, November 2008

Rundell JR, Amundsen K, Rummans T, et al: Toward defining the scope of psychosomatic medicine practice: psychosomatic medicine in an outpatient, tertiary-care practice setting. Psychosomatics 49:487–493, 2008

Saravay SM, Lavin M: Psychiatric comorbidity and length of stay in the general hospital: a review of outcome studies. Psychosomatics 35:233–252, 1994

Shakin Kunkel EJ, Monti DA, Thompson TL II: Consultation, liaison, and administration of a consultation-liaison psychiatry service, in The American Psychiatric Publishing Textbook of Consultation-Liaison Psychiatry: Psychiatry in the Medically Ill, 2nd Edition. Edited by Wise MG, Rundell JR. Washington, DC, American Psychiatric Publishing, 2002, pp 13–23

Simon GE, Walker EA: The primary care clinic, in The American Psychiatric Publishing Textbook of Consultation-Liaison Psychiatry: Psychiatry in the Medically Ill, 2nd Edition. Edited by Wise MG, Rundell JR. Washington, DC, American Psychiatric Publishing, 2002, pp 917–925

Worley LLM, Levenson JL, Stern TA, et al: Core competencies for fellowship training in psychosomatic medicine: a collaborative effort by the APA Council on Psychosomatic Medicine, the ABPN Psychosomatic Committee, and the Academy of Psychosomatic Medicine. Psychosomatics 50:557–562, 2009

2

Medicolegal Issues

We begin this chapter with a legal disclaimer: The authors of this book are not lawyers, and the information in this chapter does not constitute legal advice. The views expressed in this chapter come from clinically active psychosomatic medicine (PM) psychiatrists, not legal experts. Laws vary from state to state, legal precedents change, and hospitals have their own policies (e.g., do-not-resuscitate orders). Therefore, clinicians must become familiar with pertinent general legal concepts, state laws, and hospital policies.

No substitute exists for good faith, common sense, excellent documentation, and a high standard of medical care (Shouton et al. 1991; Wright et al. 1996). Core competencies delineated by PM professional organizations emphasize that a high degree of knowledge about confidentiality, capacity, and other medicolegal concepts is an expected skill and competency of a PM psychiatrist (Bronheim et al. 1998; Worley et al. 2009). At times, however, a clinician might find it helpful or necessary to consult an attorney who understands the legal implications of these concepts as they apply to medical practice.

Definitions

- *Advance directives*—health care documents (i.e., living will, durable power of attorney, or health care proxy) executed by competent individuals to

13

state their health care preferences and values and/or to designate substitute health care decision makers in the event of future incompetence.

- *Capacity*—a clinician's determination, through examination, that an adult patient has the ability to understand and participate in decisions regarding his or her medical care.
- *Confidentiality*—ethical and legal duty not to disclose information obtained in the course of evaluating or treating the patient without the patient's express or implied permission.
- *Guardianship*—appointment by the court of a person to be legally responsible for the care and management of an incompetent person. (In most jurisdictions, a *conservator* is granted control of the individual's estate, whereas a *guardian* is granted control of the individual's person, or body.)
- *Health Information Portability and Accountability Act (HIPAA)*—federally codified set of standards with safeguards to protect privacy of patients and their health records.
- *Incompetency*—a court determination that a patient lacks the mental capacity to understand the nature of an act.
- *Informed consent*—voluntary agreement by a competent person after full disclosure of facts needed to make a decision.
- *Right to refuse treatment*—the right to determine what is or is not done to one's body (also called the right of self-determination).
- *Seclusion and restraint*—interventions that involve isolating the patient and/or use of physical or chemical immobilization.

Patient Confidentiality

Impact of HIPAA

Trust between a patient and physician is the foundation upon which a shared healing aim is built. HIPAA (Mermelstein and Wallack 2008; Office for Civil Rights 2002) has codified standards related to protection of patient privacy and confidentiality of inpatient and outpatient health records. These federal standards have had a significant impact on the practice of medicine in general and on the practice of consultation in particular (Mermelstein and Wallack 2008). A patient has the right to have confidential communications withheld from outside parties unless he or she gives written authorization to release that information (but there are exceptions, as noted in "Statutory Exceptions to Confidentiality" below).

Balance Patient Privacy Against Consultee Need to Know

Consultation work requires a balance between safeguarding patient privacy and answering a consultee physician's questions. This work is unique in that the patient is not the primary customer. Once a consult is generated, the answer is given to the consultee. The consultee can accept or reject the opinion and recommendations of the consultant. In this balancing act, the consultant should do the following:

1. *Discuss flow of information.* Consulting psychiatrists should be clear with patients at the beginning of the consultation about the flow of information.
2. *Communicate on a "need-to-know" basis.* Psychiatrists do not have the authorization to speak to hospital staff members about all matters revealed by the patient (Simon 2002). Psychiatrists should only provide information sufficient to enable the staff to function effectively on the patient's behalf. Rarely is it necessary to disclose intimate details about the patient's life.

Obtain Patient Permission Before Speaking With Family or Friends

A psychiatrist performing a consultation should not speak to a patient's family or significant other without the patient's permission. Fortunately, the patient's refusal to allow the physician to contact the family or significant other is uncommon. If the patient refuses, the patient's reasons should be documented in a clear note in the medical record.

Statutory Exceptions to Confidentiality

Although laws and regulations vary from one jurisdiction to the next, there are general exceptions to the absolute right to confidentiality (Simon 2002; Simon et al. 2005). These include the following:

- Child abuse
- Competency proceedings
- Court-ordered examination

- Danger to self or others
- Patient as a litigant
- Civil commitment proceedings
- Appropriate communications with other health care providers involved in the patient's care

Informed Consent and Right to Direct Medical Treatment

Definition of Informed Patient

Informed consent requires an informed patient. An informed patient is one who can understand the information provided and is capable of making a reasoned judgment about the treatment or procedure, regardless of whether others agree with the decision.

Exceptions to Informed Consent Requirement

Emergencies

When the physician administers appropriate treatment in a medically emergent situation in which the patient or other people are endangered, and when obtaining either the patient's consent or that of someone authorized to provide consent for the patient has proved impossible, the law typically "presumes" that consent was granted. This presumption is not universal, however, and there are exceptions, such as when a Jehovah's Witness patient plainly refuses a blood transfusion (Ferrando et al. 2010).

Incompetency

Only a competent person can provide informed consent. When the patient does not have the capacity to provide consent, it is obtained from a substitute decision maker.

Therapeutic Privilege

This exception is the most difficult to apply. Informed consent is not required if a psychiatrist, usually in concert with the consultee, determines that a complete disclosure of possible risks and alternatives might have a deleterious effect on a patient's health and welfare. This may not be a common clinical event in a consultation-liaison setting. The clinician should do the following:

- Carefully document the rationale supporting this determination.
- Consider obtaining a second opinion from a respected colleague.

Waiver

A patient may voluntarily waive his or her right to information (e.g., the patient does not want information on possible negative surgical outcomes).

Signing Out Against Medical Advice

Leaving a hospital or emergency department against medical advice (AMA) is the right of any competent patient, as long as he or she understands the nature and consequences of the act (Groves and Vaccarino 1987). AMA discharges constitute about 1% of all hospital dismissals. They commonly occur when patients are experiencing conflict in the doctor-patient relationship, are too anxious about their medical condition or treatment to engage in the treatment, have personal or work pressures to leave the hospital, or have an addictive disorder that has not been adequately diagnosed or treated in the hospital (e.g., nicotine withdrawal or cocaine craving). The clinician should do the following:

1. *Understand that the standard of capacity to sign out AMA will vary* depending on the risk-benefit ratio in a particular situation.
2. *Look for communication problems.* A threat or an attempt to sign out AMA often signifies a communication problem between the patient and the staff. Patients who leave AMA often return to the hospital if the physician has not explicitly denied further care.
3. *Document patient capacity and understanding.* If the patient is not a danger to self or others and demonstrates capacity in the context of the risks involved, the psychiatrist cannot do much more than try to ensure adequate documentation.
   - *Request that patients sign an AMA form.* A patient is requested but not required to sign the hospital's AMA form before departure. If the patient refuses to sign the form, the clinician should simply write on the

form, "Patient refused to sign form" or "Patient departed without signing the AMA form," and then sign and date the document.

- *Document the circumstances in the medical record.* Regardless of whether the patient signs an AMA form, the situation should be documented in the medical record, along with the annotated AMA form, detailing the recommendations made to the patient about further hospitalization and the possible risks of premature discharge.

Do-Not-Resuscitate and Do-Not-Intubate Orders

Patients who require cardiopulmonary resuscitation (CPR) or intubation to support breathing in a respiratory arrest usually have not thought about or expressed a preference about its use, and others have no time to think about the consequences of reviving a patient at the time of a cardiac arrest. Ideally, patients will have signed do-not-resuscitate (DNR) or do-not-intubate (DNI) orders before the necessity arises.

Exceptions to DNR and DNI Orders

A competent patient has the right to reject resuscitative treatment. That right is rarely overruled (Simon 2002; Simon et al. 2005), except in specific or narrow circumstances, including the following:

1. *When rights of a spouse or child take precedence.* At times, the rights of a dependent spouse or child are considered more important than the patient's decision (Miles et al. 1982).
2. *When the DNR and DNI orders are not available* and the emergency providers are unsure what the status is. In a review of medical incident reports in which emergency medical services were called to long-term care facilities, resuscitation was attempted in 21% of residents who had requested DNR status (Becker et al. 2003).
3. *When a cardiopulmonary arrest occurs during hemodialysis.* In such cases, resuscitation may be attempted in some hospitals even when a DNR order exists (Ross 2003).
4. *When families or guardians intervene legally.* When a competent patient either requests or declines resuscitation and later becomes incompetent, a court may be required to reverse the patient's original decision (Miles et al. 1982). In some states, the family or significant other, physician, and/or

hospital ethics committee can intervene to resuscitate the patient if a chance of recovery exists.

5. *When a patient is deemed to lack capacity.* If a patient has a major mental disorder (e.g., severe depression) and rejects resuscitation because he or she desires death as an "appropriate deserved" outcome, the patient is considered to lack capacity (Simon 2002; Simon et al. 2005). The consultant in this type of case would recommend that the family or significant other seek guardianship.

Documentation of DNR and DNI Orders

DNR and DNI orders should be documented in a physician order at each admission. DNR and DNI orders are typically recorded as a physician order, and the date, time, and reasons for the order are documented in the chart. Hospital CPR, DNR, and DNI policies vary considerably. Hemphill et al. (2004) studied all admissions for intracerebral hemorrhage in nonfederal hospitals in California over 2 years ($N=8,233$) and found that the percentage of patients with DNR orders varied from 0% to 70% across hospitals.

Advance Directives

The Patient Self-Determination Act requires all hospitals, nursing homes, hospices, managed care organizations, and home health care agencies to advise patients or family members of their right to accept or refuse medical care in the form of an advance directive (Simon 2002; Simon et al. 2005). A living will is an example of an advance directive. This law also states that a hospital must, if it wishes to receive Medicare and Medicaid payments (Greco et al. 1991), do the following:

1. Develop policies about advance directives.
2. Ask all patients admitted to the hospital if they have advance directives and enter those into the chart.
3. Give patients information about advance directives.
4. Educate the staff and community about advance directives.

Power of Attorney

Definition

A durable power of attorney empowers a trusted family member or other agent to make health care decisions. This document is much broader and more flexible than a living will, which covers just the period of a diagnosed terminal illness and specifies only that no extraordinary treatment be used to prolong life.

Revoking or Overriding a Power of Attorney

A patient may revoke a power of attorney document or a health care proxy, sometimes even when reasonable evidence indicates that the patient is incompetent (Simon 2002; Simon et al. 2005). If the patient is grossly confused and is an immediate danger to self and others, the physician is on firm medical and legal ground to temporarily override a patient's treatment refusal if it varies from written wishes or directions expressed by a designated power of attorney. Generally, however, it is better to seek a court order for treatment than to risk legal entanglement by attempting to enforce an advance directive's original terms if a patient has expressed the desire to revoke it.

Capacity

Competency Versus Capacity

In general, *competency* refers to some minimal mental, cognitive, or behavioral ability, trait, or capability required to perform a particular legally recognized act or to assume a legal role (Simon 2002; Simon et al. 2005). Determination of incompetency is a judicial decision, whereas *incapacity* refers to a clinical opinion that is rendered by a consulting psychiatrist (or other clinician) (Leo 1999; Mishkin 1989). Evaluation of capacity is a core skill of PM psychiatrists (Worley et al. 2009). Consultations to "evaluate competency" are actually evaluations for capacity.

- *Incapacity does not prevent treatment.* It merely means that the clinician must obtain substitute consent on the patient's behalf.
- *The determination of capacity is not an all-or-none phenomenon.* For example, a patient may be judged incompetent by the court to manage financial affairs but still may be considered competent to refuse a medical procedure.
- *Most patients are found to have capacity when capacity has been questioned* (Farnsworth 1990; Mebane and Rauch 1990).

- *Most capacity consults are requested* because a patient refuses treatment or disposition (e.g., transfer from the hospital to a nursing home) or threatens to leave the hospital AMA (Farnsworth 1990; Masand et al. 1998; Mebane and Rauch 1990).
- *Some capacity consults are to confirm a patient's capacity to give informed consent.* Because the patient's mental status can change from one hour to the next, repetitive examinations are often necessary.

Elements of Capacity Evaluation

A flexible approach to assessment of capacity is important for the consultation psychiatrist to understand and apply (Roth et al. 1977; Simon et al. 2005). The matrix commonly used to organize the elements of capacity evaluation has stood the test of time and is still valid. It is based on two variables:

1. The treatment's risk-benefit ratio
2. The patient's decision regarding treatment

Capacity Threshold

Capacity can be evaluated at different thresholds, depending on the patient's clinical situation (Magid et al. 2006).

High Threshold to Establish Capacity

Patient refuses low-risk, high-benefit intervention. For example, a patient has a gangrenous leg, and amputation is proposed to save the patient's life. The danger (potential risk) of this procedure to the patient is relatively low, and the benefits are high. Therefore, if the patient refuses amputation, a rigorous (high) threshold to establish capacity is applied. Failure to pass this competency test, indicating that the patient lacks capacity, would lead the psychiatrist to recommend that the physician and the patient's family or significant other pursue court action to appoint a surrogate decision maker.

Patient consents to a high-risk intervention with low or high benefit. Consent to a heart transplant requires a stringent (high) threshold to establish competency because of the high mortality and morbidity associated with the procedure.

Low Threshold to Establish Capacity

Patient consents to low-risk, high-benefit intervention. If the patient consents to amputation, a lenient (low) threshold to establish competency is used.

Patient refuses high-risk, low-benefit intervention. If a patient declines a surgical procedure that is quite risky (e.g., a Whipple procedure in a patient with pancreatic cancer), a lenient (low) threshold to establish competency is applied.

Capacity Documentation

Documentation of capacity should be precise. The clinician should write exact quotations in the medical record whenever possible, especially if the patient is refusing potentially life-saving or life-altering treatment. In some cases, the clinician may want a witness present who can verify that the details of the interview were reported accurately in the medical record.

Documentation of cognitive examination is necessary but not sufficient. Impairment on a mental status examination (e.g., a Mini-Mental State Examination score of 18) is insufficient to declare a patient incompetent to make medical decisions. Such tests measure cognitive ability, not the ability to make decisions (Leo 1999). The consulting psychiatrist should use open-ended questions (e.g., "Tell me about your current medical condition"), avoid yes-no questions, and pursue or clarify vague answers.

The clinician should document patient understanding about the decision.

- Does the patient understand the current medical condition?
- Can the patient discuss the expected course of the medical condition, with and without treatment?
- Does the patient articulate an understanding about the recommended treatment and the risks and benefits of treatment?
- Does the patient understand the alternatives, when appropriate?

Encourage Documentation of Wishes While Patient Has Capacity

When the chance of future incompetency is high (e.g., when a patient has Alzheimer's disease or cancer with brain metastasis), the consulting psychiatrist should urge the patient and family or significant other to discuss the patient's preferences. The patient, while still competent, can prepare a living will or a durable power of attorney.

Guardianship

Legal Establishment of Substitute Decision Maker

For individuals who are judicially determined to be unable to act for themselves, guardianship establishes a substitute decision maker (Leo 1999). In general, the appointment of a guardian is limited to situations in which the individual's decision-making capacity is so impaired that he or she is unable to care for personal safety or provide necessities such as food, shelter, clothing, and medical care, and the impairment is considered permanent. Some states have a provision for emergency or temporary guardianship (e.g., 60 or 90 days), after which a second judicial hearing is conducted to determine whether to remove the guardianship or convert it to permanent status.

Standard of Proof for Incompetency

The standard of proof required for a judicial determination of incompetency is clear and convincing evidence. Although the law does not assign percentages to proof, clear and convincing evidence is in the range of 75% certainty (Simon 2002; Simon et al. 2005). The process required to adjudicate incompetence and assign a guardian can be burdensome, costly, and lengthy (Burruss et al. 2000).

Specific Versus General Guardianship

A *specific guardian* is authorized to make decisions about a particular subject area, such as major or emergency medical procedures. A *general guardian,* by contrast, has total control over another individual's person, estate, or both (Sales et al. 1982).

Choice of Guardian

Clear advantages are associated with having a family member as the substitute decision maker (Leo 1999). First, appointment of a family member as guardian maintains the integrity of the family unit and relies on those who are most likely to know the patient's wishes. Second, this arrangement is more efficient and less costly. Having a family member as guardian is not always possible, however. Sometimes no family member is available, or family members prefer not to play that role. In rare cases, there may be grounds for concern that a family member will exploit the responsibility; in such situations, the court may determine that an incompetent person's best interests will be served by appointment of a guardian *ad litem,* commonly an attorney, social worker, or certified public advocate.

Involuntary Hospitalization

Substantive Criteria for Statutory Commitment

There are three main substantive criteria for statutory commitment (although some states have additional provisions). An individual must be determined to be one or more of the following (Simon 2002; Simon et al. 2005):

- Mentally ill
- Dangerous to self or others
- Unable to provide for basic needs (i.e., gravely disabled)

Legal Commitment

Commitment is a legal decision, not a medical one. Clinicians do not legally commit patients; only a court can do that. A consulting psychiatrist merely initiates a medical certification that brings the patient before the court, which usually occurs after a brief evaluation in the hospital (Simon 2002; Simon et al. 2005).

Role of Consulting Psychiatrist in Involuntary Holding of Patients

Consulting psychiatrists must play an active role when patients are held involuntarily in a medical or surgical unit. Two types of patients are held involuntarily in these units: 1) patients who may or may not have a psychiatric disorder but require involuntary medical treatment because they lack capacity to refuse it and 2) patients being held for psychiatric reasons (e.g., an overdose patient is recovering in an intensive care unit until he or she can be transferred to inpatient psychiatric care). In the latter circumstance, patients cannot be transferred immediately to a locked psychiatric unit to be held for evaluation. Consulting psychiatrists must play active roles in educating the physicians and nursing staff of a medical or surgical unit regarding procedures related to safely holding patients for further evaluation, which may lead to a commitment hearing.

Involuntary Hospitalization and Commitment Laws

Laws governing involuntary hospitalization and commitment vary from state to state. A psychiatrist providing consultations to other physicians needs to be knowledgeable about local commitment laws and procedures, as well as local mental health treatment resources. For example, states have different laws and regulations that govern how long a patient may be held for a safety evaluation in preparation for a legal commitment hearing.

Seclusion and Restraint

Safety of Patient and Others

Legal and ethical expectations are that the minimum amount of seclusion and restraint should be used to protect the safety of patients and staff. Courts hold that seclusion and restraint are appropriate only when a patient presents an imminent risk of harm to self or others and when a less restrictive alternative is not available (Simon 2002; Simon et al. 2005).

Documentation Requirements

Documentation requirements are precise and not negotiable. Every hospital actively monitors and strives to minimize restraint and seclusion. Seclusion and restraint must be implemented by a written order from an appropriate medical official. Because jurisdictions and hospitals may vary in implementation procedures, psychiatrists need to be thoroughly familiar with local policies.

1. The examining physician must document the following:
   - Reasons for seclusion or restraint
   - Details of the patient's behavior
   - Details of the examination
   - Types of restraint needed (e.g., two-point, waist-belt, vest, medication)

2. Orders must be confined to specific, time-limited periods.
   - The patient's physical and mental condition must be regularly reviewed and documented.
   - Extension of the original order must be reviewed and reauthorized.

Prescribing Medications for Nonapproved Uses

Absence of a U.S. Food and Drug Administration (FDA) indication does not necessarily mean that no evidence base exists for the use of a drug for a specific clinical reason. The FDA evaluates only the clinical indications requested by a pharmaceutical company. Failure to indicate other uses typically means that the FDA did not receive a request to review related data. The FDA applies the principle that good medical practice requires that a physician prescribe medication according to the best information available. Prescribing an FDA-approved medication for a nonapproved purpose does not violate federal law (Macbeth et al. 1994). However, the physician who deviates from approved FDA indications has a responsibility to document the rationale for the practice.

Consultation psychiatrists frequently recommend or prescribe medications for uses not approved by the FDA. For example, no drug is currently approved by the FDA for the treatment of delirium; however, several drugs, mainly antipsychotics, are used. Prescribing drugs for nonapproved uses should be based on sound knowledge of the drugs, firm scientific rationale, and medical data (Simon 2002; Simon et al. 2005).

The threshold for informed consent is heightened when a medication is prescribed for a nonapproved use. The situation is often urgent, and the patient may lack capacity. Recommendations to administer drugs for nonapproved indications require documentation of patient or family education and a rationale for the recommendation. Many hospitals have developed algorithms or clinical protocols for treatment of conditions such as delirium, based on evidence-supported clinical practice guidelines. These protocols help standardize clinical practice and may buttress clinicians' medicolegal status when prescribing drugs for nonapproved indications.

Malpractice

Documentation

Documentation is important when malpractice is alleged. When a medicolegal issue arises or might arise at some future time, detailed documentation in the patient's medical record is of paramount importance. Fear that the patient will read the record should not preclude documentation. In fact, the consultation and notes should be written with the expectation that the patient will read the medical record.

Establishing Malpractice

Four elements are necessary to establish malpractice. Each involves the consideration of a question.

1. *The standard of care can be established.* Would a reasonable, careful, and prudent physician behave in the same or a similar way?
2. *The physician breached the standard of care.* Did the physician breach that standard of care in this specific case?
3. *The patient sustained an injury.* Was the patient demonstrably injured?
4. *The physician's behavior caused the injury.* Did the physician's unreasonable, careless, or inappropriate behavior cause that injury?

References

Becker LJ, Yeargin K, Rea TD, et al: Resuscitation of residents with do not resuscitate orders in long-term care facilities. Prehosp Emerg Care 7:303–306, 2003

Bronheim HE, Fulop G, Kunkel EJ, et al: Practice guidelines for psychiatric consultation in the general medical setting. Psychosomatics 39:S8–S30, 1998

Burruss JW, Kunik ME, Molinari V, et al: Guardianship applications for elderly patients: why do they fail? Psychiatr Serv 51:522–524, 2000

Farnsworth MG: Competency evaluations in a general hospital. Psychosomatics 31:60–66, 1990

Ferrando SJ, Levenson JL, Owen JA: Infectious diseases, in Clinical Manual of Psychopharmacology in the Medically Ill. Edited by Ferrando SJ, Levenson JL, Owen JA. Washington, DC, American Psychiatric Publishing, 2010, pp 371–404

Greco PJ, Schulman KA, Lavizzo-Mourey R, et al: The Patient Self-Determination Act and the future of advance directives. Ann Intern Med 115:639–643, 1991

Groves JE, Vaccarino JM: Legal aspects of consultation, in Massachusetts General Hospital Handbook of General Hospital Psychiatry, 2nd Edition. Edited by Hackett TP, Cassem NH. Littleton, MA, PSG Publishing, 1987, pp 591–604

Hemphill JC 3rd, Newman J, Zhao S, et al: Hospital usage of early do-not-resuscitate orders and outcome after intracerebral hemorrhage. Stroke 35:1130–1134, 2004

Leo RJ: Competency and the capacity to make treatment decisions: a primer for primary care physicians. Prim Care Companion J Clin Psychiatry 1:131–141, 1999

Macbeth JE, Wheeler AM, Sither JW, et al: Legal and Risk Management Issues in the Practice of Psychiatry. Washington, DC, Psychiatrists Purchasing Group, 1994

Magid M, Dodd ML, Bostwick JM, et al: Is your patient making the "wrong" treatment choice? Curr Psychiatry 5:13–20, 2006

Masand PS, Bouckoms AJ, Fischel SV, et al: A prospective multicenter study of competency evaluations by psychiatric consultation services. Psychosomatics 39:55–60, 1998

Mebane AH, Rauch HB: When do physicians request competency evaluations? Psychosomatics 31:40–46, 1990

Mermelstein HT, Wallack JJ: Confidentiality in the age of HIPAA: a challenge for psychosomatic medicine. Psychosomatics 49:97–103, 2008

Miles SH, Cranford R, Schultz AL: The do-not-resuscitate order in a teaching hospital. Ann Intern Med 96:660–664, 1982

Mishkin B: Determining the capacity for making health care decisions, in Issues in Geriatric Psychiatry (Advances in Psychosomatic Medicine Series, Vol 19). Edited by Billig N, Rabins PV. Basel, Switzerland, Karger, 1989, pp 151–166

Office for Civil Rights, Department of Health and Human Services: Standards for privacy of individually identifiable health information: final rule. Fed Regist 67:53182–53273, 2002

Ross LF: Do not resuscitate orders and iatrogenic arrest during dialysis: should "no" mean "no"? Semin Dial 16:395–398, 2003

Roth LH, Meisel A, Lidz CW: Tests of competency to consent to treatment. Am J Psychiatry 134:279–284, 1977

Sales BD, Powell DM, Van Duizend R: Disabled Persons and the Law, Vol 1: Law, Society, and Policy Services. New York, Plenum, 1982, p 461

Shouton R, Groves JE, Vaccarino JM: Legal aspects of consultation, in Massachusetts General Hospital Handbook of General Hospital Psychiatry, 3rd Edition. Edited by Cassem NH. St. Louis, MO, Mosby–Year Book, 1991, pp 619–638

Simon RI: Legal and ethical issues, in The American Psychiatric Publishing Textbook of Consultation-Liaison Psychiatry: Psychiatry in the Medically Ill, 2nd Edition. Edited by Wise MG, Rundell JR. Washington, DC, American Psychiatric Publishing, 2002, pp 167–189

Simon RI, Schindler BA, Levenson JL: Legal issues, in The American Psychiatric Publishing Textbook of Psychosomatic Medicine. Edited by Levenson JL. Washington DC, American Psychiatric Publishing, 2005, pp 37–54

Worley LLM, Levenson JL, Stern TA, et al: Core competencies for fellowship training in psychosomatic medicine: a collaborative effort by the APA Council on Psychosomatic Medicine, the ABPN Psychosomatic Committee, and the Academy of Psychosomatic Medicine. Psychosomatics 50:557–562, 2009

Wright M, Samuels A, Streimer J: Clinical practice issues in consultation-liaison psychiatry. Aust N Z J Psychiatry 30:238–245, 1996

3

Mental Status and Cognitive Examination

The mental status examination (MSE) is the psychiatrist's stethoscope; alert observation before, during, and after an evaluation of the patient yields a reflection of mind and body function that is indispensable to accurate diagnosis and effective care. MSE results are best understood when placed in the context of the patient's history and recent behavior, physical and neurological examination, laboratory data, and collateral information. The MSE is multifaceted in that some elements rely on astute observation, whereas others are drawn from the patient's self-report, and some portions are informal and less structured, whereas others rely on formal, structured questions or tasks. Framing the examination in two general categories, the noncognitive and the cognitive, can also be helpful, although there are areas of overlap.

Noncognitive Elements of Mental Status Examination

General Appearance and Behavior

The MSE begins the moment the clinician sees the patient. The patient's physical appearance—including grooming, dress or lack thereof, posture, mannerisms, and behaviors such as eye contact, facial expression, increased or decreased body movements, pacing, tremors, and choreiform or dyskinetic movements—shape impressions of a patient's demeanor and shed light on his or her mental function and psychological state at that particular time. Observation can provide valuable corroboration of a patient's story, or raise doubt either when a patient demonstrates a paucity of emotional investment in the symptoms described or when a patient denies any distress but is riddled with nervousness. The clinician should describe observations without the use of jargon.

Speech

Speech is disrupted by psychological factors and brain disease, particularly when the latter involves dominant-hemisphere insults. Speech is commonly described in terms of the following characteristics, as demonstrated by the examples provided:

- *Rate*—the pressured speech of the manic patient on high-dose steroids; the retarded speech of the depressed patient
- *Volume*—the loud speech of the angry patient; the soft, trailing speech of the patient with Parkinson's disease
- *Articulation*—the strained, distorted sounds with which a poststroke patient strives to forge once-familiar words; the slurred speech of the intoxicated patient; the mumbled words of a patient who hopes the examiner will give up and leave
- *Rhythm and fluency*—the long latent pauses in the speech of patients who are depressed or obsessive; the stuttering or the staccato-like bursts of words from an anxious patient
- *Prosody* (i.e., vocal inflection)—the emphatic embellishments of the histrionic patient; the flat monotone of an individual who has suffered a right parietal stroke
- *Other abnormalities of speech*—mutism (which may be a hysterical reaction to extreme stress, an expression of catatonia, or the result of neurological injury); aphonia or dysphonia (e.g., a patient may speak only in a hoarse whisper, caused by ninth cranial nerve or vocal cord disease or dissociative phenomena); paraphasias; echolalia (which can have either organic or other origins)

Thought Process

Thought process is assessed by observing the patient's speech and behavior. When the clinician asks the patient a question, how does the patient respond? Does the patient provide an answer that is directly responsive to the question asked (linear and goal-directed response), or meander through a circuitous account before eventually answering (circumstantial response), or ramble ever further afield (tangential response)? The pattern of thoughts is also an important reflection of thought process. The patient's thoughts may move extremely rapidly from one idea to another (flight of ideas); may skip linking connections, leaving the listener scrambling to follow the patient's line of reasoning (loose associations); or may stop suddenly (thought blocking).

Thought Content

The patient's thought content or major themes reflect the patient's immediate and prevailing concerns, including obsessional preoccupation, suicidal or homicidal ideation, misperceptions, and irrational beliefs. The patient's behavior also sheds light on thought content. A patient who is reluctant to talk and acts very suspiciously is usually paranoid, even if he or she denies it. The importance of observed behavior in the assessment of thought content is illustrated by a patient who denies misperceptions but is seen responding to hallucinations. Disorders of perception include the following:

- *Illusions*—misinterpretations of a real sensory experience.
- *Delusions*—fixed false beliefs not attributable to cultural or religious beliefs.
- *Ideas of reference*—incorrect interpretations that events have direct reference to oneself.
- *Hallucinations*—sensory perceptions in the absence of an external stimulus. Hallucinatory perception can be auditory, visual, tactile, olfactory (smell), gustatory (taste), or kinesthetic (body movement). Although cultural variations occur, hallucinations that occur in an awake individual are almost always symptomatic of a pathological process.
  1. *Auditory hallucinations* are more typically seen in primary psychiatric disorders.
  2. *Visual hallucinations* are typically associated with brain dysfunction, although they also occur in nonpsychiatric patients with severe recent visual loss and in some patients with schizophrenia (Bracha et al. 1989).

3. *Tactile hallucinations* may occur during substance-induced withdrawal delirium and are often experienced after a limb amputation. "Phantom limb" sensation, the feeling that the amputated limb is still present, occurs in most patients who undergo amputation. Over time, the tactile hallucinations diminish and usually completely disappear.

4. *Olfactory, gustatory, or kinesthetic hallucinations* are rare and are most commonly experienced by patients with partial seizures (Lishman 1998).

Mood

Mood is the patient's pervasive and sustained emotional state. Terms used to describe mood include *euthymic, dysphoric, depressed, elevated, euphoric, expansive,* and *irritable.* Some clinicians record both a patient's subjective description of his or her mood and the physician's objective assessment of that patient's mood, using the patient's conduct and demeanor throughout the examination to form a considered judgment. (An alternate perspective to that described here is that some clinicians define *mood* as the patient's expression of how he or she feels and *affect* as the objective assessment of mood by the examiner.)

Affect

Affect is to *mood* as *weather* is to *climate.* The parameters used to describe affect—the patient's moment-to-moment emotional states—are range, intensity, lability, reactivity, and consonance or appropriateness.

- *Affective range* may be full (i.e., the patient shows a wide range of emotional states during the interview) or narrow. The latter is sometimes distinguished as *restricted* when the patient's affect is impassive or *constricted* when the range is narrow but confined on the affective spectrum (e.g., "constricted at the dysphoric [or gleeful] end of the spectrum").
- *Affective intensity* can vary greatly across patients, from the rage seen in a patient with borderline personality disorder to the flat expression often observed in a patient with Parkinson's disease.
- *Affective lability* (i.e., extremely rapid emotional shifts) may imply a toxic or medical etiology but is also observed in some patients with prominent characterological struggles and bipolar disorder.

- *Affective reactivity* (i.e., the patient's capacity to register an emotional response, such as gratitude for empathy or a smile at shared humor) offers a clue to thought process and content as well as available emotional energy with which the patient engages his or immediate surroundings.
- *Affect that is either appropriate or inappropriate* to the topics under discussion is another important observation.

Suicidality and Homicidality

Suicidality and homicidality reside in the patient's thought content but are commonly recorded separately for ease of reference in light of their salience. A patient's wish and/or subsequent ideation may be active (deliberate cognitive engagement with the act and its consequences) or passive (e.g., thinking "If God would take me, it would be a relief"). The ideation, even if active, may or may not give rise to acknowledged intent. Also, intent may or may not mature into a specific plan, sometimes with attached contingencies. Lastly, active ideation leading to intent and a plan may yet be in the planning stage or may have already precipitated action.

Insight and Judgment

Insight is present if the patient realizes that a problem exists, that his or her thinking and behavior may contribute to that problem, and that he or she may need assistance. Judgment is an individual's ability to correctly anticipate the consequences of his or her behavior and to conduct himself or herself in a culturally acceptable way. Although judgment is often inferred by the patient's answer to a question, such as, "What would you do if you found a stamped, addressed envelope lying next to a mailbox?" the fact that a patient would put the aforementioned envelope in the mailbox does not mean that judgment is unimpaired, especially if that patient has just walked into the hospital hallway naked and recently urinated in the corner of his room. Thus, more useful questioning tests the patient's judgment relevant to his or her situation, such as asking a patient with diabetes what she would do if her glucose exceeds 400, or asking an elderly patient who is living alone what he would do if he runs out of medicine on the weekend. Recent behavior is the best way to gauge a patient's judgment.

Cognitive Elements of Mental Status Examination

General Considerations

Cognitive impairment occurs frequently in elderly patients who are medically ill, especially those who are hospitalized. Unless it is severe, this impairment often is not recognized by nonpsychiatric physicians and medical personnel (Laurila et al. 2004). The consulting psychiatrist also may miss the cognitive impairment if he or she depends too much on conversation during the interview to identify impairments and does not formally test brain function. Just as a cardiologist uses stress testing to reveal cardiac ischemia, the consulting psychiatrist must deliberately stress brain function to confidently uncover cognitive compromise. In performing an MSE, the clinician should keep in mind several important considerations:

1. *Be aware of inherent challenges.* Assessing a patient's mental status in the hospital environment can be difficult. Hospital rooms are noisy, and privacy is often lacking. Interruptions and distractions—such as intravenous alarms, a roommate who is groaning or loudly talking with visitors, and a harried nurse or phlebotomist who must have immediate access to the patient—are common. In addition, the patient is ill, often frightened, and frequently sleep deprived; sometimes, a patient has not seen a psychiatrist before and was not told about the consultation.

2. *Optimize patient performance.* Before the examination begins, the psychiatrist should ensure that the patient has his or her usual sensory aids (e.g., glasses, hearing aid). Whenever possible, roommates and others, including family members, should be asked to leave the room during the examination, thereby providing some privacy and preventing significant others from answering for the patient when specific questions are asked.

3. *Test the whole brain.* Tests of right-hemisphere, or nondominant, brain function are as important as more traditional tests of verbal function, which are the domain of the left hemisphere. The psychiatrist who asks the patient to remember verbal items but does not have the patient draw and recall shapes essentially ignores testing an important part of the brain's function (Ovsiew 1992).

4. *Respect the value of assessment.* Residents are often tempted to sheepishly preface a structured MSE by saying, "I just have a few silly questions for you now. I ask everyone these questions." Most patients are too polite to inquire why someone would ask "silly questions" as part of a serious evaluation, much less ask them of everyone. Rightly understood, the questions are no more silly than an internist feeling the quality of the carotid pulse wave or probing the depth of pretibial edema with a thumb.

Level of Consciousness and Orientation

Psychiatric consultation is often requested for patients who have a rapid or recent change in mental status. In many instances, these patients are either lethargic or agitated following surgery, have developed an infection or started taking a new medication, or have significant changes in metabolic status. In addition to changes in arousal, such patients often have hallucinations and altered thought content. The psychiatrist should gauge the patient's situational awareness by directly asking about orientation to self, place, and time. Intervals of time are difficult for delirious or demented patients to track but can easily be assessed by asking the patient how long he or she has been in the hospital. Serial measurement of orientation provides valuable longitudinal and treatment outcome data. The clinician should not rely on a medical chart entry stating "alert and oriented × 4." That usually means that the patient is arousable and generally cooperative; it does not mean that the patient's orientation was tested or that he or she is not delirious.

Attention

The capacity to direct and maintain one's attention while screening out extraneous and irrelevant stimuli is a fundamental yet highly complex cognitive function. Inattention (the breakdown of selective attention) and distractibility are common and clinically significant neuropsychiatric symptoms. Inattention also can complicate the entire evaluation process (Mesulam 1985). For example, an inattentive patient will frequently fail tests of memory or calculation on the basis of inattention alone. Standard tests for attention include digit span, spelling a five-letter word backward, reciting the months of the year backward, or subtracting serial 7s (or 3s for those who cannot do 7s).

Language

Language disturbances, specifically aphasias, refer to defects in word choice, comprehension, and syntax. The clinician should consider whether the patient's language is fluent and whether the words the patient chooses form a unified whole and make sense. Next, comprehension must be tested, which is particularly important when a patient is on a ventilator and normal speech is not possible. The clinician can ask yes-no questions, such as, "Do you put on your socks before your shoes?" "Is there a tree in this room?" and "Can an elephant ride a tricycle?" to establish comprehension and avoid being fooled by an interactive but uncomprehending patient.

Memory

The clinician should ask the patient to remember four unrelated items, such as tulip, bottle, courage, and olive. The patient should immediately repeat all four words to ensure that he or she has properly heard, understood, and registered them. After about 3 minutes of conversation or examination, the clinician should ask the patient to repeat the words. If the patient cannot recall the words, the clinician should give the patient clues to determine whether the words were not encoded into memory or were encoded but are difficult to retrieve. Patients who did not learn the words are not aided by prompting, whereas patients who learned the words but have difficulty accessing them usually will recall with prompting. Testing right-brain function is accomplished by asking the patient to copy three geometric shapes and then, after several minutes, to draw them from memory. In some situations, the clinician can hide three objects in the room while the patient is watching, and then ask the patient to find them later in the interview.

Abstraction

Educational level is a strong determinant of a person's ability to abstract. The clinician usually conducts bedside testing by asking the patient to interpret proverbs, such as, "The image maker does not worship the gods" or "The golden hammer breaks the iron door." Selecting an unfamiliar proverb is preferable because it reduces the likelihood of an automatic response (Sims 2003). The patient need not reply with a definitive interpretation, because the assessment has more to do with the patient's approach than with the "correctness" of his or her answer. Concrete interpretations are more commonly given by individuals with less than a high school education, schizophrenia (whose interpretations are also often bizarre), and dementia. The ability to abstract can also be assessed more subtly by observing the patient's response to and use of figures of speech, analogies, and metaphors.

Screening Tools for Bedside Cognitive Assessment

Several bedside examinations can be used to screen patients for cognitive dysfunction. For nonpsychiatric physicians who do not typically perform a formal MSE or for medical students who are learning to treat mental status problems, screening MSEs are useful. In addition, serial screening MSEs are often used to follow up the clinical course of a patient with delirium, especially in response to treatment. Also, the score obtained from a screening MSE may influence a physician who doubts that the patient is cognitively impaired but believes "hard data." For the consultation psychiatrist, however, a screening MSE is only one part of a more extensive cognitive examination.

Advantages and Disadvantages

Advantages of most bedside screening tools include the following:

- Brief time requirements (can be completed in 5–10 minutes)
- Structured format
- Simple administration and scoring
- Minimal effort required of medical patients

Disadvantages of most bedside screening tools include the following:

- Failure to identify focal deficits
- Failure to identify mild global deficits
- Dependence on education (risk of false negatives in well-educated patient with deficits and of false positives in patients with limited education)
- False sense of security when score indicates "normal" function

Commonly Used Bedside Cognitive Screening Tools

Mini-Mental Status Examination

The Mini-Mental Status Examination (MMSE) is probably the most widely used and best-known screening MSE (Folstein et al. 1975). The MMSE takes about 5 minutes to administer, can be administered serially to monitor a patient's clinical course, and is a reliable and valid MSE for medical patients (Nelson et al. 1986). A score of 20 or less may indicate impairment (Folstein et al. 1975); however, Mungas (1991) proposed that scores of 0–9 correspond to severe cognitive impairment, 10–20 to moderate impairment, 21–24 to mild impairment, and 25–30 to questionable impairment or intact function. A high score on the MMSE is insufficient to declare that the patient has normal cognitive function.

Short Test of Mental Status

The Short Test of Mental Status (STMS) was developed to be more sensitive than the MMSE for assessing problems of learning and recall in patients with early and mild dementia (Kokmen et al. 1987, 1991). Additionally, the STMS includes items that allow an improved evaluation of abstract reasoning and mental agility in comparison with the MMSE (Tang-Wai et al. 2003).

Montreal Cognitive Assessment

The Montreal Cognitive Assessment (MoCA; available at www.mocatest.org) is a 30-item test that can be administered in 10 minutes and was developed to better discriminate between mild cognitive impairment and normal function (Nasreddine et al. 2005). The MoCA also contains elements, such as a modified Trail Making Test, that help assess executive function.

Addenbrooke's Cognitive Examination

Addenbrooke's Cognitive Examination–Revised (ACE-R) is a detailed bedside cognitive screening test that requires the clinician to read from a copy of the test during administration (Miosha et al. 2006). The ACE-R can be administered in 15–20 minutes. The instrument, on which patients can score up to 100 points, assesses complex language and executive function, as well as visuospatial ability. The ACE-R is more sensitive to early deficits in Alzheimer's disease and frontotemporal dementia compared with the MMSE, and has a role in screening patients whose results on the MMSE are ambiguous (Mathuranath et al. 2000).

Other Useful Tests of Cognitive Function

The consultation psychiatrist may encounter patients for whom the administration and interpretation of more focal cognitive tests will yield increased diagnostic clarity. Lishman's (1998) classic text has an excellent detailed discussion of cognitive function and psychometric tests. A few clinically helpful examples are described below. Observing the patient while he or she attempts to draw, calculate, name, or recall is quite informative regarding both brain function and personality style.

Tests Requiring No Accompanying Specialized Kit

Clock Drawing Test

The Clock Drawing Test is a very useful bedside test and is part of a basic MSE. Many examiners hand the patient a blank sheet of paper and ask the patient to draw the entire clock, including the circle; however, patients often draw a small circle and scribble numbers inside. This makes assessment of dyspraxia impossible, especially if the patient is mildly impaired. For this reason, the clinician might choose instead to give the patient a sheet of paper with a large circle already drawn on it and then say, "Write the numbers as if this circle is the face of a clock." After the patient is partially finished with the task, the psychiatrist should interject, "When you finish, draw the hands of the clock so that the time says 15 minutes past 10 o'clock." The clinician can simplify the task by naming an easier time (e.g., 3 o'clock). This task is easy to administer and is instructive, particularly for documenting constructional apraxia and, therefore, early dementia (Esteban-Santillan et al. 1998) or delirium (Trzepacz et al. 2011). Visuospatial errors are more common in patients with right-hemisphere damage; by contrast, left-hemisphere injury is more likely to result in time setting errors (Tranel et al. 2008). More than a dozen methods are used to score the Clock Drawing Test (Colombo et al. 2009). A practical bedside approach is to observe the following principal components of the patient's product (Freund et al. 2005):

- *Numbers*. Are all 12 numbers present, inside the clock face, and without omission or duplication?
- *Spacing*. Are the numbers spaced (nearly) equally from one another and the edge of the circle?

- *Time.* Are there two clock hands that are at least approximating the instructed time? (Further, the patient should not resort to additional markings, such as arrows pointing to an intended number or the time written out in digital clock format, such as "10:15.")

Frank Jones Story

The Frank Jones story tests the patient's ability to conceptualize a situation and to solve a problem (Bechtold et al. 2001). The patient is asked to explain the following story: "I have a friend by the name of Frank Jones whose feet are so big that he has to put on his pants by pulling them over his head." The psychiatrist should watch the patient's immediate response closely to see whether the patient instantly smiles or appears puzzled and confused. Then the psychiatrist asks the patient, "Can Mr. Jones do that?" A patient with normal cognitive function will chuckle and explain in an understandable way why it is impossible. When patients with cognitive difficulties hear the story, they often do not laugh because they do not "get it." They are also unable to rationally explain their response. Patients with delirium may smile (they seem to understand), but their explanations often are bizarre (e.g., "Well, maybe he can if he unzips his fly" or "I guess so if he takes off his shoes").

Set Test

The Set Test is an assessment of verbal fluency designed to screen elderly patients for dementia (Isaacs and Kennie 1973). The patient is asked to name 10 items from each of four categories: fruits, animals, colors, and towns. (A useful mnemonic to recall the four categories is FACT.) The patient is asked to name 10 fruits, then 10 animals, and so on. The score is the total number of items correctly named, with a maximum score of 40. For patients ages 65 and older, scores lower than 15 are clearly abnormal and indicate impairment. This test is not timed, and it should not require such patience that the examiner is tempted to forgo its use. The Set Test is a challenging distraction after the examiner has presented four words for the patient to recall later and is a sensitive indicator of frontal lobe dysfunction. The test also introduces the opportunity for a patient to unwittingly demonstrate perseveration, another clue that the patient might have frontal deficits.

Vigilance Test

The vigilance test (Strub and Black 1985; Wong et al. 2010) measures the patient's ability to sustain attention. For example, the psychiatrist reads—at a rate of one letter per second—a series of 60 letters, in which 18 are the letter *A*, and the patient is asked to raise his or her hand each time the letter *A* is read. Two or more errors are considered abnormal.

Tests That Require Accoutrements

Bender-Gestalt Test

The Bender-Gestalt Test (Bender 1938) examines the patient's ability to copy designs. During a full protocol, nine designs are presented, one at a time, and the patient is asked to copy them. Errors suggest brain dysfunction, and error-free performance strongly supports the absence of brain disease. Visual memory can be tested by asking the patient to reproduce the figures from memory after a brief period has elapsed. A clinician can select and carry three or four of these cards for bedside testing.

Blessed Dementia Scale

The Blessed Dementia Scale has two parts, which are used separately or together (Blessed et al. 1968). One part measures the patient's ability to perform everyday activities, and the second part measures the patient's performance on an information-memory-concentration test. Information about daily activities is provided by a knowledgeable family member or close friend. The Blessed Dementia Scale does not have a cutoff score to establish the diagnosis of dementia. Instead, an increasing score correlates with worsening dementia.

The Marie Three Paper Test

The Marie Three Paper Test provides a quick assessment for comprehension and receptive aphasia (Lishman 1998). Three different-sized pieces of paper are placed in front of the patient. The patient is asked to take the biggest piece and hand it to the examiner, take the smallest piece and throw it to the ground, and take the middle-sized piece and place it in his or her pocket or underneath the hospital bed pillow.

Trail Making Test

The Trail Making Test has two parts, each consisting of several circles distributed on a sheet of paper (Reitan 1958). In Part A, the circles contain numbers, and the patient is asked to connect the numbers in sequence by drawing a line as quickly as possible from one circle to the next. In Part B, each circle contains either a number or a letter. The patient is asked to connect the circles, alternating between numbers and letters (i.e., 1, A, 2, B, etc.). Parts A and B are timed, and age-corrected norms are available. More than one error on either test is usually significant.

Tests of Executive Function

The term *executive function* refers to an array of mental skills used to initiate, maintain, and organize the flow of information and to coordinate actions. Examples of these processes include attention allocation, goal maintenance, and other functions that stabilize performance. Several of the tests already mentioned, such as the Trail Making Test Part B, the Set Test, and the Clock Drawing Test, are used to test executive function. The following are additional bedside methods of assessing this critical contribution of the frontal lobes (Kipps and Hodges 2005).

Letter and Category Fluency

To assess letter fluency, the patient is asked to list as many words as possible in 1 minute that begin with a given letter of the alphabet (F, A, and S are common examiner choices), excluding proper names and sequential word derivatives (e.g., *nut, nuts, nutter*). A score of 15 words per letter is normal. Category fluency is assessed by asking the patient to list as many names of animals as possible in 1 minute. Young adults can typically list 20 animals; 15 is considered a low average score, and a score of 10 or less confirms impairment. Patients with executive dysfunction typically perform poorly in both letter and category fluency, and individuals with subcortical or frontal pathology usually have particular difficulty with letter fluency. By contrast, patients with Alzheimer's disease are likely to have more prominent impairment with category fluency.

Go–No Go Evaluation of Impulsivity

In the go–no go evaluation, the patient is instructed, "Tap your fingers [on your lap/bed/table] once when I tap once, but do not tap at all when I tap twice." The examiner proceeds with a series of taps, randomly alternating single and double taps. This challenge can be heightened by inverting the instructions before a second trial (i.e., telling the patient to withhold tapping in response to a single tap of the examiner, but to tap once when the examiner taps twice). Impulsivity is believed to indicate a failure of response inhibition. The patient who is unable to regulate taps as instructed and instead responds as if cued by the examiner's activity demonstrates probable inferior frontal pathology.

Cognitive Estimates

Patients with executive dysfunction do not estimate effectively and may give unusual or even bizarre answers to estimation questions. The clinician can easily present estimation questions that give the appearance of arising naturally from the clinician's conversation with a patient (e.g., "Yes, this is a large hospital. Big buildings are interesting. What do you think is the height of the Empire State Building?" or "You mentioned you have a daughter in Dallas. How many hours do you think it would take to drive to Detroit?").

Similarities

Inferential reasoning is often hobbled in patients with frontal lobe impairment. The examiner can evaluate this reasoning by asking the patient to explain the similarity between two conceptually equivalent objects; the task can be made progressively more challenging by moving from obvious pairs, such as "bananas and strawberries," to more complicated pairs, such as "concertos and mosaics."

Three-Step Luria

The left frontal lobe is believed to enable motor sequencing. This executive function can be assessed with the Luria three-step test (Weiner et al. 2011), in which the patient is asked to demonstrate an ongoing, unbroken, three-step sequence of a fist on the thigh, followed by an upright hand with the edge of the hand contacting the thigh, followed by an open palm on the thigh, then back to the fist, and so on. The examiner typically illustrates this sequence first for two or three cycles to be sure the patient understands what is expected.

Neurological Examination

A basic bedside neurological examination can provide illuminating information about any patient with cognitive dysfunction, suspected somatoform or conversion disorder with neurological complaints, or malingering. The examination does not need to be time consuming. Often, the patient's history suggests deficits and helps focus the examination.

Basic Neurological Examination

In a basic neurological examination, the clinician should do the following:

1. *Check deep tendon reflexes* for symmetry. Check for the presence of a Babinski reflex (extension of the great toe, with flexion and splaying of the other toes, when the sole of the foot is firmly stroked). Some clinicians also check for primitive reflexes (snout, grasp, glabellar, and palmomental).
2. *Check muscle strength* for asymmetry, weakness, tone, or embellishment.
3. *Observe gait and associated arm movements,* when possible.
4. *Examine cranial nerve function.*
5. *Check the distribution of any sensory complaints.*
6. *Check for signs of meningeal irritation,* such as neck stiffness, headache, Kernig's sign (inability to straighten the leg when the hip is flexed to 90 degrees), or Brudzinski's sign (flexion of the hips and knees when the neck is fixed).

Consultation Psychiatrist as Neuropsychiatrist

Knowledge of brain-behavior relationships and familiarity with neurological terminology is useful for psychiatrists to function well as consultants in the hospital setting. The list below contains a few commonly used neurological terms. The prefix *a-* means complete loss of ability (e.g., *aphasia* is the loss of ability to comprehend or express speech), and the prefix *dys-* means an impaired ability, as in the following examples:

- *Dysarthria*—disturbance of articulation of speech caused by muscle dysfunction
- *Dysbulia*—decrease in willpower
- *Dyscalculia*—impaired ability to do mathematical calculations
- *Dysgnosia*—impaired ability to recognize the importance of sensory impressions
- *Dysgraphia*—impaired ability to express thought in writing
- *Dyslexia*—impaired ability to read
- *Dysphasia*—impaired ability to comprehend, elaborate, or express speech
- *Dyspraxia*—impaired ability to use objects correctly
- *Dysprosody*—impaired pitch, rhythm, and variation of speech

References

Bechtold KT, Horner MD, Labbate LA, et al: The construct validity and clinical utility of the Frank Jones story as a brief screening measure of cognitive dysfunction. Psychosomatics 42:146–149, 2001

Bender L: A Visual-Motor Gestalt Test and Its Clinical Use. New York, American Orthopsychiatric Association, 1938

Blessed G, Tomilinson BE, Roth M: The association between quantitative measures of dementia and of senile change in the cerebral gray matter of elderly subjects. Br J Psychiatry 114:797–811, 1968

Bracha HS, Wolkowitz OM, Lohr JB, et al: High prevalence of visual hallucination in research subjects with chronic schizophrenia. Am J Psychiatry 146:526–528, 1989

Colombo M, Vaccaro R, Vitali SF, et al: Clock Drawing Interpretation Scale (CDIS) and neuropsychological functions in older adults with mild and moderate cognitive impairments. Arch Gerontol Geriatr 49 (suppl 1):39–48, 2009

Esteban-Santillan C, Praditsuwan R, Ueda H, et al: Clock drawing test in very mild Alzheimer's disease. J Am Geriatr Soc 46:1266–1269, 1998

Folstein MF, Folstein SE, McHugh PR: "Mini-Mental State": a practical method for grading the cognitive state of patients for the clinician. J Psychiatr Res 12:189–198, 1975

Freund B, Gravenstein S, Ferris R, et al: Drawing clocks and driving cars: use of brief tests of cognition to screen driving competency in older adults. J Gen Intern Med 20:240–244, 2005

Isaacs B, Kennie AT: The Set Test as an aid to the detection of dementia in old people. Br J Psychiatry 123:467–470, 1973

Kipps CM, Hodges JR: Cognitive assessment for clinicians. J Neurol Neurosurg Psychiatry 76 (suppl 1):i22–i30, 2005

Kokmen E, Naessens JM, Offord KP: A short test of mental status: description and preliminary results. Mayo Clin Proc 62:281–288, 1987

Kokmen E, Smith GE, Petersen RC, et al: The Short Test of Mental Status: correlations with standardized psychometric testing. Arch Neurol 48:725–728, 1991

Laurila JV, Pitkala KH, Strandberg TE, et al: Detection and documentation of dementia and delirium in acute geriatric wards. Gen Hosp Psychiatry 26:31–35, 2004

Lishman WA: Organic Psychiatry: The Psychological Consequences of Cerebral Disorder, 3rd Edition. Oxford, UK, Blackwell Scientific, 1998

Mathuranath PS, Nestor PJ, Berrios GE, et al: A brief cognitive test battery to differentiate Alzheimer's disease and frontotemporal dementia. Neurology 55:1613–1620, 2000

Mesulam M-M: Attention, confusional states, and neglect, in Principles of Behavioral Neurology. Edited by Mesulam M-M. Philadelphia, PA, FA Davis, 1985, pp 125–140

Miosha E, Dawson K, Mitchell J, et al: The Addenbrooke's Cognitive Examination Revised (ACE-R): a brief cognitive test battery for dementia screening. Int J Geriatr Psychiatry 21:1078–1085, 2006

Mungas D: In-office mental status testing: a practical guide. Geriatrics 46:54–66, 1991

Nasreddine ZS, Phillips NA, Bédirian V, et al: The Montreal Cognitive Assessment, MoCA: a brief screening tool for mild cognitive impairment. J Am Geriatr Soc 53:695–699, 2005

Nelson A, Fogel BS, Faust D: Bedside cognitive screening instruments: a critical assessment. J Nerv Ment Dis 174:73–83, 1986

Ovsiew F: Bedside neuropsychiatry: eliciting the clinical phenomena of neuropsychiatric illness, in The American Psychiatric Press Textbook of Neuropsychiatry, 2nd Edition. Edited by Yudofsky SC, Hales RE. Washington, DC, American Psychiatric Press, 1992, pp 89–126

Reitan RM: Validity of the Trail Making Test as an indicator of organic brain damage. Percept Mot Skills 8:271–276, 1958

Sims ACP: Eliciting the symptoms of mental illness, in Symptoms in the Mind: An Introduction to Descriptive Psychopathology, 3rd Edition. Edinburgh, UK, Saunders, 2003, pp 25–37

Strub RL, Black FW: The Mental Status Examination in Neurology, 2nd Edition. Philadelphia, PA, FA Davis, 1985

Tang-Wai DF, Knopman DS, Geda YE, et al: Comparison of the Short Test of Mental Status and the Mini-Mental State Examination in mild cognitive impairment. Arch Neurol 60:1777–1781, 2003

Tranel D, Rudrauf D, Vianna EP, et al: Does the Clock Drawing Test have focal neuroanatomical correlates? Neuropsychology 22:553–562, 2008

Trzepacz PT, Meagher DJ, Leonard M: Delirium, in The American Psychiatric Publishing Textbook of Psychosomatic Medicine, 2nd Edition. Edited by Levenson JL. Washington, DC, American Psychiatric Publishing, 2011, pp 71–114

Weiner MF, Hynan LS, Rossetti H, et al: Luria's three-step test: what is it and what does it tell us? Int Psychogeriatr May 4, 2011 [Epub ahead of print]

Wong CL, Holroyd-Leduc J, Simel DL, et al: Does this patient have delirium? Value of bedside instruments. JAMA 304:779–786, 2010

4

Personality and Response to Illness

Personality is a fairly consistent but individual worldview that shapes a person's emotional experience of life and the subsequent—often predictable—set of behaviors that characterize a person's management of day-to-day living. These long-term traits are generally stable and usually ego-syntonic; only a minority of individuals have a style so inflexible and maladaptive as to cause significant interpersonal impairment or subjective distress (i.e., a personality disorder). In a hospital, however, two additional factors are at work. First, the patient is obliged to interact within a confined, often unfamiliar, psychological and literal space in which friction and collision are commonplace. Second, even the proverbial well-adjusted person who is medically ill is confronted with new stressors that can disturb the usual balance between needs, longings, external reality, and conscience. Medical illness and hospitalization present the patient with a strange, demanding environment that may destabilize personality function. Under severe stress, many individuals regress (unconsciously, in an attempt to "retreat" to former, more familiar, and seemingly more secure psychological ground). Most individuals are resilient and cope well with an illness or injury, but when personality is strained and a patient's behavior bends beyond its usual boundaries, treatment might be complicated or the patient's cooperation with the medical or nursing staff might be hindered. In these cases, the consultation-liaison psychiatrist is often called. From the patient's perspective, the psychiatrist's arrival may add insult to injury; the psychiatrist is unexpected and unwelcome in a setting with limited privacy that is already littered with unpleasant surprises and pain, and his or her uninvited presence has uncertain meaning.

The Person

Whether the patient has a serious acute illness prompting urgent hospital admission, has already been in the hospital for 2 months, or is referred for outpatient evaluation in the context of a new medical diagnosis, several factors shape the patient's perspective on his or her situation and life when he or she encounters the psychiatrist. The more aware the consulting psychiatrist can become of the role of these factors for an individual patient, the better equipped the psychiatrist will be to offer the patient and the requesting physician effective recommendations. These factors include the disease itself; the patient's premorbid personality and past history; and the individual's spiritual and existential strengths or struggles, and the experience of illness and suffering introduced by the disease—often molded by the presence or absence of supportive family, friends, or other networks of support.

Nature of the Disease

Disease is no respecter of persons. Pauper or president may experience loss of control of basic bodily functions, such as eating, sleeping, walking, breathing, or bladder and bowel control.

The disease may be common or rare. The diagnosis may have been established immediately and easily, or it may remain uncertain even after tertiary referral and extensive testing. The disease may be traceable in the family tree or an unknown intruder; its boundaries may be distinct, or the disease may bring a lifetime of uncertainty. Effects of the disease may mean that the patient can no longer drive or can no longer bowl. Some diseases gnaw and nag, whereas others threaten life. The effects may be unseen or may draw covert stares in public. Whatever the current dimensions of the disease, for most patients, there was a day when the disease had no place in their lives, and now their story of life will not be complete without inclusion of the disease.

Acute Versus Chronic Disease

The disease may be acute or chronic. An acute disease presents particular intrapsychic challenges that cause a patient to contemplate what the disease means for him or her at this moment and whether he or she can exert any control. Chronic disease involves additional interpersonal factors, in that the patient tries to see himself or herself through the eyes of others, including their reactions and expectations.

Collateral Factors

Collateral factors, such as medical and toxic conditions, can independently produce profound personality change.

- *Acute conditions,* particularly central nervous system insults, can either change personality traits or magnify preexisting ones. The family of a patient with a secondary personality syndrome, for example, may report that the patient is "not himself." Appropriate social behavior often disappears. Apathy, suspiciousness, affective instability, poor impulse control, and a change in demeanor can occur.
- *Chronic pain or chronic illness* can lead to maladaptive chronic behavior patterns (e.g., expectation of disappointment and rejection).
- *Medications* used to treat medical and neurological disease may also have direct effects on a patient's experience and behavior.

Personality and Past History

A patient's behavior during times of severe stress does not necessarily reflect long-term personality dysfunction or the presence of a personality disorder. Patients with personality disorder do not commonly seek mental health treatment for the behavior itself, although they may try to find relief from the emotional distress that is provoked by their style; the patterns of behavior are ingrained, stable, and "comfortable." More commonly, someone else, such as a family member or hospital staff, wants the patient's behavior to change, especially when the behavior complicates medical management. Patients with personality disorders also affect the physician's and staff's abilities to respond appropriately, leading the medical team members to demonstrate nontherapeutic behaviors, such as avoiding the patient, not responding to a change in symptoms, or assigning the patient's care to the least skilled member of the team. In this way, countertransference can influence the patient's clinical outcome.

- *Personality patterns.* Personality patterns are a mosaic of traits, in which particular "colors" or combinations often predominate. The more common patterns are described with further detail below (see "Personality Patterns of Patients").
- *Past history.* Patients perceive their current medical difficulties through a lens shaped not only by prior psychiatric illness but also by previous experiences with general medical hospitalizations.

Meaning of Illness

Disease, personality, and spiritual or existential perspective each play a role in the patient's subjective experience of the medical plight that has pushed the patient to a physician's office or a hospital. One approach to assessing what meaning the patient attributes to an illness is to review the following common themes (Rowland 1989):

- *Distance*—disruption, separation, or loss of close relationships
- *Dependence*—necessity of relying on others for care and support
- *Disability*—interruption in the trajectory of life and day-to-day achievement
- *Disfigurement*—physical changes that distort body image and integrity
- *Death*—threat of final closure of personal connection with family and friends

Personality Patterns of Patients

Personality may be viewed as a constellation of characteristic assumptions, interpretive framework, and behavioral responses that emerge over time from a person's biological propensities, developmental context, life experience, and view of the future (Ursano et al. 2002). Behaviors associated with personality are characteristically ego-syntonic; because they feel "natural," the individual may not understand why his or her actions distress others. Trauma and medical illness often induce psychological regression and can exacerbate personality dysfunction. The following descriptions of personalities, as well as the possible psychological factors that may drive patient behavior in the medical setting and the common responses among medical staff, are drawn from multiple sources, each of which will reward the reader who reflects on the original manuscript (Geringer and Stern 1986; Groves 1978; Groves and Muskin 2011; Kahana and Bibring 1964; Leigh and Reiser 1992; Levenson et al. 2000; Miller 2001; Nash et al. 2009; Perry and Viederman 1981; Strous et al. 2006).

Dependent, Demanding Patients

Dependent, demanding patients communicate an urgent, intense, and persistent insistence on exceptional attention to assuage their anxiety and deep uncertainty regarding their acceptability and security. They seem to act as though they cannot tolerate the current stress without a perpetual demonstration that their medical team will be as omnipresent and solicitous as the imagined "perfect mother" of a helpless infant. Unmet demands often provoke anger, occasionally depression or apathy, and less commonly a paradoxical and impulsive demand to leave the hospital.

- *Perceived threat.* Patient fears being neglected, overlooked, dismissed, or abandoned.
- *Clinician response.* The physician may initially feel gratified and enhanced by the patient's profuse expression of need and appreciation, but when the patient's hunger for reassurance proves insatiable, the physician may feel overwhelmed, irritated, and angry. The physician must avoid withdrawing from the patient or responding to the patient's demands by withholding support and punitively curtailing responses. Rather, the physician is more likely to calm the patient's fears through neutral and judicious reassurance, sensible limits accompanied by clear statements of continuing commitment to care, mobilization of other resources, and rewarding of the patient's efforts toward independence.

Orderly, Controlling Patients

Orderly, controlling patients have concluded that the vicissitudes of life, not to mention the raw risk of impulsive or rebellious behavior, are best kept in check by hypertrophied thinking, lest action break away and shame the owner. Accordingly, these patients are likely to be self-disciplined, fastidious, orderly, earnest, and given to serious concern with right and wrong. These patients may respond to the anxious uncertainties that accompany illness by redoubling their determination to suppress emotion, exhibit responsibility, practice self-restraint, and find refuge in inflexible (i.e., immutably true) perceptions of how details should be approached. This behavior may set the stage for vigorous critique of perceived shortcomings by the staff.

- *Perceived threat.* The patient fears loss of control over life, including impulses, emotions, and body (not far removed from a fear of helplessness).
- *Clinician response.* The physician may initially admire the patient's apparent stoic, impervious response to stress, but if the patient responds to perceived impotence by obstinate complaining and contentious accusations, the physician must avoid responding with blanket reassurances and impressionistic optimism. Rather, communicating respect for the patient's high regard for responsibility and autonomy, the physician will reinforce predictable routine where possible and look for opportunities to give the patient choices to restore some sense of control. Furthermore, the physician can engage such a patient's interest in detail and desire to understand by offering ample data and explanation of the illness, and then enlist the patient's collaboration in care, such as by having the patient record specific symptoms or responses to particular interventions. The physician should remember to recognize the patient's attentive participation in subsequent encounters.

Dramatizing, Emotional Patients

Dramatizing, emotional patients unwittingly feel that a close relationship with the physician or medical team is likely to prove more soothing than physician knowledge and skill. Achieving an intense, idealized connection becomes important to reinforce a sense of desirability and prove one's femininity or masculinity. Female patients are often effusive and sometimes overtly seductive.

Male patients flirt with female nurses and physicians, perhaps peppering their conversation with stories that exaggerate their courage or manliness. Unfortunately, the patient's eagerness for a special relationship often evokes anxiety, discomfort, and distancing in others, and these reactions in turn serve to aggravate the patient's fear of diminishing physical appeal. In working with these patients, the medical team members (including multiple shifts of nurses) often find that they are of two minds: some rally to reassure these colorful, emotional patients, whereas others are angered by the patients' behavior.

- *Perceived threat.* The patient fears loss of attractiveness, admiration, or affection.
- *Clinician response.* The physician may respond to the patient's expression of keen personal warmth with charmed interest, fascination, or attraction. The patient often provides his or her history with flourishes that suggest unique vitality. The impressionistic history, with a diffusion of detail, may exasperate the physician who is striving to build a precise and sequential clinical story. The challenge for the physician is to acknowledge the patient's anxieties and encourage the patient to discuss his or her fears while maintaining clear boundaries; responding with a respectful balance of personal concern and professional formality will model the reassuring stance that the patient finds so difficult to provide for himself or herself. Further underscoring the imperative of explicit boundaries, these patients often have a tangled sexual or relational past and may perceive intimacy when no such offer is intended.

Long-Suffering, Complaining Patients

Long-suffering, complaining patients often present their self-sacrificing resignation to life's adversities and disappointments with apparent humility and modesty, but a different angle reveals a patina of exhibitionistic relief, if not muted pleasure. Close examination may eventually reveal a propensity to willingly forgo comfort, sometimes choosing service or difficulty—perhaps with unconscious choreography—that invites misfortune. Such a patient longs for acceptance, care, and a relationship, but at some level feels unworthy or too guilty to receive this without purchasing it with self-sacrifice and heartache. Accepting reassurance or, worse yet, experiencing resolution of symptoms would jeopardize the economy whereby this patient negotiates the complex relationship of affliction and gratification.

- *Perceived threat.* The patient fears the potential loss of deserved punishment or the pleasure of pain.
- *Clinician response.* The physician may respond to the patient's account of misery and suffering with earnest efforts to comfort or frame the patient's tribulations in a redemptive light, only to be put off, frustrated, and possibly eventually angered by a patient who answers any encouragement or hope with increased complaint. The unaware physician may doubt his or her effectiveness and begin to feel as impotent as the patient's accentuation of unending hardship suggests. The physician who appreciates the dynamic at work understands that the patient who laments, "It's not easy, Doctor," will successfully resist any encouragement but will find consolation when the physician shares the patient's pessimism and grimly applauds the patient's sacrifice and perseverance. Recovery poses a deep dilemma for these patients, so much so that cooperation with treatment may be undermined, either covertly or openly. The astute physician will downplay potential treatment benefit and suggest that the treatment is an additional burden that the patient must endure, not for his or her own sake, but to garner some relief for concerned family members or to enable the patient to continue to serve others sacrificially.

Guarded, Suspicious Patients

Guarded, suspicious patients are particularly fearful of being placed in a vulnerable position where they could, without warning, be exposed, used, or hurt. When ill, the fundamentally suspicious person is at a particular disadvantage; not only does dependence on the medical team magnify this patient's fear of being found defenseless, but he or she cannot trust the physician to act in the patient's best interests and may therefore withhold relevant history. It feels like a no-win situation for the patient, confirming his or her perspective that the world is more often than not oppressive and persecutory, and that relationships with people (i.e., physicians and nurses) are dangerous.

- *Perceived threat.* The patient fears that harm will result from invasive, exploitative medical care.

• *Clinician response.* The physician may try to win over such a patient with generous attention, but this effort will more likely stir the patient's fear and guardedness even further, prompting the physician to become defensive when the patient lashes out, perhaps attributing malicious motives to the medical team. When the patient persists in quarrelsome attribution of negative intentions, the physician may feel repeatedly accused and attacked, and thus torn between defending the team or nursing staff and overlooking the patient's exaggerations and oversensitivity. The physician may ease the patient's anxiety by identifying perceived suspiciousness as "sensitivity," acknowledging the patient's criticisms by observing, "I can see how you would feel that way given the circumstances." Although disputing either the patient's feelings or the perceived facts that fuel the patient's accusations is never useful, commiserating—from a distance—about the inconveniences of impersonal hospital policies may be useful. The physician should avoid undue warmth and ambiguity, both of which arouse distrust. A useful tactic is for the physician to advise this patient as far in advance as possible about forthcoming diagnostic tests, being candid about details. The physician should strive for an objective, neutral presentation of recommended procedures to avoid provoking unnecessary resistance when the patient concludes that a physician's preference for one option over another is evidence that the patient is being manipulated.

Superior, Critical Patients

Superior, critical patients see themselves as powerful, all-important, and brimming with self-confidence, although some of these patients partially obscure this reality with a feigned, patronizing humility. The inevitable jostling between such a patient's urgent need to be superior in every domain and the loss of an idealized body image, not to mention function, that accompanies illness places these patients in a precarious plight. Anxious and feeling acutely endangered, such patients may come across to the medical team as snobby, condescending, or grandiose. They may hint that they are privy to elusive and exclusive knowledge, and they often relish detailing their achievements and prowess, whether physical, financial, or otherwise. Such a patient, when threatened by disease, often dismisses the value of "lesser" members of the staff, so that the patient can reinforce his or her foundering sense of grandeur by noting that the situation can only be addressed by a senior, eminent physician.

- *Perceived threat.* The patient fears the shameful loss of self-identity as perfect and invulnerable.
- *Clinician response.* The physician may momentarily be pleased to be involved in the care of a very important person, if indeed the patient is such, but this reaction typically fades quickly and is replaced by feelings of inferiority as the patient "name-drops" and points out the physician's shortcomings, whether obliquely by inquiring about particular details of the physician's educational pedigree or directly by noting alleged details that reveal substandard care. The physician's irritation may grow to anger and an urge to take advantage of his or her knowledge of medicine and the function of the hospital to counterattack and "trim down to size" the patient's entitlement. The astute physician resists this urge; reframes the patient's entitlement as deserving of the best advice, care, and outcome; and enlists the patient's adherence to treatment recommendations in the service of this deserved prerogative. An additional challenge for the physician is to avoid excessive humility, a quality that may be so foreign to the patient's personal experience that it will succeed only in awakening the patient's fear that he or she is under the care of an incompetent. A secure, confident physician will comfortably create room for the patient to show off and even complement the patient's strengths.

Seclusive, Aloof Patients

Seclusive, aloof patients give the impression of disinterest in everyday events, preferring solitary activities and sometimes appearing socially awkward or inhibited. They find solace in detachment, and their inner tranquility is best sustained by absorption in themselves and things familiar to them, occasionally expressed by solitary immersion in unusual fringe interests. This deep reluctance to engage the world and risk a loss of equilibrium may translate into considerable delay in seeking medical attention. Such patients may succeed in muting the anxiety one expects to accompany certain diagnoses or procedures so thoroughly that they appear conspicuously unconcerned. Close friends are few, if they exist at all, and even family may allow that the patient has been a loner, and perhaps eccentric.

- *Perceived threat.* The patient fears intrusion, obligatory interaction, and loss of privacy.

- *Clinician response.* The physician may feel ill at ease or question his or her skills of communication and empathy because the patient seems difficult to engage and conversations show no sign of establishing a connection. The physician may suspect depression or conclude that the patient's desire to preserve a "circle of distance" reflects indifference toward the medical problem; however, either interpretation is likely wrong. The challenge for the physician is to respect the patient's stance of "unsociability" while maintaining a gentle, quiet interest in the patient that accepts the absence of any reciprocal effort. Beneath the unemotional, seemingly imperturbable exterior, these patients may have a history of repeated disappointments in early life that taught them to regard the love of others as fickle and untrustworthy. The physician, then, should try to honor the patient's preference for privacy, but not to the extremity of allowing the patient to withdraw completely.

Impulsive, Acting-Out Patients

Impulsive, acting-out patients are intolerant of frustration, acute distress, pain, and the necessity of either sustained collaboration or delayed gratification. Sometimes even minor discomfort, delay, or frustration will leave the patient feeling overwhelmed by unbearable impotence. The patient will demand immediate relief but rail against attempted intervention if it involves further time or a procedure. The patient may curse, kick an IV pole, or demand to sign out against medical advice. Such a patient seems devoid of the capacity to deliberate; the patient may reach decisions immediately and later express remorse and explain that he or she acted "without thinking."

- *Perceived threat.* The patient fears loss of comfort and consequent disintegration.
- *Clinician response.* The physician may react to this patient with reflexive dislike, concluding that the patient is choosing to throw a childish temper tantrum that warrants forceful, adult discipline. By viewing the behavior as possibly reflecting a defect in executive brain function, the physician will find greater tolerance for the patient, and thereby more emotional "elbow room" to select constructive interventions. Judicious but proactive use of anxiolytic and analgesic medications may avert untimely and disruptive

eruptions of anger that often only delay treatment. Firm, but not punitive, limit setting may actually reassure such patients that they will not be allowed to utterly "fall to pieces." The physician might recruit the presence of family or a trusted friend to shore up the patient's sense of safety.

Idealizing, Provocative Patients

Idealizing, provocative patients often seek to secure their self-esteem and yearning for stability by searching for relationships that shower them with attention and apparent singular commitment. The urgent longing to feel valued in relationships, coupled with an amplified capacity to misinterpret, sets the stage for intense, idealized perceptions. However, the inverse is also true: any disappointment or perception of slight can unleash devastating doubt and explosive rage. Feeling massively violated, such patients may be convinced that yesterday's uniquely compassionate hero is today's persecutory monster. Tumult spreads like contagion.

- *Perceived threat.* The patient fears that attachment, although desperately desired, may prove all-consuming.
- *Clinician response.* The physician may initially endeavor to go the extra mile in response to the patient's provocative style and lament that he or she was misunderstood by a prior insensitive and hurried physician, who, the patient may imply, simply did not display the attentive sagacity so clearly present now. The physician may warm to the patient's generous praise and unwittingly allow overly optimistic expectations to blossom in the patient's imagined construction of a special connection. Disappointment is assured, may be triggered by imperceptible snubs, and will lead to distracting upheaval. The physician may avoid disruptive commotion by conducting himself or herself with consistent, caring clarity regarding necessary limits and boundaries and by ensuring that the team communicates with a united voice to the patient.

Cold, Deceitful Patients

Cold, deceitful patients may arouse suspicion and distaste from the outset, or may assume a calculated charm that hides their true personality until they have achieved their objective. These individuals have no regard for accepted rules of fair play and consider the clinical encounter as one more relationship, however brief, to exploit for social, legal, financial, or medicinal benefit. Some of these patients may be confirmed criminals, and a few are dangerous. Unprincipled and sometimes devoid of conscience, such a patient may threaten violence to self or hint at violence to another when he or she thinks it will bend the physician to favorable action.

- *Perceived threat.* The patient believes that every relationship is a prelude to betrayal, whether accomplished by foil or seduction.
- *Clinician response.* The physician may overlook early clues to the source of the patient's inappropriate demands, unconsciously preferring to avoid confrontation. Most physicians resist being used and, even more so, abused. When the antisocial patient's effort to exploit becomes apparent, the physician may be tempted to retaliate; however, even a liar who has exaggerated his or her symptoms for personal gain may have an illness that warrants medical attention. Physicians must stow their anger or disgust, which may otherwise contaminate their medical reasoning. Special requests from the patient (e.g., for a letter to court or a particular prescription) are best answered in a straightforward, calm and firm manner that relies on observation of fact and medical judgment, and the physician should avoid showing personal antipathy for the impropriety of the patient's demand. Argument is never constructive. The physician should respect his or her own fear, and if he or she feels uncomfortable, should suspend the examination until safety can be ensured.

Timid, Apprehensive Patients

Timid, apprehensive patients may be prone to private self-critique and may feel either undeserving or unworthy of pressing for medical attention. They may be willing to downplay any symptoms in the hope of dodging or deferring knowledge of a medical diagnosis that may provoke fresh anxiety and uncertainty. Some of these patients may have a dysthymic propensity that inclines them to doubt that help or hope could be in store; they may reason that any malady that does not utterly incapacitate them is best borne silently. Such a perspective may collude with the patient's anxiety to protect himself or herself from further uncomfortable contact with the medical profession and the risk of discovering additional reasons for anxiety.

- *Perceived threat.* The patient fears confirmation of his or her unfit, marginal, and onerous status.
- *Clinician response.* The physician may allow time constraints to conspire with the patient's innately hesitant style and gloss over meek responses without summoning the patience and deliberate effort to extract a full, cohesive history from the patient. Occasionally, such patients will provide more detail, with less censorship, on a written questionnaire than in an interview. The careful physician will guard against betraying impatience or irritation, lest the patient feel confirmed in his or her misgivings and seek an early exit from the examination. The physician must be alert to subtle clues of minimization or underreporting of symptoms and may seek family for collateral history.

Common Defenses in Medical Patients

Understanding a patient's defenses is one way to identify his or her behavioral tendencies during times of stress. The consulting psychiatrist must remember that patients under the stress of hospitalization and severe illness use less "mature" defenses that are nevertheless adaptive for the patients. Even if the defenses cause problems for the patient care unit or clinic, these defenses are the patient's best available coping tools and, unless dangerous, should initially be supported. Attempts to remove psychological defenses are almost always counterproductive. A frontal assault on a patient's less mature defenses usually makes matters worse, causing intense fear, despair, anger, or even psychosis. If the consulting psychiatrist's interventions can reduce anxiety and discomfort, the patient should be able to return to more characteristic, hopefully mature, defenses. A patient's defensive style may stir powerful feelings among the medical team; these feelings may prompt the consultation request and may provide important diagnostic information for the consulting psychiatrist. The following are a sampling of mature, neurotic, and immature defenses that may be encountered in medical patients (Groves and Muskin 2011; Vaillant 1971).

Mature Defenses

- *Anticipation*—arranging whatever details are open to control to maximize the odds of coping effectively

- *Humor*—giving open voice to "unacceptable feelings" by diluting the intensity with irony, self-deprecation, or a surprising punch line
- *Suppression*—conscious distraction from ruminating about a coming diagnostic procedure

Neurotic Defenses

- *Displacement*—changing subjects when asked to talk about the illness or injury
- *Isolation of affect*—discussing a diagnosis or serious prognosis devoid of any expression of anxiety, fear, or dysphoria
- *Rationalization*—constructing a plausible, but typically untrue (in this instance), reason for being untroubled by medical issues at hand
- *Repression*—unintentional, unconscious forgetting of a frightening, painful, or threatening experience or reaction

Immature Defenses

- *Denial*—steadfastly refusing to recognize threatening medical realities
- *Passive aggression*—"forgetting" to follow instructions (e.g., for urine collection or for avoiding food or liquid intake), thus indirectly expressing anger and thwarting a caregiver's efforts
- *Projection*—ascribing intolerable motives, thoughts, or impulses to the medical team
- *Splitting*—resorting to categorization of some caregivers as "all good" and others as "all bad" to manage conflicting feelings

Helping the Patient Cope Constructively

Optimal management of maladaptive stress responses is not possible without an understanding of how the patient sees himself or herself with this illness at this time. Armed with this information, the consultant can recommend the most appropriate psychopharmacological, psychotherapeutic, and unit management interventions. Therefore, after receiving a consult on a patient with personality or coping style problems, the psychiatrist must do the following:

1. Identify and attempt to reverse any remediable organic factors.
2. Carefully consider whether other psychiatric disorders are present.
3. Clarify the patient's style of personality functioning and past responses to stressors.
4. Try to understand the meaning of the illness and hospitalization to the patient.
5. Whenever possible, strive to engage the patient in ways that strengthen resilience.
6. Recommend indicated somatic therapies, recognizing that in many conditions, the foregoing steps may yield more immediate benefit than do medications.

References

Geringer ES, Stern TA: Coping with medical illness: the impact of personality types. Psychosomatics 27:251–261, 1986

Groves JE: Taking care of the hateful patient. N Engl J Med 298:883–887, 1978

Groves MS, Muskin PR: Psychological responses to illness, in The American Psychiatric Publishing Textbook of Psychosomatic Medicine, 2nd Edition. Edited by Levenson JL. Washington, DC, American Psychiatric Publishing, 2011, pp 45–70

Kahana RJ, Bibring GL: Personality types in medical management, in Psychiatry and Medical Practice in a General Hospital. Edited by Zinberg NE. New York, International Universities Press, 1964, pp 108–123

Leigh H, Reiser MF: The patient's personality, in The Patient: Biological, Psychological, and Social Dimensions of Medical Practice, 3rd Edition. New York, Plenum Medical Book Company, 1992, pp 383–399

Levenson H, Servis M, Hales RH: Brief psychodynamic therapy in the medically ill, in Psychiatric Care of the Medical Patient, 2nd Edition. Edited by Stoudemire A, Fogel BS, Greenberg D. New York, Oxford University Press, 2000, pp 17–30

Miller MC: Personality disorders. Med Clin North Am 85:819–837, 2001

Nash SS, Kent LK, Muskin PR: Psychodynamics in medically ill patients. Harv Rev Psychiatry 17:389–397, 2009

Perry S, Viederman M: Management of emotional reactions to acute medical illness. Med Clin North Am 65:3–14, 1981

Rowland JH: Developmental stage and adaptation: adult model, in Handbook of Psychooncology. Edited by Holland JC, Rowland JH. New York, Oxford University Press, 1989, pp 25–43

Strous RD, Ulman AM, Kotler M: The hateful patient revisited: relevance for 21st century medicine. Eur J Intern Med 17:387–393, 2006

Ursano RJ, Epstein RS, Lazar SG: Behavioral responses to illness: personality and personality disorders, in The American Psychiatric Publishing Textbook of Consultation-Liaison Psychiatry: Psychiatry in the Medically Ill, 2nd Edition. Edited by Wise MG, Rundell JR. Washington, DC, American Psychiatric Publishing, 2002, pp 107–125

Vaillant GE: Theoretical hierarchy of adaptive ego mechanisms. Arch Gen Psychiatry 24:107–118, 1971

5

Suicidality

Suicidal statements made by medical-surgical patients usually lead to prompt psychiatric referral. Inpatient consultation-liaison services work with patients who have attempted suicide and been hospitalized in an intensive care unit or general medical unit. Occasionally, even a hospitalized medical-surgical patient attempts or completes a suicide. Outpatient consultation services work with patients whose medical conditions may be associated with thoughts of suicide or of life as not worth living. Suicidality assessment is an integral part of almost every psychosomatic medicine consultation.

Epidemiology

Completed Suicides

General Population

- Suicide is the eleventh leading cause of death in the United States and accounts for over 33,000 documented deaths per year (Centers for Disease Control and Prevention 2007).
- The most successful suicide method is firearms, followed by hanging and self-poisoning (Juurlink et al. 2004).

- The elderly account for approximately 25% of suicides, although they account for only 10% of the population (Bostwick and Levenson 2005).
- Suicides among whites occur at twice the rate as nonwhites (excepting Native Americans) (Bostwick and Levenson 2005).
- The male-to-female ratio for suicide is 3:1 (Runeson and Asberg 2003). Men tend to use more violent means, such as shooting, hanging, and jumping from high places.
- Loss of a partner increases the risk for suicide (Bostwick and Levenson 2005). Divorced men have four times the suicide rate of married men, and divorced women have three times the rate of married women.

Medical-Surgical Patients

- Physical disease is an independent suicide risk factor, present in 25%–75% of people who commit suicide (Kontaxakis et al. 1988).
- Medical-surgical patients who commit suicide may have experienced a recent loss of emotional support; anger may be a predominant affect.
- The reported suicide rate in most hospitals is lower than in the general population. Access to means of suicide is more difficult in hospitals, and patients who give clear warning signs are usually promptly attended to.
- Jumping is the most successful suicide method for general hospital patients (Bostwick and Levenson 2005).
- Most general hospital patients who commit suicide have chronic, painful, or disfiguring illnesses (Sanders 1988). They also have a high frequency of psychiatric illness, particularly mood disorders and alcohol use disorders. Interpersonal problems with family members and ward staff are common.
- Institutional response is important. A suicide in a hospitalized patient can be devastating. Successful organizational management of the aftermath of an in-house suicide includes the formation of a multidisciplinary leadership team (Ballard et al. 2008).

Attempted Suicides

General Population

- The ratio of suicide attempts to completions is about 10:1 (Bostwick and Levenson 2005).

- A 3:1 female-to-male ratio exists for suicide attempts, in contrast to the 3:1 male-to-female ratio for completed suicides (Bostwick and Levenson 2005).
- Suicide attempts are a common reason for admissions to general hospitals. For example, 1%–2% of all admissions to emergency departments and 1%–5% of all admissions to medical intensive care units are drug overdose patients (Bostwick and Levenson 2011).
- Drugs used in nonlethal suicide attempts are commonly available: benzodiazepines, alcohol, nonnarcotic analgesics, antidepressants, barbiturates, and antihistamines. Overdoses of acetaminophen, with its potential liver toxicity and over-the-counter availability, are particularly likely to result in a medical-surgical or psychiatric admission.

Medical-Surgical Patients

- Although not well studied, the rate of attempted suicide in general hospital settings is estimated at 24 per 100,000 patients per year (Sanders 1988).
- The most frequent psychiatric diagnosis in attempters is personality disorder, in contrast to depression and alcoholism in patients on medical-surgical services who complete suicide (Sanders 1988).
- A recent history of loss of emotional support is common.
- Wrist slashing and drug overdose are the most common nonlethal suicide attempt methods in hospitals (Sanders 1988).

Clinical Assessment

Psychiatric Risk Factors Associated With Increased Suicide Risk

Psychiatric Diagnoses

Based on psychological autopsies, 95% of patients who completed suicides had psychiatric diagnoses. Of these individuals, 40% had mood disorders, 20%–25% had alcoholism, 10%–15% had schizophrenia, and 20%–25% had personality disorder (Litman 1989).

Past Attempts

History of a suicide attempt is an important predictor of future suicide risk. One of every 100 suicide attempt survivors will die by suicide within 1 year after the index attempt, a suicide risk approximately 100 times that of the general population (Hawton 1992).

Psychological Factors

Suicide is often a response to a loss, real or metaphorical. Fantasies of revenge, punishment, reconciliation with a rejecting object, relief from the pain of loss, or reunion with a dead loved one may be evident (Furst and Ostow 1979). Holidays and anniversaries of important days also increase suicide risk.

Medical Disorders Associated With Increased Suicide Risk

Terminal Illness

Reviews of death certificates indicate that about 5% of suicide completers have a terminal illness (Murphy 1986); however, this rate may underrepresent the true prevalence. Physicians may misstate causes of death on death certificates to help patients' families avoid adverse financial and psychosocial consequences.

Medical Disorders With Specific Risk

Suicide rates higher than those in the general population are reported in patients with congestive heart failure, chronic obstructive pulmonary disease, urinary incontinence, chronic pain, Alzheimer's disease, diabetes, cancer, and HIV, as well as in patients undergoing renal dialysis (Bostwick and Levenson 2011; Juurlink et al. 2004; Polednak 2007; Pompili et al. 2009; Voaklander et al. 2008). The fear of pain, disfigurement, and loss of function from cancer, HIV, and chronic renal failure can precipitate suicide, particularly early in the patient's course.

Treatment and Management

Identify the Risk Level

Initial management decisions may be difficult because patients are often ambivalent about suicide. In outpatient medical-surgical screening for suicidality, many times more patients may meet organizational criteria for mental health referral for further suicidality assessment than are actually suicidal (Shemesh et al. 2009). Patients demonstrate a gradation of risk. Most patients examined are at "some risk." Information from a third party often helps the clinician gain other perspectives on a patient's situation. The clinician should always err on the side of safety. The response of both patient and third party to the treatment plan gives some indication of the patient's resilience and of the social resources available to aid in recovery from the suicidal crisis.

Protect the Patient

Arrange for Psychiatric Hospitalization

If the patient's suicide potential is substantial, he or she should be hospitalized, voluntarily or involuntarily.

Secure the Surroundings

If the patient requires medical hospitalization, once he or she is admitted to the hospital, the patient's room should be secured (Bostwick and Levenson 2011). The staff must do the following:

1. *Remove dangerous articles* (i.e., anything that a patient could potentially use for self-injury, such as sharp objects or material that could be fashioned into a noose). Access to means of suicide is associated with likelihood of successful suicide completion in an impulsive in-hospital attempt (Bostwick and Rackley 2007).
2. *Search luggage and possessions.*
3. *Monitor all objects coming into the room* that are potential weapons (e.g., the cutlery on the dinner tray).
4. *Assertively address agitation.* Agitation and anger are two emotional states associated with likelihood of successful suicide completion in an impulsive in-hospital attempt (Bostwick and Rackley 2007).
5. *Provide constant observation* (e.g., by using a sitter).

Establish Capacity When Patients Reject Life-Prolonging Treatments

A patient may decline life-prolonging treatments that complicate the natural course of death and dying. This may sometimes be seen as a suicidal act. The consulting psychiatrist should establish capacity for decision making in the context of a suicidality assessment. Reality testing and rationality of explanation for a decision to avoid life-prolonging treatments or technology are component parts of this multiaxial assessment (Bostwick and Cohen 2009; Sullivan and Youngner 1994).

Document Communications

The psychiatric consultant must carefully document the clinical diagnosis and treatment plan in the patient's chart. Frequent updates and reassessments of suicide potential and the treatment plan are necessary. The consultant's chart notes should identify the level of risk, clearly state the plan, and report the interval at which the consultant will return to continue the assessment and recommend modifications to the plan (Bostwick and Levenson 2011). The consultant should also arrange follow-up care for the patient before discharge and detail this care in the chart so that it is part of the inpatient's discharge plan.

Remove Risk Factors

Treat Psychiatric Disorders

- *Mood disorders.* Depressed patients receiving treatment should be observed for a period of increased suicide risk during early phases of treatment.
- *Substance-related disorders.* Alcohol and drug abuse is underdiagnosed among medically ill patients, including patients in the general hospital.
- *Psychosis.* The consulting psychiatrist should ask about command hallucinations and treat psychotic symptoms.
- *Delirium.* Any remediable causes of cognitive impairment must be removed.

Provide Medical Psychotherapy

Brief psychotherapy may be quite helpful for some suicidal patients, especially when dealing with themes of loss. The psychiatrist or psychotherapist should approach such patients with an accepting, supportive, empathic, and concerned manner and attempt to develop a therapeutic alliance. The patient's family should be involved, whenever possible. The clinician should make an effort to reestablish or strengthen the patient's connections to friends or community social service agencies.

Manage Patient in Emergency Department and Outpatient Setting

According to Davidson (1993), the emergency department or outpatient clinic setting is acceptable for outpatient management if the suicidal patient has the following:

- Satisfactory impulse control
- No psychosis or intoxication
- No specific plan or easily accessible means for suicide
- Accessible social supports to which he or she is willing to turn
- The capacity for establishing rapport with the consultant

References

Ballard ED, Pao M, Horowitz L, et al: Aftermath of suicide in the hospital: institutional response. Psychosomatics 49:461–469, 2008

Bostwick JM, Cohen LM: Differentiating suicide from life-ending acts and end-of-life decisions: a model based on chronic kidney disease and dialysis. Psychosomatics 50:1–7, 2009

Bostwick JM, Levenson JL: Suicidality, in The American Psychiatric Publishing Textbook of Psychosomatic Medicine. Edited by Levenson JL. Washington, DC, American Psychiatric Publishing, 2005, pp 219–234

Bostwick JM, Levenson JL: Suicidality, in The American Psychiatric Publishing Textbook of Psychosomatic Medicine, 2nd Edition. Edited by Levenson JL. Washington, DC, American Psychiatric Publishing, 2011, pp 199–218

Bostwick JM, Rackley SJ: Completed suicide in medical/surgical patients: who is at risk? Current Psychiatry Reports 9:242–246, 2007

Centers for Disease Control and Prevention: 20 leading causes of death, United States, 2007. WISQARS Leading Causes of Death Reports, 1999–2007. Office of Statistics and Programming, National Center for Injury Prevention and Control. Data Source: National Center for Health Statistics (NCHS), National Vital Statistics System. 2007. Available at: http://webappa.cdc.gov/sasweb/ncipc/leadcaus10.html. Accessed April 6, 2011.

Davidson L: Suicide and aggression in the medical setting, in Psychiatric Care of the Medical Patient. Edited by Stoudemire A, Fogel BS. New York, Oxford University Press, 1993, pp 71–86

Furst S, Ostow M: The psychodynamics of suicide, in Suicide: Theory and Clinical Aspects. Edited by Hankoff LD, Einsidler B. Littleton, MA, PSG Publishing, 1979, pp 165–178

Hawton K: Suicide and attempted suicide, in Handbook of Affective Disorders, 2nd Edition. Edited by Paykel ES. New York, Guilford, 1992, pp 635–650

Juurlink DN, Nerrman N, Szalai JP, et al: Medical illness and the risk of suicide in the elderly. Arch Intern Med 164:1179–1184, 2004

Kontaxakis VP, Christodoulou GN, Mavreas VG, et al: Attempted suicide in psychiatric outpatients with concurrent physical illness. Psychother Psychosom 50:201–206, 1988

Litman RE: Suicides: what do they have in mind? in Suicide: Understanding and Responding. Edited by Jacobs D, Brown HN. Madison, CT, International Universities Press, 1989, pp 143–154

Murphy GE: Suicide and attempted suicide, in The Medical Basis of Psychiatry. Edited by Winokur G, Clayton PJ. Philadelphia, PA, WB Saunders, 1986, pp 562–579

Polednak AP: Suicide among breast cancer patients who have had reconstructive surgery: a population-based study. Psychosomatics 48:178–179, 2007

Pompili M, Lester D, Innamorati M, et al: Quality of life and suicide risk in patients with diabetes mellitus. Psychosomatics 50:16–23, 2009

Runeson B, Asberg M: Family history of suicide among suicide victims. Am J Psychiatry 160:1525–1526, 2003

Sanders R: Suicidal behavior in critical care medicine: conceptual issues and management strategies, in Problems in Critical Care Medicine. Edited by Wise MG. Philadelphia, PA, JB Lippincott, 1988, pp 116–133

Shemesh E, Annunziato RA, Rubinstein D, et al: Screening for depression and suicidality in patients with cardiovascular illnesses. Am J Cardiol 104:1194–1197, 2009

Sullivan MD, Youngner SJ: Depression, competence, and the right to refuse lifesaving medical treatment. Am J Psychiatry 151:971–978, 1994

Voaklander DC, Rowe BH, Dryden DM, et al: Medical illness, medication use and suicide in seniors: a population-based case control study. J Epidemiol Community Health 62:138–146, 2008

PART II

Syndromes

6

Anxiety

Anxiety in medically ill patients has various causes. Anxiety can be a reaction to the stress of illness or hospitalization, a manifestation of a medical or psychiatric disorder, a result of substance abuse or withdrawal, or an adverse effect of a medication (Miller and Massie 2006).

Anxiety is associated with medical morbidity. The impact of anxiety disorders on function and outcome in persons with chronic medical illness is not as well studied as the impact of depression. Available evidence, however, suggests that anxiety may have as great an impact as depression in terms of risk, outcomes, and measures of morbidity (Roy-Byrne et al. 2008). Kessler et al. (2003) reported that anxiety disorders had an association equal to or greater than that of depression with four chronic medical conditions: hypertension, arthritis, asthma, and ulcers. Anxiety often amplifies somatic symptoms (e.g., tachycardia, dyspnea, pain) and worsens outcomes (Roy-Byrne et al. 2008).

Anxiety is associated with health care utilization. Anxiety accounts for up to 10% of all visits to physicians (Colon and Popkin 2002). Anxiety symptoms are easily mistaken for cardiac arrhythmia, asthma, cerebrovascular disease, coronary disease, an endocrine disorder, or vertigo. Consequently, patients with anxiety disorders are frequently referred for expensive and unnecessary examinations, such as ambulatory electrocardiographic monitoring, cardiac catheterization, and pheochromocytoma testing (Simon and Walker 1999). Anxiety severity also correlates with frequency of health care use, health care cost, and length of hospital stay, even when accounting for illness severity (Colon and Popkin 2002; Epstein and Hicks 2011; Levenson et al. 1992; Saravay et al. 1991).

Epidemiology

General Population

Anxiety disorders are among the most common psychiatric disorders. The lifetime prevalence of anxiety disorders is 25%; the 12-month prevalence is 17% (Colon and Popkin 2002; Epstein and Hicks 2011). Compared with men, women are at twice the risk for having a current anxiety disorder.

Medically Ill Patients

Patients with chronic medical conditions have a 50% higher lifetime prevalence of an anxiety disorder (Wells et al. 1988). Panic disorder is present in 3–10 times more patients with asthma than in the general population (Colon and Popkin 2002). When panic disorder is treated in medical patients, hospitalization rates decline (Katon 1984).

Biology of Anxiety

Neurotransmitters

Basic science and clinical research implicate noradrenergic, serotonergic, and γ-aminobutyric acid (GABA) systems, and possibly glucocorticoid neuropeptides, in the genesis of normal and pathological anxiety.

Neurophysiology

Patients with anxiety disorders appear to have unstable autonomic nervous systems, hypersensitive respiratory control mechanisms, and hypersensitive central nervous system (CNS) carbon dioxide (CO_2) chemoreceptors (Colon and Popkin 2002).

Neuroanatomy

Pharmacological challenge studies and functional CNS imaging suggest that key CNS structures that are important in producing normal and pathological anxiety include the locus coeruleus, amygdala, hippocampus, temporal lobes, and frontal lobes. Projections from the amygdala and hypothalamus modulate autonomic and endocrine responses associated with regulation of vigilance and anxiety; amygdala stimulation in humans induces anxiety and fear (Colon and Popkin 2002).

Anxiety Disorders

Secondary Anxiety (Toxic or Metabolic Etiologies)

Anxiety Secondary to General Medical Condition

Anxiety due to a general medical condition exists when a patient has pathological anxiety that is an integral part of the pathophysiology of a medical illness or metabolic syndrome (e.g., anxiety caused by a hyperthyroid state). Sometimes, the diagnosis is finalized only after the fact, when removing the medical etiology remediates the anxiety or panic symptoms. Even then, relations between organic and reactive aspects of an overall anxiety syndrome are complex; having a medical condition causally related to a secondary anxiety syndrome does not rule out reactive anxiety.

Anxiety Induced by Substance

Substance-induced anxiety disorder is diagnosed when the anxiety symptoms are linked to substance intoxication or withdrawal. The symptoms must emerge within a month of substance intoxication or withdrawal.

Causes of Secondary Anxiety

Causes of secondary anxiety are numerous, as demonstrated in the following list. (Examples are given for each category.)

- *Cardiovascular conditions* (e.g., angina, cardiac dysrhythmia, cerebrovascular insufficiency, congestive heart failure, hypovolemia, left ventricular assist device, myocardial infarction, syncope, paroxysmal atrial tachycardia, valvular disease)

- *Metabolic conditions* (e.g., anemia, hyperkalemia, hyperthermia, hyponatremia)
- *Endocrine conditions* (e.g., carcinoid syndrome, hyperadrenalism, hyperthyroidism, hypocalcemia, hypoparathyroidism, pheochromocytoma)
- *Neurological conditions* (e.g., encephalitis, postencephalitic syndromes, Huntington's disease, multiple sclerosis, neurosyphilis, restless legs syndrome, seizure disorder [especially temporal lobe epilepsy], stroke, vascular headaches)
- *Respiratory conditions* (e.g., asthma, chronic obstructive pulmonary disease, pneumonia, pneumothorax, pulmonary edema, pulmonary embolus, ventilator dependence)
- *Drugs and withdrawal* (e.g., alcohol and its withdrawal, aminophylline/ theophylline, amphetamine, anticholinergics, antidepressants, caffeine, calcium channel blockers, cannabis, cocaine, digitalis toxicity, ephedrine, epinephrine, hallucinogens, insulin, levodopa, lidocaine, methylphenidate, antipsychotics (akathisia), phenylephrine, procaine, procarbazine, pseudoephedrine, salicylates, sedative-hypnotic withdrawal, steroids, sympathomimetics, thyroid preparations, yohimbine)

Generalized Anxiety Disorder

Generalized anxiety disorder (GAD) is characterized by excessive anxiety plus apprehensive expectations about events or activities. A patient's incessant worry is difficult to control and commonly evokes restlessness, fatigue, irritability, muscle tension, and sleep dysfunction (American Psychiatric Association 2000). When encountered in psychosomatic medicine, GAD is often an established condition that is exacerbated or unmasked in the outpatient or inpatient medical-surgical setting. Patients with GAD often have other psychiatric disorders. Motor tension, which may include trembling and twitching, is a routine part of GAD. Age at onset is usually the 20s or 30s.

Panic Disorder

Patients with primary panic disorder have recurrent, unexpected panic attacks, followed by worry, concern, and behavior changes related to the attacks (American Psychiatric Association 2000). The attacks are not due to a general medical condition or the direct effects of a substance. Panic disorder is underrecognized, underdiagnosed, and undertreated in outpatient medical settings. Panic disorder was present in about 35%–45% of the patients with chest pain whose cardiac catheterizations indicated normal coronary arteries (Colon and Popkin 2002).

Agoraphobia Without Panic Disorder

Patients with agoraphobia are not seen in medical-surgical settings for the simple reason that they rarely leave home unless there is a life-threatening emergency or unless their family or an outreach program brings them to medical attention.

Specific Phobias and Social Anxiety Disorder

Specific phobias and social anxiety disorder are usually hidden by the patient and are seldom identified by the primary care physician (Colon and Popkin 2002), unless the degree of impairment is pronounced or interferes with clinical care, such as when a claustrophobic patient cannot tolerate the magnetic resonance imaging procedure or when phobias involve blood, injection, general anesthesia, or injury. Patients often delay seeking medical attention because of avoidance associated with specific phobias.

Obsessive-Compulsive Disorder

Ego-dystonic obsessions and irresistible compulsive behaviors can produce somatic manifestations. For example, patients can develop dermatoses from frequent washing, and scarring from scratching. Obsessive-compulsive disorder (OCD) is highly comorbid with major depressive disorder and other anxiety disorders. Primary OCD, when it appears or recurs during a hospitalization or an outpatient workup for a new medical problem, may be aggravated by the stress, uncertainty, and loss of control experienced by patients. Secondary obsessive-compulsive syndromes occur in several neuropsychiatric conditions, including Tourette syndrome and epilepsy, and after head injury.

Acute Stress Disorder

Acute stress disorder (ASD) involves exposure to a life-threatening event that produces dissociative symptoms, reexperiencing of the trauma, avoidance of associated stimuli, increased arousal, and significant distress or social or occupational impairment (American Psychiatric Association 2000). Symptoms must last for more than 2 days but no more than 4 weeks and emerge within 1 month of the trauma. The symptoms are not substance induced and do not result from metabolic aspects of a general medical condition, although a life-threatening medical condition can certainly be the stressor associated with the psychological symptoms. ASD identifies patients at risk for posttraumatic stress disorder (PTSD); 50% of individuals with ASD go on to develop PTSD.

Posttraumatic Stress Disorder

A diagnosis of PTSD requires that a life-threatening trauma is persistently re-experienced, that the duration of the symptoms is longer than 1 month, that emotional numbing and increased arousal are present, and that stimuli linked to the trauma are avoided (American Psychiatric Association 2000). The experience of hospitalization or severe illness can trigger reexperiencing phenomena, nightmares, strong emotions, and autonomic arousal. A PTSD diagnosis should alert the clinician to the potential presence of comorbid psychiatric disorders, especially substance-related disorders, mood disorders, and panic disorder. PTSD risk is elevated when a person has traumatic brain injury. Traumatic stress disorders and their treatment are discussed in more detail in Chapter 19, "Disaster and Terrorism Casualties."

Adjustment Disorder With Anxiety

Adjustment disorder is a maladaptive response to an identifiable stressor. For many patients, the stressors are the medical illness, the clinic or hospital environment, and the treatment. Common sources of anxiety include uncertainty regarding medical diagnosis or prognosis; fears of amputation, loss of functional capacities, dependency, pain, or death; the potential impact of illness on the ability to work, perform essential household functions, or maintain income; and discomfort in the hospital due to being alone or entrusting one's care to strangers.

Health Anxiety

Definition

Health anxiety is worry or fear about having or getting a serious disease. There is a substantial focus on somatic symptoms, checking for signs of physical illness, and efforts to get reassurance from loved ones and the health care system.

Prevalence

In the U.S. general population, 3%–10% of individuals have significant health anxiety (Abramowitz and Braddock 2008); up to 30% of the population experience intermittent or milder fears about health.

Causes

The etiology of pathological health anxiety may be multifactorial in an individual patient. Causes may include genetically anxious temperament, early negative childhood experiences, social learning and modeling, and previously stressful experiences with illness and death (Abramowitz and Braddock 2008).

Differential Diagnosis

When pathological anxiety is present, the symptoms may be due to situational stress, a primary anxiety disorder, or a medical or toxic etiology. Several important questions must be answered when differentiating among causes of pathological anxiety:

1. *What past and family historical data are present?* Past or family history of a primary anxiety disorder increases the probability that current signs and symptoms are manifestations or recurrences of a primary anxiety disorder.
2. *Is there an identifiable potential medical or toxic cause for the anxiety?* The differential diagnosis of anxiety disorders includes a wide range of physical illnesses and psychoactive substances. Evaluation directed toward the body system most prominently affected by anxiety symptoms (e.g., gastrointestinal, respiratory) may provide diagnostic evidence for the etiology.
3. *What other potential psychiatric disorders are present?* Anxiety disorders are sometimes mistaken for other psychiatric disorders, especially agitated depression. Anxiety disorders usually have an earlier age at onset and are less episodic than mood disorders. Anxiety disorders frequently coexist with other psychiatric disorders, especially depression and substance-related disorders.
4. *What does the mental status examination show?* The mental status examination differentiates agitated delirium and psychotic disorders from anxiety disorders. The akathisia that occasionally occurs with antipsychotics can resemble anxiety.

Treatment and Management

Anxiety Disorder Due to General Medical Condition or Substance

When a remediable etiology for an anxiety syndrome is found, the clinician should reverse it, unless medically impossible or contraindicated. Unless anxiety symptoms are self-limited, treatment is indicated.

Acute Anxiety and Generalized Anxiety Disorder

Benzodiazepines

Benzodiazepines are effective anxiolytics. Few features make them potentially dangerous, especially with short-term use, in medically ill hospitalized patients. However, tolerance, dependence, and accident proneness present limitations to long-term use of benzodiazepines for some patients in the ambulatory setting. In patients without a history of previous addiction or risk factors for it, iatrogenic addiction is seldom a concern. Table 6–1 summarizes clinical and pharmacodynamic information about the most commonly used benzodiazepines. Dosages for elderly and medically ill patients should start lower than those for physically healthy younger patients.

Importance of half-life.   Agents with longer half-lives (e.g., diazepam, clonazepam) can be administered less frequently and may be easier to taper after prolonged use than agents with shorter half-lives. However, the former are more likely to accumulate in patients who have impaired hepatic function or who are taking multiple medications. Agents with shorter half-lives reach steady state much more rapidly and are eliminated more quickly, making them reasonable options for the short-term management of anxiety.

Lorazepam and oxazepam.   Lorazepam and oxazepam are metabolized by glucuronidation, have no active metabolites, and are better suited for patients with liver impairment or patients taking multiple medications.

Alternate routes of administration.   Among benzodiazepines, only lorazepam and midazolam are reliably absorbed when administered intramuscularly. Lorazepam, midazolam, and diazepam can be given intravenously, and lorazepam can be absorbed sublingually.

Adverse effects.   The most common side effect of benzodiazepines is sedation. Dizziness, weakness, anterograde amnesia (correlated with decreasing duration of action), nausea, and impaired motor performance are also reported. Tolerance can develop with chronic use. Withdrawal syndromes occur if dosage is reduced rapidly.

Buspirone

Advantages in medically ill patients.   Buspirone has advantages in medically ill patients because it is not sedating, has few drug interactions, and has no known abuse potential. Buspirone may be a particularly desirable choice in treating chronic anxiety in patients with severe chronic lung disease because it does not cause respiratory depression (Garner and Eldridge 1989).

Efficacy.   Evidence indicates that buspirone may be effective for GAD for some patients. Buspirone is not useful in the treatment of acute anxiety because its onset of therapeutic response requires 2–4 weeks or possibly longer. Buspirone is not effective as a primary treatment for panic disorder.

Dosage.   The average total daily dosage of buspirone is 30 mg, but the initial dosage is 5 mg twice daily, which can be increased by 5 mg/day every 3–4 days.

Adverse effects.   The adverse effects of buspirone include nausea, vomiting, headache, and dizziness. Buspirone can produce serotonin syndrome when taken with monoamine oxidase inhibitors (MAOIs) or with other medications that increase serotonin activity (Fait et al. 2002). It also can displace less firmly protein-bound drugs such as digoxin.

Antidepressants

Antidepressants, especially selective serotonin reuptake inhibitors (SSRIs) and serotonin-norepinephrine reuptake inhibitors (SNRIs), are effective in the treatment of GAD and other anxiety disorders (Gorman and Kent 1999). Most patients obtain some benefit within 2 weeks, with additional improvement over the next 6–8 weeks of treatment (Schatzberg 2003). Duloxetine, citalopram, paroxetine, sertraline, and venlafaxine have been approved by the U.S. Food and Drug Administration (FDA) for treatment of GAD.

Table 6–1.   Benzodiazepines in medical-surgical patients

Generic name	Trade name	Onset	Duration of action	Usual therapeutic dosage range (mg/day)[a]	Approximately equivalent anxiolytic dosage (mg)	Approximately equivalent hypnotic dosage (mg)
Alprazolam	Xanax	Intermediate	Short	2–8	0.5	1
Chlordiazepoxide	Librium	Intermediate	Long	15–150	10	25
Clonazepam	Klonopin	Intermediate	Long	1–3	1	1
Clorazepate	Tranxene	Rapid	Long	15–60	7.5	15
Diazepam	Valium	Rapid	Long	5–40	5	10
Estazolam	ProSom	Rapid	Intermediate	1–2	—	1
Flurazepam	Dalmane	Rapid to intermediate	Long	15–30	—	30
Lorazepam	Ativan	Intermediate	Intermediate	1–6	1	2
Midazolam	Versed	Rapid	Very short	0.1 mg/kg	2	2
Oxazepam	Serax	Intermediate to slow	Intermediate	30–120	15	30
Prazepam	Centrax	Slow	Long	20–60	10	20
Quazepam	Doral	Rapid	Long	7.5–15	—	15

Table 6–1.   Benzodiazepines in medical-surgical patients (*continued*)

Generic name	Trade name	Onset	Duration of action	Usual therapeutic dosage range (mg/day)[a]	Approximately equivalent anxiolytic dosage (mg)	Approximately equivalent hypnotic dosage (mg)
Temazepam	Restoril	Intermediate to slow	Short	15–30	15	30
Triazolam	Halcion	Intermediate	Short	0.125–0.5	—	0.5

[a]Doses for elderly and medically ill patients are often lower.

Source.   Adapted from Fair ML, Wise MG, Jachna JS, et al.: "Psychopharmacology," in *The American Psychiatric Publishing Textbook of Consultation-Liaison Psychiatry: Psychiatry in the Medically Ill,* 2nd Edition. Edited by Wise MG, Rundell JR. Washington, DC, American Psychiatric Publishing, 2002, pp. 939–987. Copyright, American Psychiatric Publishing, Inc. Used with permission.

Antipsychotic Medications

Antipsychotics may be beneficial in the medical setting when anxiety is accompanied by extreme fear, agitation, or delirium, although this is an off-label use. For example, 0.5 mg of haloperidol two or three times per day can markedly reduce the extreme fear that patients sometimes experience when they are being weaned from a ventilator. Low-dose antipsychotics can be useful in treating secondary anxiety disorders and other secondary psychiatric disorders resulting from high-dose steroids. Patients who are medically ill and have severe, refractory anxiety or panic or those in whom sedation from benzodiazepine agents cannot be tolerated also may benefit from a cautious trial of antipsychotics. The treating physician usually checks an electrocardiogram and observes the patient for acute dystonia, akathisia, and signs of neuroleptic malignant syndrome.

Beta-Blockers

Beta-blockers help control some peripheral sympathetic nervous system symptoms of anxiety, such as palpitations and sweating. The psychological components of anxiety are not ameliorated. Adverse effects of beta-blockers include bradycardia, hypotension, and fatigue.

Medical Psychotherapy

Supportive psychotherapy.   Supportive psychotherapy can help patients cope with acute stressors during a hospitalization or series of clinic visits.

Cognitive-behavioral therapy.   Cognitive-behavioral therapy (CBT) has demonstrated efficacy in treatment of anxiety disorders, including in medically ill patients (Kunik et al. 2008; Welkowitz et al. 1991). CBT involves active exploration, clarification, and testing of the patient's perceptions, beliefs, and self-perpetuating pathological behavior patterns.

Psychodynamic psychotherapy.   Common psychodynamic themes in patients with anxiety are loss, real and metaphorical physical threats, and lack of control. The clinician needs to address potential factors in the hospital environment that may be associated with the hospitalized patient's anxiety. These include intrusive medical procedures, sleep deprivation, financial stressors, noise, loss of privacy, and medical uncertainty.

Behavior therapies. Behavior therapies provide an opportunity for reduction of acute anxiety, enhancement of the patient's sense of mastery, and clarification of measurable goals. Behavioral interventions commonly used in psychosomatic medicine include relaxation techniques, systematic exposure and desensitization, biofeedback, meditation, hypnosis, and establishing graded goals with simple reinforcement schedules.

Panic Disorder

Benzodiazepines

Alprazolam and clonazepam are approved by the FDA for treatment of panic disorder; they may be most useful when rapid control of attacks is necessary. A significant limitation of alprazolam in chronic treatment of panic is the potential for dependence, withdrawal, and rebound symptoms on discontinuation and between doses. Discontinuation of alprazolam should be very gradual. Clonazepam has a longer half-life than alprazolam (24–48 hours); it is quite sedating for many patients.

Antidepressants

Four antidepressants (fluoxetine, paroxetine, sertraline, and venlafaxine) have received FDA approval for use in treating panic disorder. After a 2-week single-blind placebo lead-in, 168 patients with panic disorder entered a 10-week double-blind phase in which they were randomly assigned to treatment with either sertraline or placebo. Compared with placebo-treated patients, patients receiving the SSRI experienced decreases in frequency, severity, and duration of panic attacks (Pohl et al. 1998). Antidepressant dosages used for panic are similar to those used for depression, but higher dosages are frequently necessary for complete control of panic attacks, including the elimination of limited-symptom panic attacks. Tricyclic antidepressants, trazodone, and MAOIs are also efficacious, but panic disorder is an off-label usage. Bupropion is not effective in treating panic disorder. Chapter 10, "Mood Disorders," contains information on normal antidepressant dosages and potential adverse effects.

Antipsychotic Medications

Antipsychotics can be effective for rapid relief of acute panic attacks that endanger life or medical status. Parenteral haloperidol, in dosages of 2–5 mg (or higher if needed), can help control attacks, but this is an off-label use.

Other Medications

Propranolol blocks some peripheral manifestations of panic attacks. Clonidine is effective in decreasing symptoms in some patients.

Medical Psychotherapy

Explaining panic disorder to the patient as a part of supportive psychotherapy is helpful and reassuring. Behavioral, cognitive-behavioral, and relaxation therapies are effective primary or adjunctive treatments for panic disorder (Kunik et al. 2008). Cognitive-behavioral approaches emphasize the combination of symptom control (especially breathing) and cognitive restructuring to give physical symptoms a noncatastrophic interpretation. Use of medication and psychotherapy together is particularly efficacious, especially for patients with severe panic disorder.

Specific Phobia and Social Anxiety Disorder

The treatment of choice for specific phobia is graded exposure. In the hospitalized patient, exposure treatments do not have to be in vivo. Imagery-based exposure that uses a graded hierarchy of anxiety-producing stimuli is also effective (Hollander et al. 1988). Social anxiety in the outpatient setting is amenable to treatment with SSRIs and SNRIs. Paroxetine, sertraline, and the extended-release version of venlafaxine are approved by the FDA to treat social anxiety disorder and are superior to placebo, although overall, fewer than half of patients respond favorably (Stein et al. 1999).

Obsessive-Compulsive Disorder

Clomipramine is a potent serotonin reuptake blocker but is not well tolerated because of side effects. Two-thirds of patients with OCD who take clomipramine can expect significant symptomatic improvement; some patients have almost complete remission (Hollander et al. 1988). SSRIs are also effective for obsessive-compulsive symptoms, and they lack anticholinergic and sedating side effects. Three SSRI antidepressants—fluoxetine, paroxetine, and sertraline—are approved by the FDA for treating OCD. OCD treatment is enhanced when medication is combined with behavioral treatments, such as graded exposure and response prevention techniques.

Acute Stress Disorder and Posttraumatic Stress Disorder

Patients may have experienced traumatic events that resulted in hospitalization (e.g., motor vehicle accidents) or events that occurred in medical facilities (e.g., cardiac arrests). The mainstay of treatment of ASD and PTSD is CBT-based group and individual psychotherapy, along with antidepressant medication. Detailed discussion of the treatment of ASD and PTSD appears in Chapter 19, "Disaster and Terrorism Casualties."

Health Anxiety

Antidepressants and antianxiety medications may address some of the physiological manifestations of health anxiety. The primary psychological treatment shown to be effective for health anxiety is CBT. The goals of treatment (Abramowitz and Braddock 2008) are to help the patient do the following:

1. Decrease specific behaviors, such as frequent checking of the body for symptoms and asking for reassurance about health
2. Overcome avoidance of situations related to illness
3. Learn to face worries about illness realistically
4. Learn to reduce fear associated with thoughts about health and death
5. Accept the reality of ultimate death and resolve to enjoy life to its fullest
6. Improve relaxation and stress management skills
7. Improve physical conditioning

References

Abramowitz J, Braddock A: Treatment of Health Anxiety and Hypochondriasis: A Biopsychosocial Approach. Ashland, OH, Hogrefe & Huber, 2008

American Psychiatric Association: Diagnostic and Statistical Manual of Mental Disorders, 4th Edition, Text Revision. Washington, DC, American Psychiatric Association, 2000

Colon EA, Popkin MK: Anxiety and panic, in The American Psychiatric Publishing Textbook of Consultation-Liaison Psychiatry: Psychiatry in the Medically Ill, 2nd Edition. Edited by Wise MG, Rundell JR. Washington, DC, American Psychiatric Publishing, 2002, pp 393–415

Epstein SA, Hicks D: Anxiety disorders, in The American Psychiatric Publishing Textbook of Psychosomatic Medicine, 2nd Edition. Edited by Levenson JL. Washington DC, American Psychiatric Publishing, 2011, pp 241–260

Fait ML, Wise MG, Jachna JS, et al: Psychopharmacology, in The American Psychiatric Publishing Textbook of Consultation-Liaison Psychiatry: Psychiatry in the Medically Ill, 2nd Edition. Edited by Wise MG, Rundell JR. Washington, DC, American Psychiatric Publishing, 2002, pp 939–987

Garner SJ, Eldridge FL: Buspirone, an anxiolytic drug that stimulates respiration. Am Rev Respir Dis 139:945–950, 1989

Gorman JM, Kent JM: SSRIs and SNRIs: broad spectrum of efficacy beyond major depression. J Clin Psychiatry 60 (suppl 4):33–38, 1999

Hollander E, Liebowitz MR, Gorman JM: Anxiety disorders, in The American Psychiatric Press Textbook of Psychiatry. Edited by Talbott JA, Hales RE, Yudofsky SC. Washington, DC, American Psychiatric Press, 1988, pp 443–491

Katon W: Panic disorder and somatization: review of 55 cases. Am J Med 77:101–106, 1984

Kessler RC, Ormel J, Demler O, et al: Comorbid mental disorders account for the role impairment of commonly occurring chronic physical disorders: results from the National Comorbidity Survey. J Occup Environ Med 45:1257–1266, 2003

Kunik ME, Veazey C, Cully JA, et al: COPD education and cognitive behavioral therapy group treatment for clinically significant symptoms of depression and anxiety in COPD patients: a randomized controlled trial. Psychol Med 38:385–396, 2008

Levenson JL, Hamer RM, Rossiter LF: Psychopathology and pain in medical inpatients predict resource use during hospitalization but not rehospitalization. J Psychosom Res 36:585–592, 1992

Miller K, Massie MJ: Depression and anxiety. Cancer J 12:388–397, 2006

Pohl RB, Wolkow RM, Clary CM: Sertraline in the treatment of panic disorder: a double-blind multicenter trial. Am J Psychiatry 155:1189–1195, 1998

Roy-Byrne PP, Davidson KW, Kessler RC, et al: Anxiety disorders and comorbid medical illness. Focus 6:467–485, 2008

Saravay SM, Steinberg MD, Weinschel B, et al: Psychological comorbidity and length of stay in the general hospital. Am J Psychiatry 148:324–329, 1991

Schatzberg A: Antidepressants, in Manual of Clinical Psychopharmacology, 4th Edition. Edited by Schatzberg AF, Cole JO, DeBattista C. Washington, DC, American Psychiatric Publishing, 2003, pp 37–157

Simon GE, Walker EA: The consultation psychiatrist in the primary care clinic, in Essentials of Consultation-Liaison Psychiatry. Edited by Rundell JR, Wise MG. Washington, DC, American Psychiatric Press, 1999, pp 513–520

Stein MB, Fyer AJ, Davidson JRT, et al: Fluvoxamine treatment of social phobia (social anxiety disorder): a double-blind, placebo-controlled study. Am J Psychiatry 156:756–760, 1999

Welkowitz LA, Papp LA, Cloitre M, et al: Cognitive-behavior therapy for panic disorder delivered by psychopharmacologically oriented clinicians. J Nerv Ment Dis 179:472–476, 1991

Wells KB, Golding JM, Burnham MA: Psychiatric disorder in a sample of the population with and without chronic medical conditions. Am J Psychiatry 145:976–981, 1988

7

Delirium

Definition

Delirium is a global dysfunction in cerebral metabolism that generally has an acute onset; is often reversible; may be persistent; and is associated with significant mortality, morbidity, and health care cost.

Recognition

Delirium is underrecognized, even in settings where it is common. Palliative care physicians and nurses identify patients with rating scale–confirmed delirium only 44% of the time (Fong et al. 2009).

Consultation Effectiveness

Psychiatric consultation can improve outcomes for patients with delirium. General hospital patients with delirium who receive psychiatric consultations, compared with those who do not, have a lower readmission rate (33% vs. 50%, $P=0.01$) and lower likelihood of discharge to a nursing home (21% vs. 36%, $P=0.02$) (Mittal et al. 2006).

Epidemiology

Incidence

The prevalence of delirium is 1%–2% in the community but 15%–25% among patients in the general hospital and 30%–80% among patients in the intensive care unit (ICU) (Fong et al. 2009). Delirium incidence in the hospital varies widely by setting. Prevalence and incidence are highest in complex care settings, such as postoperative, intensive care, and palliative care settings (Fong et al. 2009; Franco et al. 2001; Robinson et al. 2009; Siddiqi et al. 2006).

Mortality

Mortality in delirium patients is estimated to be 15%–30% in the hospital and up to 40% over 1 year in elderly patients with delirium (Inouye 2006; Tennen and Rundell 2008).

One-Year Mortality

The relative risk for mortality in elderly patients with delirium and age-matched control subjects without delirium is 3.44 (95% confidence interval, 1.18–3.77). This effect is sustained over 12 months, adjusted for covariates (McCusker et al. 2002).

Accelerated Death

Delirium may also hasten death among patients who die from other causes, especially cancer. Among Mayo Clinic psychiatrically consulted medical-surgical inpatients who died within a year of hospitalization, the mean time to death was 122 days for patients with delirium and 218 days for patients without delirium (Tennen and Rundell 2008). Patients with cancer and delirium who died had a mean time to death of 60 days.

Morbidity

The more severe the delirium is, the poorer the outcome for the patient (Marcantonio et al. 2002). The agitation or lethargy associated with delirium can produce significant medical complications, including decreased oral intake, pulmonary emboli, aspiration, and decubitus ulcers (Fong et al. 2009).

Health Care Costs

After adjusting for preexisting risk factors, researchers have found that delirium is an independent determinant of duration of hospital stay, duration of ICU stay, rate of postdischarge institutionalization, nursing time per patient per day, and higher per-day hospital costs (Fong et al. 2009; Franco et al. 2001; Inouye 2008; Maldonado et al. 2009; Robinson et al. 2009; Siddiqi et al. 2006). For patients with delirium, significant increases in medical costs result from additional consultations, nursing, and support services such as laboratory testing and pharmacy (Fick et al. 2005; Millbrandt et al. 2004).

Predisposing Factors

Common Risk Factors

Several common risk factors predispose patients to delirium (Inouye 2006; Robinson et al. 2009):

- Age over 65 years
- Dementia (two-thirds of delirium patients have underlying dementia)
- Visual or hearing impairment
- Dehydration or malnutrition
- Multiple medications
- Multiple medical conditions
- Impaired functional status

Relationship of Predisposing Factors to Delirium Etiology

Delirium in higher-vulnerability patients (i.e., those with more risk factors predisposing to delirium) is often the result of mild precipitants, such as urinary tract infections and dehydration, which are treatable. By contrast, delirium in lower-vulnerability patients (who tend to be resistant to mild precipitants) is more likely to be the result of serious insults, such as head trauma, which are not treatable.

Assertive management of remediable etiologies in vulnerable patients, such as elderly individuals with dementia, can result in robustly positive responses. Figure 7–1 summarizes the relationship between patient vulnerability and severity of precipitating factors in delirium.

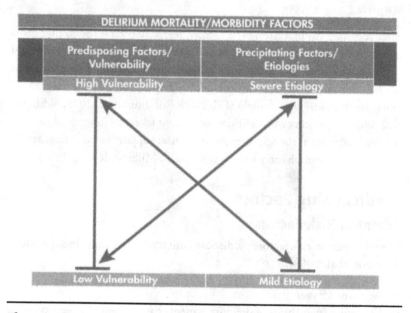

Figure 7-1.   Relationship between vulnerability and etiology in delirium.

Precipitating Factors and Etiologies

Delirium always has at least one etiology, often remediable or partly remediable. Development of delirium is a complex interaction between predisposing factors, context of care, and precipitating factors. Dozens of precipitants of delirium have been reported; the more frequently reported are listed below.

Toxic Etiologies

Toxic etiologies of delirium that are related to substances or poisons and associated abstinence syndromes include the following:

- *Medications* (Table 7-1)—normal dosages of medications may produce toxicity when polypharmacy results in hepatic enzyme inhibition or when an individual is a slow metabolizer at one of the cytochrome P450 enzymes.
- *Substances of abuse*—cocaine, amphetamines, cannabis, sedative-hypnotics.

Table 7–1. Common medications associated with delirium

Analgesics: meperidine, opiates

Antibiotics: acyclovir, ganciclovir, amphotericin B, interferon, cephalosporins, rifampin, isoniazid, ciprofloxacin

Anticholinergics: antihistamines, antispasmodics, atropine, benztropine, scopolamine, tricyclic antidepressants, trihexyphenidyl, belladonna alkaloids

Anticonvulsants: phenobarbital, phenytoin, valproic acid

Antineoplastic drugs: methotrexate, tamoxifen, vinblastine, vincristine, asparaginase, aminoglutethimide

Antiparkinsonian drugs: amantadine, bromocriptine, L-dopa

Cardiac drugs: beta-blockers, captopril, clonidine, digitalis, lidocaine, mexiletine, methyldopa, quinidine, tocainide, procainamide

Corticosteroids

Sedative-hypnotics: barbiturates, benzodiazepines

Sympathomimetics: amphetamine, cocaine, ephedrine, epinephrine, phenylephrine, theophylline

Others: cimetidine, disulfiram, lithium, metrizamide, ranitidine, quinacrine

- *Withdrawal syndromes*—alcohol, drug withdrawal delirium.
- *Poisons*—pesticides, solvents, lead, mercury.

Metabolic Etiologies

Delirium may result from neuropsychiatric effects of hypermetabolic or hypometabolic states, including but not limited to the following:

- *Acid-base balance abnormalities*—acidosis, alkalosis
- *Electrolyte disturbances*—hyponatremia, hyperkalemia, hypokalemia
- *Organ failure consequences*—hepatic failure (e.g., serum ammonia elevation), renal failure (elevated creatinine)
- *Burns*—electrolyte disturbances, acid-base problems, organ failure
- *Vitamin deficiencies*—vitamin B_{12}, folate, niacin, thiamine
- *Endocrinopathies*—hyperadrenalism, hypoadrenalism, hyperthyroidism, hypothyroidism, hyperglycemia, hypoglycemia

Central Nervous System Conditions and Events

The following central nervous system (CNS) conditions and events can contribute to delirium:

- *CNS trauma*—closed head injury, postoperative states, heatstroke, severe burns
- *Structural lesions*—stroke, CNS tumors (primary and metastatic), subdural hematoma, hydrocephalus, abscess, hemorrhage
- *Vasculitis*
- *Limbic encephalitis*
- *Seizure disorders*—including complex partial seizures and partial status epilepticus
- *Hypertensive encephalopathy*

Hypoxic Etiologies

Delirium can be caused by conditions or events, including the following, that decrease delivery of oxygen to the CNS:

- *Anemia*—including acute blood loss
- *Carbon monoxide*
- *Hypotension*
- *Pulmonary failure*
- *Cardiac failure*—congestive heart failure, myocardial infarction, arrhythmia, shock

Inflammatory Etiologies

Inflammatory etiologies of delirium include the following:

- *CNS infections*—meningitis, encephalitis
- *CNS effects of systemic infections*—syphilis, HIV, hepatitis, sepsis

Clinical Characteristics

Core Features

Delirium has a core set of clinical features that are virtually always present, and other signs and symptoms that are occasionally present (American Psychiatric Association 2000; Cole et al. 2007). Cole et al. (2007) used the Confusion Assessment Method (CAM; Inouye et al. 1990) to assess the frequency of core features among 290 medical inpatients older than 65 years diagnosed with delirium. Table 7–2 lists the frequency of various delirium symptoms in this population.

In addition, Cole et al. (2007) used a delirium rating measure to screen elderly patients admitted to medical services. The patients were studied over the course of their admissions. Three DSM-IV-TR symptoms—orientation to person, hyperactivity, and inattention—were associated with recovery in these patients. The authors recommended that these three symptoms be emphasized when screening elderly medical inpatients for delirium.

Table 7–2. Frequency (%) of symptoms in an elderly medical inpatient population diagnosed with delirium

Confusion Assessment Method (CAM) item*	Percentage identified
Acute onset*	100
Inattention*	100
Disorientation*	100
Fluctuation*	100
Memory impairment*	99
Psychomotor changes (agitation or retardation)	87
Altered level of consciousness*	59
Altered sleep-wake cycle	59
Perceptual disturbance*	25

Note. *Indicates DSM-IV-TR criteria item.
Source. Adapted from Cole et al. 2007.

Prodromal and Subsyndromal States

Some patients manifest mild to moderate prodromal and subsyndromal delirium symptoms, such as restlessness, anxiety, irritability, distractibility, or sleep disruption. How to differentiate subsyndromal symptoms from prodromal ones is not yet known, suggesting that assertive evaluation for potential delirium etiologies is important when these early or milder symptoms and signs emerge.

Psychomotor Variations

Patients with delirium may be hyperkinetic (psychomotor agitation), hypokinetic (somnolent or stuporous), or mixed (alternating between hyperkinetic and hypokinetic).

Frequency

Hyperkinetic delirium represents 15%–45% of delirium cases, hypokinetic delirium 20%–30%, and mixed delirium 25%–50% (J.R. Rundell, "Review of 129 Articles Between 2000 and 2008 Discussing Frequency, Mortality and Morbidity of Delirium in Inpatient Medical-Surgical Facilities," unpublished data, 2009). Variation in reported proportions can be accounted for by differences in clinical setting, patient populations, and definitions used.

Prognosis

Hypokinetic delirium patients have the worst prognosis in terms of illness severity, length of stay, mortality, and morbidity (J.R. Rundell, "Review of 129 Articles Between 2000 and 2008 Discussing Frequency, Mortality and Morbidity of Delirium in Inpatient Medical-Surgical Facilities," unpublished data, 2009). Hypokinetic delirium is more likely than hyperkinetic delirium to be underrecognized and undertreated.

Complications

The higher frequency of medical-surgical complications in patients with hypokinetic delirium may be partly due to their being more severely ill to begin with (Rundell 2008), and partly due to a higher risk of nosocomial infections, falls, venous thromboses, pressure sores, and aspiration because of the hypokinesis.

Temporal Course

Initial Phase of Delirium

Three features of the temporal course of acute delirium are characteristic and assist in differential diagnosis:

- Abrupt acute or subacute onset of symptoms
- Fluctuation of symptom severity during an episode—relatively lucid intervals alternating with more severe symptoms
- Subsyndromal or prodromal signs and symptoms

Persistence of Cognitive Dysfunction

Jackson et al. (2004) reviewed seven prospective studies of patients who developed delirium as inpatients and were compared over time (median 2 years) with control patients without delirium. Four studies showed that patients with delirium had lower scores over time on cognitive measures, and three studies found a higher incidence of dementia in patients with a history of delirium.

Characteristic Neuropsychiatric Impairments on Mental Status Examination

Impaired Attention and Concentration

The patient with delirium has difficulty sustaining attention and is usually either distractible or unable to focus.

Impaired Short-Term Memory

In the presence of impaired attention and registration, memory difficulties in patients with delirium are secondary unless a patient has preexisting dementia. After recovering from delirium, some patients are amnestic for the entire episode, others have islands of memory, and a few will recall the entire episode.

Disorientation

Disorientation to time and place is typical in patients with delirium.

Changes in Level of Consciousness

Level of consciousness varies from hyperalert in a patient with hyperkinetic delirium to stuporous or comatose in a patient with severe hypokinetic delirium.

Impaired Visuospatial Skills

Patients with delirium often have visuoconstructional impairment and have difficulty drawing simple geometric designs or drawing more complex figures such as a clock face. Clock face drawing requires input from the following:

- Nondominant parietal cortex for overall spatial proportions and relations
- Dominant parietal cortex for details such as numbers or hands
- Prefrontal cortex for understanding the concept of time

Disturbed Executive Functions

Many higher-level executive functions are dependent on the prefrontal cortices and are affected by delirium. These functions include switching mental sets, abstraction, sequential thinking, verbal fluency, and judgment (Trzepacz 1994).

Disorganized Thought Processes

Patients with delirium often have disorganized thought patterns. The severity of the thought disturbance can range from tangentiality and circumstantiality to loose associations. At the most severe level of thought disorganization, speech may resemble a fluent aphasia (Wise and Trzepacz 1999).

Impaired Language and Speech

Language and speech impairments in patients with delirium range from mild dysarthria or mumbling to dysphasia or muteness. Word-finding difficulty, dysnomia with paraphasias, and reduced comprehension are common.

Perceptual Disturbances

The patient with delirium often experiences misperceptions, usually illusions or hallucinations. Perceptual disturbances can be auditory or visual; visual illusions and hallucinations are more common than auditory.

Diagnosis

Components of Diagnostic Assessment

1. *History.* Establishing a time line is vital to understanding temporal associations of potentially related medical conditions or events. Although

temporality does not equate to causality, it raises the index of suspicion and helps prioritize evaluation and management recommendations.

2. *Physical and neurological examination, including vital signs.*
3. *Medication review.* Dosage initiation or changes should be correlated with behavior changes.
4. *Mental status examination.* The clinician should use standardized formats that can be repeated over time (e.g., clock drawing, Mini-Mental State Examination).
5. *Electrocardiogram.*
6. *Chest X ray.*
7. *Electroencephalogram and lumbar puncture, if indicated.*
8. *Laboratory tests.* The following should be tested: electrolytes, glucose, calcium, liver function, renal function, magnesium, complete blood count, serum drug levels, urine drug levels, and oxygen saturation or arterial blood gases.

Differential Diagnosis

The differential diagnosis of delirium is extensive. Delirium may have multiple etiologies. Francis et al. (1990) found that 55% of elderly patients with delirium had a single definite or probable etiology, and the remaining 45% had an average of 2.8 etiologies per patient.

Differentiating delirium from dementia and depression is particularly important because considerable comorbidity among these three conditions ("the 3 *Ds*") exists (Trzepacz et al. 2011; see Table 7–3).

Electroencephalogram Findings

Almost all cases of delirium show diffuse slowing (delta waves) on the electroencephalogram. Although other electroencephalographic patterns are suggestive of particular delirium etiologies (Kennard et al. 1945; Trzepacz 1994), none are pathognomonic.

Diagnostic Instruments

Several instruments are available that measure a broad range of symptoms of delirium and can be used for screening purposes or to quantitate symptom severity over time.

Table 7–3. The 3 Ds: delirium, dementia, and depression

	Delirium	Dementia	Depression
Onset	Acute or subacute	Chronic	Subacute/variable
Course	Fluctuating	Progressive	Variable
Reversibility	Common	Rare	Remission
Orientation	Impaired	Impaired late	Clear
Attention	Impaired	Impaired late	Impaired
Memory	Impaired	Impaired	Intact
Hallucinations	Usually visual	Visual or auditory	Auditory
Delusions	Fleeting/fragmented	More fixed	Mood congruent

Source. Adapted from Trzepacz et al. 2011.

Confusion Assessment Method

The CAM (Inouye et al. 1990) is an algorithm of four cardinal symptoms of delirium intended for use in high-risk settings by nonpsychiatric clinicians. The CAM can be supplemented by more intensive interviews to diagnose delirium.

Delirium Rating Scales

The Delirium Rating Scale (DRS; Trzepacz et al. 1988) and the substantially revised DRS-R-98 (Trzepacz et al. 2001) can help distinguish delirium from dementia, schizophrenia, depression, and other medical conditions; it is available in several languages.

Memorial Delirium Assessment Scale

The Memorial Delirium Assessment Scale (MDAS; Breitbart et al. 1996) is a 10-item severity rating scale that is used after a patient has been diagnosed with delirium and in serial examinations.

Prevention

Prevention is the most effective delirium management principle. Attention to the following six factors, all of which can be addressed by nursing staff in the general hospital, reduces delirium frequency (15% vs. 10%), number of delirium episodes, and delirium duration (Inouye et al. 1999):

1. *Frequent orientation*
2. *Noise reduction protocol*—attention to a quiet environment, and normalizing lighting for as normal a sleep-wake cycle as possible
3. *Early mobilization*—encouraging ambulation and mobility as soon as possible, especially after surgery, and continuing on a regular and increasing basis
4. *Visual aids*—ensuring that spectacles are on the patient's head and not on the bedside stand
5. *Hearing aids*—ensuring that patients with hearing aids are wearing them
6. *Hydration*—assertive attention to intake, output, and serum electrolytes

Management and Symptomatic Treatment

Management and symptomatic treatment of delirium have two separate and important goals. The first is critical and bears directly on the survival of the patient: to identify and reverse, when possible, the reason(s) for the delirium. The second is to reduce neuropsychiatric symptoms of delirium with environmental and pharmacological interventions (American Psychiatric Association 1999).

Identification and Reversal of Remediable Etiologies

Careful attention to diagnostic assessment, as summarized in the "Diagnosis" section earlier in this chapter, is important to identify remediable etiologies. Construction of a time line to identify and prioritize potentially related medical conditions or events is a key component of this assessment.

Reduction of Symptoms

Environmental Management of Delirium Signs and Symptoms

Preventive measures, implemented by the entire health care team, can be effective once delirium has occurred or when a prodrome is evident. The need to use pharmacological symptomatic treatment indicates a failure of prevention. The health care team can apply the following measures, which may obviate the need for pharmacotherapy in some patients and reduce pharmacotherapy requirements in others:

1. Monitor vital signs, fluid intake and output, and oxygenation.
2. Avoid sleep interruptions whenever possible.
3. Place the patient in a room near the nursing station.
4. Arrange for a sitter if safety is a potential issue.
5. Maintain the bed in a low position; exercise caution with the use of side rails.
6. Avoid placing delirious patients in a room together.
7. Encourage presence of family members; educate patients and families about delirium.
8. Provide familiar objects and visual cues, such as family photos, clocks, and calendars.

9. Provide adequate lighting, including a night-light at night.
10. Minimize transfers; perform procedures in the patient's room when possible.
11. Maximize staff continuity and familiarity.
12. Reduce excessive environmental stimuli.
13. Repeatedly orient the patient to staff, surroundings, and situations.
14. Make sure glasses and hearing aids are used.
15. Use mechanical restraints only as a last resort, when potential danger to patient or others cannot be addressed by other environmental measures or by chemical restraint.

Pharmacological Management of Delirium Signs and Symptoms

Medications are used when an etiology of delirium is not immediately remediable and when hyperactive signs and symptoms produce clinical or safety complications. Antipsychotics are most commonly used; the most frequently used nonantipsychotic medication is lorazepam, which may be administered instead of or along with an antipsychotic.

There is scant evidence to support the use of psychotropic medications in managing hypoactive delirium.

Evidence base for antipsychotic medication treatment of delirium target symptoms.   There are more than a dozen studies of pharmacological management of delirium symptoms conducted in well-designed prospective paradigms that included severity ratings and structured assessments (Seitz et al. 2007). No double-blind, placebo-controlled clinical trials have been conducted; giving placebo medications to patients with such a potentially lethal condition may be unethical.

• *Equivalent clinical responses*—Clinical improvement of delirium signs and symptoms has been reported with the medications studied: chlorpromazine, haloperidol, quetiapine, olanzapine, and risperidone. No clinical benefit has been demonstrated for one antipsychotic medication over another in terms of target symptoms of delirium, although the medications have different adverse effects (Fong et al. 2009).
• *Lorazepam versus haloperidol*—A 2004 review identified nine studies comparing haloperidol with lorazepam. In the only double-blind study, halo-

Table 7–4.   Antipsychotic medication management of delirium symptoms: average daily dosages

Medication	Average daily dosage (range)
Haloperidol (all forms)	5.9 mg (0.5–30 mg)
Oral haloperidol	3.2 mg (0.5–20 mg)
Intramuscular haloperidol	6.5 mg (0.5–17.5 mg)
Intravenous haloperidol	7.3 mg (0.5–30 mg)
Olanzapine	6.2 mg (2.5–20 mg)
Quetiapine	100.4 mg (12.5–1,000 mg)
Risperidone	2.8 mg (0.25–35 mg)
Ziprasidone	101.8 mg (20–160 mg)

Source.   Adapted from Rundell 2008.

peridol was found to be more effective. The other eight studies were open-label and found the two drugs to be similar in efficacy (Khasati et al. 2004). Lorazepam was more likely to cause sedation and worsening of symptoms; haloperidol was more likely to have QTc prolongation. The authors concluded that haloperidol would be a superior first choice, although lorazepam, either alone or in combination with haloperidol, would be an acceptable alternative, particularly for patients with cardiac risks.

Medication management guidelines.

- *Frequently used antipsychotic medications*—At Mayo Clinic, the five antipsychotic medications most frequently used in pharmacological management of delirium symptoms are haloperidol, olanzapine, quetiapine, risperidone, and ziprasidone (Rundell 2008) (see Table 7–4). Haloperidol has a number of clinical advantages, including its availability as a parenteral formulation, its low cost, and decades of experience in seriously ill patients. Other antipsychotics have advantages for particular subgroups of patients with delirium (e.g., patients with Parkinson's disease and other movement disorders, patients with severe insomnia).

- *Antipsychotic medication dosages*—Dosage ranges vary among all medications used. Starting dosages are often difficult to determine. At Mayo Clinic, daily dosage ranges for frequently used antipsychotic medications administered in the inpatient medical-surgical setting vary considerably (Rundell 2008), as shown in Table 7–4.
- *Haloperidol for hyperactive delirium symptoms*—Starting doses and administration guidelines (Mayo Clinic Delirium Workgroup 2007 [unpublished]) for haloperidol in the management of hyperactive delirium symptoms are provided in Table 7–5.

Table 7–5. Haloperidol management of hyperactive delirium: starting doses and administration guidelines

Starting doses

Agitation level

  Mild: 0.5–2.5 mg

  Moderate: 2.5–5.0 mg

  Severe: 5.0–10.0 mg

Administration guidelines

For elderly patients, use a starting dose about half that recommended in Table 7–4.

Allow 30 minutes between parenteral doses and 60 minutes between oral doses before readministering.

Check QT and QTc intervals if haloperidol is newly initiated or changed from another antipsychotic.

For continued agitation, double the previous dose and monitor patient's vital signs.

Once the patient is calm, add the total milligrams of haloperidol required; administer the same number of milligrams over the next 24 hours.

If the patient remains calm, reduce the dose by 50% every 24 hours.

To convert haloperidol from intravenous to oral dosage, double the intravenous total daily dosage and administer orally in two or three divided doses.

Source. Mayo Clinic Delirium Workgroup 2007 (unpublished).

Morbidity and Mortality Risks Associated With Antipsychotic Medications

All antipsychotic medications may prolong the QT or QTc interval, but some increase it more than others do. Most antipsychotic medications, including all atypical antipsychotics, carry a black box warning regarding reports of increased mortality in elderly patients with dementia-related psychosis who are treated with antipsychotics. Although the relevance of studies that support the black box warnings to short-term use for delirium symptoms is unclear, clinicians need to be aware of findings from these studies.

Associations Between Antipsychotic Medication Use and Mortality

Fifteen of 17 antipsychotic medication trials of ziprasidone showed higher mortality in treated patients than in nontreated patients; most deaths were due to cardiac events (U.S. Food and Drug Administration 2005). A subsequent review suggested elevated mortality for patients taking any antipsychotic medication (Gill et al. 2007). Although statistically significant, absolute elevations of mortality risk are slight (e.g., 0.2%–2.2% absolute risk differences in the landmark review by Gill et al. 2007). None of these studies were done in the specific setting of delirium treatment.

Potential Reasons for Association Between Antipsychotic Medications and Mortality

A number of possible reasons, apart from cardiac concerns, may explain the association between antipsychotic medications and elevated mortality, especially in elderly patients with dementia. Sedation may lead to elevated risk for choking, aspiration, and deep vein thromboses. Hypotension may lead to fall and fracture risk.

Practice Guideline Recommendations

Although absolute causality has not been established, the presence of elevated mortality risk suggests the importance of following the American Psychiatric Association's (1999) recommendation to check electrocardiograms before and after initiating or changing an antipsychotic medication in a delirious hospitalized patient.

Prolongation of QT or QTc Interval

Caution should be exercised when the patient's baseline QT interval is greater than 436 milliseconds or the QTc is greater than 475 milliseconds, or when a prior dose caused prolongation of the QTc interval from baseline (Tisdale et al. 2007). Evidence indicates that monitoring either the uncorrected QT interval or the QTc interval may be helpful; Tisdale et al. (2007) found that each was equally accurate in predicting haloperidol-associated torsade de pointes in a review of ICU patients.

Risk of Torsade de Pointes

Prolonged cardiac conduction is associated with development of torsade de pointes. The precise risk and frequency of torsade de pointes following antipsychotic administration is unknown.

- Reported frequency varies between 1/2,500 and 1/25 depending on clinical setting (e.g., general medical unit or ICU treating overdose patients). In one report of 1,100 consecutive ICU patients, intravenous haloperidol was implicated in inducing torsade de pointes tachyarrhythmia in 4 patients (Wilt et al. 1993).
- Associated factors found to be present in patients who develop torsade de pointes include preexisting advanced heart disease, doses of haloperidol >35 mg over 24 hours, baseline elevated QTc interval, baseline bradycardia, personal or family history of sudden death or syncope (suggestive of familial long QT syndrome), concurrent use of other QT-prolonging medications, hypokalemia, and hypomagnesemia (Tisdale et al. 2007).

Medication Management Alternatives

Administration of small doses of intravenous lorazepam, particularly in patients whose symptoms have not responded to haloperidol alone, often helps to reduce agitation and decrease the amount of antipsychotics required. Benzodiazepines are the symptomatic treatment of choice in the setting of alcohol or benzodiazepine withdrawal associated with delirium. Propofol, midazolam, and sometimes dexmedetomidine are used for short-term or emergent behavioral control when other alternatives in the ICU setting have been ineffective.

References

American Psychiatric Association: Practice guideline for the treatment of patients with delirium. Am J Psychiatry 156 (suppl):1–20, 1999

American Psychiatric Association: Diagnostic and Statistical Manual of Mental Disorders, 4th Edition, Text Revision. Washington, DC, American Psychiatric Association, 2000

Breitbart W, Marotta R, Platt MM, et al: A double-blind trial of haloperidol, chlorpromazine, and lorazepam in the treatment of delirium in hospitalized AIDS patients. Am J Psychiatry 153:231–237, 1996

Cole MG, McCusker J, Ciampi A, et al: An exploratory study of diagnostic criteria for delirium in older medical inpatients. J Neuropsychiatry Clin Neurosci 19:151–156, 2007

Fick DM, Kolanowski AM, Waller JL, et al: Delirium superimposed on dementia in a community-dwelling population: a 3-year retrospective study of occurrence, costs, and utilization. J Gerontol B Psychol Sci Soc Sci 60:748–753, 2005

Fong TG, Tulebaev SR, Inouye SK: Delirium in elderly adults: diagnosis, prevention, and treatment. Nat Rev Neurol 5:210–220, 2009

Francis J, Martin D, Kapoor W: A prospective study of delirium in hospitalized elderly. JAMA 263:1097–1101, 1990

Franco K, Litaker D, Locala J, et al: The cost of delirium in the surgical patient. Psychosomatics 42:68–73, 2001

Gill SS, Bronskilil SE, Normand SL, et al: Antipsychotic drug use and mortality in older adults with dementia. Ann Intern Med 146:775–786, 2007

Inouye SK: Delirium in older persons. N Engl J Med 354:1157–1164, 2006

Inouye SK: One-year health care costs associated with delirium in the elderly population. Arch Intern Med 168:27–32, 2008

Inouye SK, van Dyck CH, Alessi CA, et al: Clarifying confusion: the confusion assessment method: a new method for detection of delirium. Ann Intern Med 113:941–948, 1990

Inouye SK, Bogardus ST, Charpentier PA, et al: A multicomponent intervention to prevent delirium in hospitalized older patients. N Engl J Med 340:669–676, 1999

Jackson JC, Gordon SM, Hart RP, et al: The association between delirium and cognitive decline: a review of the empirical literature. Neuropsychol Rev 14:87–98, 2004

Kennard MA, Bueding E, Wortis WB: Some biochemical and electroencephalographic changes in delirium tremens. Q J Stud Alcohol 6:4–14, 1945

Khasati N, Thompson J, Dunning J: Is haloperidol or a benzodiazepine the safest treatment for acute psychosis in the critically ill patient? Interact Cardiovasc Thorac Surg 3:233–236, 2004

Maldonado JR, Wysong A, van der Starre PJ, et al: Dexmedetomidine and the reduction of postoperative delirium after cardiac surgery. Psychosomatics 50:206–217, 2009

Marcantonio E, Ta T, Duthie E, et al: Delirium severity and psychomotor types: their relationship with outcomes after hip fracture repair. J Am Geriatr Soc 50:850–857, 2002

McCusker J, Cole M, Abrahamowicz M, et al: Delirium predicts 12-month mortality. Arch Intern Med 162:457–463, 2002

Millbrandt EB, Deppen S, Harrison PL, et al: Costs associated with delirium in mechanically ventilated patients. Crit Care Med 32:955–962, 2004

Mittal D, Majithia D, Kennedy R, et al: Differences in characteristics and outcome of delirium as based on referral patterns. Psychosomatics 47:367–375, 2006

Robinson TN, Raeburn CD, Tran ZV, et al: Postoperative delirium in the elderly: risk factors and outcomes. Ann Surg 249:173–178, 2009

Rundell JR: Antipsychotic practice patterns among medical and surgical inpatients who receive psychiatric consultation. Presented at the annual meeting of the European Association of Consultation-Liaison Psychiatry and Psychosomatics, Bologna, Italy, June 2008

Seitz DP, Gill SS, Van Zyl LT: Antipsychotics in the treatment of delirium: a systematic review. J Clin Psychiatry 68:11–21, 2007

Siddiqi N, House AO, Holmes JD: Occurrence and outcome of delirium in medical in-patients: a systematic literature review. Age Ageing 35:350–364, 2006

Tennen G, Rundell JR: Factors associated with mortality in hospitalized medical-surgical patients requiring psychiatric consultation. Poster presented at the annual meeting of the Academy of Psychosomatic Medicine, Miami, FL, November 2008

Tisdale JE, Kovacs R, Mi D, et al: Accuracy of uncorrected versus corrected QT interval for prediction of torsade de pointes associated with intravenous haloperidol. Pharmacotherapy 27:175–182, 2007

Trzepacz PT: Neuropathogenesis of delirium: a need to focus our research. Psychosomatics 35:375–391, 1994

Trzepacz PT, Baker RW, Greenhouse J: A symptom rating scale for delirium. Psychiatry Res 23:89–97, 1988

Trzepacz PT, Mittal D, Torres R, et al: Validation of the Delirium Rating Scale–Revised-98: comparison with the Delirium Rating Scale and the Cognitive Test for Delirium. J Neuropsychiatry Clin Neurosci 13:229–242, 2001

Trzepacz PT, Meagher DJ, Leonard M: Delirium, in The American Psychiatric Publishing Textbook of Psychosomatic Medicine, 2nd Edition. Edited by Levenson JL. Washington, DC, American Psychiatric Publishing, 2011, pp 71–114

U.S. Food and Drug Administration: Public health advisory: deaths with antipsychotics in elderly patients with behavioral disturbances. April 11, 2005. Available at: www.fda.gov/Drugs/DrugSafety/PostmarketDrugSafetyInformationforPatientsandProviders/DrugSafetyInformationforHeathcareProfessionals/PublicHealthAdvisories/UCM053171. Accessed January 1, 2011.

Wilt JL, Minnema AM, Johnson RF, et al: Torsade de pointes associated with the use of intravenous haloperidol. Ann Intern Med 119:391–394, 1993

Wise MG, Trzepacz PT: Delirium (confusional states), in Essentials of Consultation-Liaison Psychiatry. Edited by Rundell JR, Wise MG. Washington, DC, American Psychiatric Press, 1999, pp 81–93

8

Dementia

Dementia is present in a substantial number of patients admitted to medical and surgical inpatient units and is associated with longer lengths of stay and higher costs for those patients than for patients without dementia. An estimated 2.4–4.5 million individuals in the United States have dementia, and if no scientific advances reduce the incidence of dementia, the prevalence is anticipated to increase to 11–18.5 million by 2050 (Holsinger et al. 2007).

Epidemiology

Prevalence

The prevalence of dementia increases with advancing age. The rate is 6%–8% in individuals ages 65 years and older, and more than 30% in those older than 85 years (Knopman et al. 2003).

Incidence and Survival

Incidence rates of dementia are about 1% per year. Survival rates for patients with dementia are lower than for individuals without dementia; however, survival is still relatively long, with a median survival of 6 years after the onset of dementia symptoms. Therefore, the prevalence rate surpasses the incidence rate (Knopman et al. 2003).

Clinical Features of Dementia
Decline and Sufficient Impairment

- The person with dementia demonstrates a decline from his or her previous level of functioning.
- The impairment is sufficient to cause disruption in social and occupational activities.

Multiple Cognitive Deficits

Multiple cognitive deficits are present that include memory impairment (the ability to learn, retain, and retrieve newly acquired information) and at least one of the following (Holsinger et al. 2007; Knopman et al. 2003):

- *Aphasia*—impaired ability to comprehend and express verbal information
- *Apraxia*—impaired ability to execute motor activities despite intact motor abilities, sensory function, and comprehension of the required task
- *Agnosia*—failure to recognize or identify objects despite intact sensory function
- *Disturbance in executive functioning*—impaired ability to perform abstract reasoning, plan for future events, solve problems, maintain focus despite distraction, and manipulate more than one idea at a time

Memory Impairment

Memory impairment as a primary feature does not encompass all dementias. For example, memory is relatively spared in primary progressive aphasia and frontotemporal dementia (Holsinger et al. 2007).

Neurological Disorders

The definition of dementia includes neurological disorders, such as head trauma, that are associated with cognitive impairment and disruption in functioning but are not progressive. The definition does not include impairment due to Axis I disorders or delirium (American Psychiatric Association 2000).

Mild Cognitive Impairment

Definition

Cognitive dysfunction without functional decline. Individuals who have cognitive dysfunction beyond what is expected for normal aging but do not have functional decline as seen in dementia are said to have mild cognitive impairment (MCI).

At least one cognitive domain affected. In MCI, cognitive dysfunction affects at least one cognitive domain, most commonly recent memory as demonstrated by impaired performance on delayed recall (referred to as the amnesic type).

Prevalence and Incidence

The reported prevalence and incidence of MCI vary widely because of inconsistencies in the way the diagnostic criteria are used and the frequency of comorbid depression. Findings from some studies have suggested that up to 60% of patients with MCI who progress to Alzheimer's disease (AD) have depression (Chertkow et al. 2008).

Risk of Progression to Dementia

The risk of progression from MCI to dementia is high. The risk of developing dementia is 5–10 times higher for individuals with MCI than for individuals with normal cognition (Knopman et al. 2003).

Risk Factors for Dementia

- *Age* is the strongest risk factor for dementia, especially for AD.
- *Baseline cognitive impairment.*
- *Family history.* The relative risk of dementia in individuals with at least one first-degree relative with AD is 3.5, and the risk is higher for female relatives than males (Green et al. 2002; van Duijn et al. 1991). Familial risk is greater for early-onset dementia (Silverman et al. 2003) and for African Americans (Green et al. 2002).

- *Genetic factors.* The allele producing the ε4 type of apolipoprotein E (APOE*E4) has the strongest evidence for a genetic risk factor in late-life nonfamilial AD (Li et al. 2008).
- *Vascular factors.* Vascular disease is a risk factor for most dementias, including AD. Diabetes mellitus, hypercholesterolemia, and tobacco smoking have been associated with a higher risk of AD, whereas hypertension, angina, and atrial fibrillation have been associated with accelerated decline in patients with AD (Viswanathan et al. 2009).
- *Other.* Lack of alcohol consumption (compared with consumption of only 1–2 drinks per day), low body mass index (<18.5), low educational attainment, and history of coronary bypass surgery may also be risk factors (Barnes et al. 2009).

Major Types of Dementia

Alzheimer's Disease

Prevalence

AD is the most common cause of dementia in elderly people. AD accounts for at least 50%–60% of all dementias, and up to 80% if combined with other pathological lesions (Knopman et al. 2003).

Pathophysiology

The accumulation of β-amyloid peptide is primary in the pathogenesis and leads to neuritic plaques. Formation of neurofibrillary tangles is considered to be secondary to the deposition of β-amyloid (Cummings 2004).

Key Diagnostic Features

The DSM-IV-TR (American Psychiatric Association 2000) diagnostic criteria for dementia of the Alzheimer's type are listed in Table 8–1. The following are important features:

- The pattern of progression varies, but most often recent memory impairment is observed first, with pervasive forgetfulness demonstrated through repetitive questions and statements.

- Deficits in executive function, such as problems with paying bills or preparing a meal, are generally seen early in the course of the disease.
- Motor and sensory deficits, incontinence, gait disturbances, and seizures are evident late in the disease (Cummings 2004).

Neuropsychiatric Symptoms

The following neuropsychiatric symptoms are common in AD:

- *Depression* prevalence estimates among patients with AD vary widely, but most estimates range from 30% to 50%, which suggests that major depressive syndrome of AD may be among the most common mood disorders of late life. A high rate of major depressive episodes occurs at or after the onset of cognitive decline (Zubenko et al. 2003).
- *Agitated or aggressive behaviors* occur in up to 70% of patients with AD.
- *Delusions or hallucinations* are seen in 30%–50% of patients with AD. Psychotic symptoms usually present in the later stages of disease.

Neuropsychiatric symptoms typically result in longer hospital stays, a higher rate of nursing home placement, increased cost, and more caregiver stress (Kales et al. 2007; Sink et al. 2005; Sultzer et al. 2008).

Dementia Due to Cerebrovascular Disease

Prevalence

The prevalence of pure vascular dementia ranges from 10% to 15%, or about one-fifth that of AD, and an additional 20% of patients have a combination of vascular dementia and AD. The definition of dementia due to cerebrovascular disease generally includes pure vascular dementia and vascular dementia combined with AD (Knopman et al. 2003).

Pathophysiology

Cerebrovascular disease is most often secondary to atherosclerotic disease or amyloid angiopathy. Rarely, autoimmune mechanisms are the etiology. Cerebral injury can be caused by large-vessel infarctions, multiple lacunar infarctions, extensive subcortical and periventricular white matter disease, and microvascular changes (American Psychiatric Association Work Group 2007).

Table 8–1. DSM-IV-TR diagnostic criteria for dementia of the Alzheimer's type

A. The development of multiple cognitive deficits manifested by both

  (1) memory impairment (impaired ability to learn new information or to recall previously learned information)

  (2) one (or more) of the following cognitive disturbances:

    (a) aphasia (language disturbance)

    (b) apraxia (impaired ability to carry out motor activities despite intact motor function)

    (c) agnosia (failure to recognize or identify objects despite intact sensory function)

    (d) disturbance in executive functioning (i.e., planning, organizing, sequencing, abstracting)

B. The cognitive deficits in criteria A1 and A2 each cause significant impairment in social or occupational functioning and represent a significant decline from a previous level of functioning.

C. The course is characterized by gradual onset and continuing cognitive decline.

D. The cognitive deficits in criteria A1 and A2 are not due to any of the following:

  (1) other central nervous system conditions that cause progressive deficits in memory and cognition (e.g., cerebrovascular disease, Parkinson's disease, Huntington's disease, subdural hematoma, normal-pressure hydrocephalus, brain tumor)

  (2) systemic conditions that are known to cause dementia (e.g., hypothyroidism, vitamin B_{12} or folic acid deficiency, niacin deficiency, hypercalcemia, neurosyphilis, HIV infection)

  (3) substance-induced conditions

E. The deficits do not occur exclusively during the course of a delirium.

F. The disturbance is not better accounted for by another Axis I disorder (e.g., major depressive disorder, schizophrenia).

Code based on presence or absence of a clinically significant behavioral disturbance:

294.10 Without behavioral disturbance: if the cognitive disturbance is not accompanied by any clinically significant behavioral disturbance.

294.11 With behavioral disturbance: if the cognitive disturbance is accompanied by a clinically significant behavioral disturbance (e.g., wandering, agitation).

Table 8–1. DSM-IV-TR diagnostic criteria for dementia of the Alzheimer's type *(continued)*

Specify subtype:

With early onset: if onset is at age 65 years or below

With late onset: if onset is after age 65 years

Coding note: Also code 331.0 Alzheimer's disease on Axis III. Indicate other prominent clinical features related to the Alzheimer's disease on Axis I (e.g., 293.83 mood disorder due to Alzheimer's disease, with depressive features, and 310.1 personality change due to Alzheimer's disease, aggressive type).

Source. Reprinted from American Psychiatric Association: *Diagnostic and Statistical Manual of Mental Disorders,* 4th Edition, Text Revision. Washington, DC, American Psychiatric Association, 2000, pp. 157–158. Used with permission.

Key Diagnostic Features

DSM-IV-TR diagnostic criteria for dementia with cerebrovascular disease are listed in Table 8–2. The following are important clinical features:

- The onset or significant worsening of cognitive impairment occurs within 3 months of a clinically recognized stroke.
- Evidence of bilateral brain infarctions that involve cortical or subcortical gray matter structures is present on neuroimaging.
- Controversy exists regarding the significance of magnetic resonance imaging (MRI)–confirmed white matter hyperintensities in the diagnosis of cerebrovascular dementia. White matter hyperintensity is a nonspecific marker for cerebrovascular disease and does not confirm the diagnosis of cerebrovascular dementia.
- A specific pattern of cognitive dysfunction is not seen with cerebrovascular dementia, although attentional and executive functioning deficits may be more prominent than short-term memory impairment.
- The prognosis is worse than that of AD. The median survival rate is 3 years (Knopman et al. 2003).

Table 8–2.   DSM-IV-TR diagnostic criteria for vascular dementia

A.   The development of multiple cognitive deficits manifested by both

   (1)   memory impairment (impaired ability to learn new information or to recall previously learned information)

   (2)   one (or more) of the following cognitive disturbances:

      (a)   aphasia (language disturbance)

      (b)   apraxia (impaired ability to carry out motor activities despite intact motor function)

      (c)   agnosia (failure to recognize or identify objects despite intact sensory function)

      (d)   disturbance in executive functioning (i.e., planning, organizing, sequencing, abstracting)

B.   The cognitive deficits in criteria A1 and A2 each cause significant impairment in social or occupational functioning and represent a significant decline from a previous level of functioning.

C.   Focal neurological signs and symptoms (e.g., exaggeration of deep tendon reflexes, extensor plantar response, pseudobulbar palsy, gait abnormalities, weakness of an extremity) or laboratory evidence indicative of cerebrovascular disease (e.g., multiple infarctions involving cortex and underlying white matter) that are judged to be etiologically related to the disturbance.

D.   The deficits do not occur exclusively during the course of a delirium.

Code based on predominant features:

290.41   With delirium: if delirium is superimposed on the dementia

290.42   With delusions: if delusions are the predominant feature

290.43   Without depressed mood: if depressed mood (including presentations that meet full symptom criteria for a major depressive episode) is the predominant feature. A separate diagnosis of mood disorder due to a general medical condition is not given.

290.40   Uncomplicated: if none of the above predominates in the current clinical presentation

Specify if: **With behavioral disturbance**

Coding note: Also code cerebrovascular condition on Axis III.

Source.   Reprinted from American Psychiatric Association: *Diagnostic and Statistical Manual of Mental Disorders,* 4th Edition, Text Revision. Washington, DC, American Psychiatric Association, 2000, p. 161. Used with permission.

Dementia of Parkinson's Disease and Dementia With Lewy Bodies

Two subtypes of dementia are dementia of Parkinson's disease and dementia with Lewy bodies (DLB). Differential diagnosis depends on whether Parkinson's disease precedes the onset of dementia (dementia of Parkinson's disease) or cognitive impairment is the predominant symptom (DLB).

Prevalence

Lewy body pathology is present in 10%–20% of patients with dementia at autopsy (Knopman et al. 2003).

Pathophysiology

Lewy inclusion bodies are seen in both cortical and subcortical regions. Pathology associated with AD may also be seen in conjunction with Lewy body pathology (American Psychiatric Association Work Group 2007).

Key Diagnostic Features

Diagnostic criteria for DLB are listed in Table 8–3. DLB is characterized by the presence of at least two of the following symptoms:

- Parkinsonism, including muscular rigidity, resting tremor, bradykinesia, postural instability, and parkinsonian gait disorder
- Prominent, fully formed visual hallucinations
- Substantial fluctuations in alertness or cognition
- Other clinical features
  1. Rapid eye movement disorder is considered by some to be a key diagnostic feature (Knopman et al. 2003).
  2. Increased sensitivity to extrapyramidal symptoms may be caused by antipsychotic medications.
  3. Psychiatric treatment is often necessary because of the high prevalence of depression in Parkinson's disease and associated psychotic symptoms (American Psychiatric Association Work Group 2007).

Table 8–3.   Diagnostic criteria for dementia with Lewy bodies

A. On the basis of evidence from a patient's history and mental status examination, dementia with cerebrovascular disease is characterized by the presence of at least two of the following impairments:

1. Impaired learning and impaired retention of new information

2. Impaired handling of complex tasks

3. Impaired reasoning ability

4. Impaired spatial ability and orientation

5. Impaired language

B. The impairments in criterion A notably interfere with work or usual social activities or relationships with others

C. The impairments in criterion A represent a notable decline from a previous level of functioning

D. Dementia with Lewy bodies is characterized by the presence of at least two of the following symptoms:

1. Parkinsonism (muscular rigidity, resting tremor, bradykinesia, postural instability, parkinsonian gait disorder)

2. Prominent, fully formed visual hallucinations

3. Substantial fluctuations in alertness or cognition

4. Rapid eye movement sleep behavior disorder

E. The impairments in criterion A do not occur exclusively during the course of delirium

F. The impairments in criterion A are not better explained by a major psychiatric diagnosis

G. The impairments in criterion A are not better explained by a systemic disease or another brain lesion

---

Note.   Rapid eye movement is an additional characteristic diagnostic feature.

Source.   Based on the Consortium on Dementia With Lewy Bodies (McKeith et al. 1996) with modifications by Knopman et al. (2003).

Frontotemporal Dementia

Prevalence

Frontotemporal dementia is relatively rare, but it accounts for 20%–50% of dementia cases with age at onset of less than 65 years (Mendez et al. 2008). Specific genetic defects have been identified, and approximately one-third of the cases are familial (American Psychiatric Association Work Group 2007).

Pathophysiology

Frontotemporal lobar degeneration is seen on gross pathology, with circumscribed and often asymmetrical lobar atrophy. The previous term of "Pick's disease" referred to frontotemporal lobar degeneration with intranuclear inclusion bodies (Mendez et al. 2008).

Key Diagnostic Features

Criteria for frontotemporal dementia are listed in Table 8–4. The following are also important features (Mendez et al. 2008):

- The primary features are changes in personality, behavior, and judgment; therefore, the presentation of patients with frontotemporal dementia can often mimic a psychiatric disorder.
- Changes in personality can range from apathy with loss of interest and initiative to elevated mood and disinhibition.
- Loss of insight occurs early in the disease; patients lack awareness into their deficits and do not appreciate the consequences of their behavior. Decreased empathy is also seen; patients appear indifferent and emotionally unresponsive.
- Disturbances in social and moral behavior include physical aggressiveness, sexually inappropriate behaviors, and loss of social manners.
- Eating behavior changes occur in about 80% of patients; changes include hyperorality, carbohydrate craving, and indiscriminate eating (including placing nonfood items in mouth).
- Repetitive acts of simple verbal and motor behaviors (e.g., hand clapping, lip smacking), as well as more complex rituals (e.g., cleaning, hoarding, checking), can develop.

Table 8–4.   American Neuropsychiatric Association consensus criteria for frontotemporal dementia

Core diagnostic features (all need to be present for diagnosis)

1. Insidious onset and gradual progression

2. Early decline in social interpersonal conduct

3. Early impairment in regulation of personal conduct

4. Early emotional blunting

5. Early loss of insight

Features that support the diagnosis

1. Decline in personal hygiene and grooming

2. Mental rigidity and inflexibility

3. Distractibility and impersistence

4. Hyperorality and dietary changes

5. Perseverative and stereotyped behavior

6. Utilization behavior

Source.   Adapted from Mendez et al. 2008 and Neary et al. 1998.

Other Clinical Features

- Relative preservation of memory is a unique feature of frontotemporal dementia. Visuospatial function can also be normal. Psychometric testing demonstrates deficits primarily in tests of executive function.
- Prefrontal or anterior temporal atrophy on computed tomography (CT) or MRI is useful in confirming frontotemporal dementia but is not necessary to make the diagnosis.

Rapidly Progressive Dementias

Creutzfeldt-Jakob disease should be considered when a patient presents with dementia of subacute onset, typically having lasted for weeks to months. Motor and cognitive symptoms are present early in the disease, and seizures may develop later. The 14-3-3 protein in the cerebrospinal fluid is a useful marker in supporting the diagnosis. Nonvasculitic autoimmune inflammatory meningoencephalopathies, such as Hashimoto's encephalopathy and Sjogren-associated encephalopathy, can be misdiagnosed as Creutzfeldt-Jakob disease, and the essential difference is that these latter dementias respond to high-dose steroids (Knopman et al. 2003).

Differential Diagnosis

The differential diagnosis of dementia syndromes is summarized in Table 8–5.

Evaluation

Figure 8–1 shows a hierarchical approach to diagnosing MCI, dementia, and the major subtypes of dementia. The components of a thorough evaluation, as described in the following subsections, are important in diagnosis.

History

- *A knowledgeable informant such as a family member, spouse, or friend is critical,* because another person often recognizes cognitive deficits and personality changes before the patient does. Collateral history from a reliable informant may be as useful as the brief screening instruments for detecting dementia, although history from an informant combined with cognitive testing is recommended.

- *Consideration should be given to interviewing the spouse or family member separately* from the patient, because the informant may not be as forthcoming with the patient present due to concerns about the patient's reactions.

- *Data on subjective memory loss as an indicator of dementia are conflicting,* with some reports indicating that memory problems correlate more closely with depressive symptoms and personality traits than with dementia (Holsinger et al. 2007).

- *Assessment of daily activities* may include questions about the patient's ability to recall recent events and conversations, to balance a checkbook, and to remember medications. Table 8–6 lists other important daily activities that should be assessed.

Table 8–5.   Differential diagnosis of dementias and subacute confusional states

Irreversible conditions

Alzheimer's disease

Dementia due to cerebrovascular disease

Dementia with Lewy bodies

Frontotemporal dementia

Progressive supranuclear palsy

Huntington's disease

Creutzfeldt-Jakob disease

Paraneoplastic limbic encephalitis

HIV-associated dementia

Potentially reversible conditions

Toxic disturbances
    Alcohol-related syndromes, including Wernicke-Korsakoff syndrome
    Medication effects

Metabolic abnormalities
    Vitamin B_{12} deficiency
    ↑↓ Thyroid level
    Hepatic or renal failure
    Electrolyte disturbances

Depressive disorders

Central nervous system infections: meningitis or encephalitis

Autoimmune and inflammatory encephalopathies
    Lupus erythematosus
    Hashimoto's encephalopathy
    Neurosarcoidosis

Brain structural lesions
    Primary or secondary brain tumors
    Subdural hematoma
    Normal-pressure hydrocephalus

Head trauma

Acute stroke

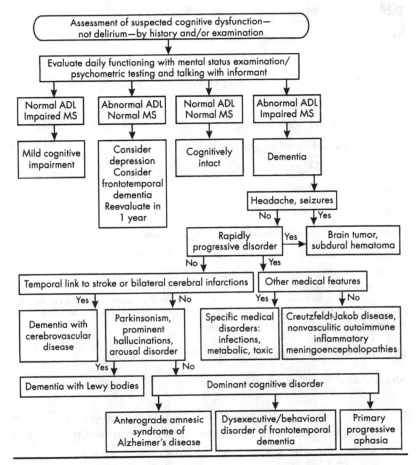

Figure 8–1. A hierarchical approach to diagnosing mild cognitive impairment, dementia, and the major subtypes of dementia.

The sequence of decisions reflects a hierarchy of importance of diagnostic information: features appearing earlier in the decision tree suggest diagnoses regardless of features assessed later.

ADL = activities of daily living necessary for independent life, including complex activities such as managing finances. MS = mental status, assessed through bedside mental status testing or formal neuropsychological evaluations.

Source. Reprinted from Knopman DS, Boeve BF, Petersen RC: "Essentials of the Proper Diagnoses of Mild Cognitive Impairment, Dementia, and Major Subtypes of Dementia." *Mayo Clinic Proceedings* 78:1302, 2003. Used with permission.

Table 8–6.   Assessment of daily activities

Recalling recent events and conversations

Keeping track of personal items (e.g., keys, wallet, purse, glasses)

Writing checks, paying bills, balancing a checkbook

Assembling tax records, business affairs, or papers

Shopping alone for clothes, household necessities, or groceries

Playing a game of skill, working on a hobby

Heating water, making a cup of coffee, turning off stove

Preparing a balanced meal

Keeping track of current events

Paying attention to, understanding, discussing a TV show, book, or magazine

Remembering appointments, family occasions, holidays, medications

Traveling out of the neighborhood, driving, arranging to take buses

Source.   Reprinted from Knopman DS, Boeve BF, Petersen RC: "Essentials of the Proper Diagnoses of Mild Cognitive Impairment, Dementia, and Major Subtypes of Dementia." *Mayo Clinic Proceedings* 78:1301, 2003. Used with permission.

Mental Status Examination

Mini-Mental State Examination

- The Mini-Mental State Examination (MMSE; Folstein et al. 1975) is the most studied of the brief cognitive tests with proven validity, but it may often be insensitive in screening for MCI and mild dementia.
- Scores need to be adjusted for age and are influenced by education.

Other Cognitive Instruments

- The Short Test of Mental Status (Kokmen et al. 1991) is similar to the MMSE, but it has added features that improve sensitivity in detecting mild cognitive deficits (Tang-Wai et al. 2003).
- Table 8–7 lists brief cognitive tests used to screen patients. Instruments that require more time but may increase accuracy include the Modified Mini-Mental State Examination (Teng and Chui 1987) and the Montreal

Cognitive Assessment (Nasreddine et al. 2005; see also Feldman et al. 2008; Holsinger et al. 2003).

Laboratory Assessment

Laboratory assessment is outlined in Table 8–7. A patient's medical comorbidities need to be considered in the determination of appropriate laboratory screening. Vitamin B_{12} levels and thyroid function tests are recommended for elderly patients suspected of having dementia, because vitamin B_{12} deficiency and hypothyroidism are not uncommon in this population and are easily treated.

Neuropsychological Testing

Table 8–7 indicates the potential uses of neuropsychological testing for patients with dementia.

Neuroimaging

Table 8–7 includes information about the use of neuroimaging for diagnostic evaluation for dementia.

- Some experts support the use of neuroimaging (noncontrast CT or MRI) for most patients during the initial evaluation of dementia to detect structural lesions such as brain neoplasms or subdural hematomas, but the yield is very low if the patient has no focal signs.
- Medial temporal lobe atrophy, specifically hippocampal atrophy or entorhinal atrophy, may support a diagnosis of AD (Knopman et al. 2001).

Treatment

Considerations for General Management

Review of Potential Contributions

A detailed review of potential contributions (e.g., infection, dehydration, pain) to a patient's neuropsychiatric symptoms is necessary before treatment is instituted, because addressing the concurrent problem may result in resolution of agitation or aggression. Other considerations include visual or auditory impairment and the level of environmental stimulation (Ballard et al. 2009a).

Table 8–7.   Diagnostic evaluation for dementia

Brief cognitive tests

Examples: Mini-Mental State Examination, Montreal Cognitive Assessment, and Short Test of Mental Status

Insufficient evidence to recommend one test over another

Failure to discriminate between dementia subtypes

Laboratory investigations

Thyroid-stimulating hormone

Serum vitamin B_{12}

Serum electrolytes

Complete blood count

Liver function tests

Serum creatinine and blood urea nitrogen

Serum calcium

Serum fasting glucose

Other tests if clinically indicated

Serum folate

Fluorescent treponemal antibody absorption

Serum HIV

Serum and urine screens for alcohol, drugs, and heavy metals

Erythrocyte sedimentation rate

Arterial blood gases

Urinalysis

Chest X ray

Electrocardiogram

Lumbar puncture

Neuropsychological testing

Not required for a diagnosis of dementia

May assist with distinguishing between normal aging, mild cognitive impairment, and dementia

May assess for other syndromes of cognitive impairment apart from dementia

May address the risk of progression from mild cognitive impairment to dementia

Table 8–7. Diagnostic evaluation for dementia *(continued)*

Neuroimaging and CSF

In some cases: structural neuroimaging with either a noncontrast CT or MRI scan in routine evaluation of dementia

Not recommended for routine use: PET imaging and SPECT

For patients with rapid deterioration in cognition, or unexplained fever or elevated white blood count: CSF examination

If Creutzfeldt-Jakob disease is suspected: CSF 14-3-3 protein

Note. CSF = cerebrospinal fluid; CT = computed tomography; MRI = magnetic resonance imaging; PET = positron emission tomography. SPECT = single-photon emission computed tomography.

Source. Adapted from Feldman et al. 2008; Knopman et al. 2001; Tang-Wai et al. 2003.

Pain

Observational studies suggest that pain is undertreated among patients with cognitive impairment. Assessment of pain in patients with dementia is a needed area of research because existing pain rating scales are designed for communicative patients (Scherder et al. 2005).

Management of Comorbid Medical Conditions

Management of comorbid medical conditions is essential. For example, control of hypertension and hyperlipidemia may stabilize vascular dementia.

Decisions Regarding Life-Prolonging Interventions

Decisions regarding life-prolonging interventions, such as intravenous fluids, antibiotics, feeding tubes, and surgery, should respect the patient's advance directive and involve collaboration with the surrogate decision makers (Cummings 2004).

Treatment of Cognitive Deterioration

Cognitive Training

The data are mixed regarding the effectiveness of cognitive training or cognitive rehabilitation in improving or maintaining cognitive and functional performance (Hogan et al. 2008). One meta-analysis showed that cognitive training had a modest effect size on learning, memory, executive function, and activities of daily living (Sitzer et al. 2006).

Cholinesterase Inhibitors

- Cholinesterase inhibitors may slow cognitive decline in patients with mild to moderate dementia.
- Available cholinesterase inhibitors include donepezil, rivastigmine, galantamine, and tacrine. Tacrine is rarely used due to hepatotoxicity.
- Side effects include nausea, vomiting, bradycardia, syncope, fatigue, and abnormal dreams (Cummings 2004).

Memantine

- Memantine, an N-methyl-D-aspartate (NMDA) receptor antagonist, is used either as monotherapy or as adjunctive therapy with a cholinesterase inhibitor for patients with moderate to severe dementia.
- Side effects include dizziness, constipation, confusion, headache, and hypertension (Hogan et al. 2008).

Other Medications

Insufficient evidence is available for the use of anti-inflammatory agents, hormone replacement therapy, or vitamin E (Cummings 2004).

Nonpharmacological Interventions for Management of Neuropsychiatric Symptoms

Because of the limited long-term efficacy and the adverse effects of pharmacological treatment, nonpharmacological interventions should be tried first in most circumstances. Most studies that have evaluated the efficacy of nonpharmacological interventions have been methodologically weak, but emerging evidence supports the use of practical psychosocial treatments (Ayalon et al. 2006).

Randomized controlled trials (RCTs) have demonstrated that intensive 6- to 12-month programs to educate staff in person-centered care resulted in decreased use of psychotropic medications in nursing homes, with no increase in patients' behavioral problems (Fossey et al. 2006). Some evidence supports the efficacy of validation therapy, a group-based treatment that focuses on empathy for the patient and respecting the individual's reality with activities that involve movement and music (Ballard et al. 2009a).

Pharmacological Treatment of Agitation and Aggression

Typical Antipsychotics

Efficacy.

- Haloperidol, the typical antipsychotic that has been studied most extensively, has been associated with modest improvement in symptoms of aggression compared with placebo but has shown minimal benefit in treating other symptoms of agitation (Ballard et al. 2009a). When adverse effects are taken into account, the risks generally outweigh the benefits, especially for long-term treatment, but this issue remains debatable.
- No data are available to suggest that one typical antipsychotic is more efficacious than another.
- RCTs have not been done to compare the efficacy of typical and atypical antipsychotics in the treatment of dementia (Sink et al. 2005).

Adverse effects.

- The U.S. Food and Drug Administration (FDA) warning in 2005 about increased mortality with the use of atypical antipsychotics for treatment of dementia in elderly patients was extended to the typical antipsychotics in 2007. The warning came after studies suggested that the mortality rates from typical antipsychotics are comparable to or higher than those from atypical antipsychotics (Gill et al. 2007; Wang et al. 2005).
- One study showed that the risk of death was increased with higher dosages. The relative risk was 1.14 with low dosages (less than the median dosage) and 1.73 with high dosages (greater than the median) (Wang et al. 2005). The absolute risk, however, is still quite low.
- Other serious adverse effects include dystonia, parkinsonism, tardive dyskinesia, and QTc prolongation.

Atypical Antipsychotics.

Efficacy.

- Atypical antipsychotics are the most commonly used pharmacological treatment for agitation and psychosis in patients with dementia.

- Most trials have studied efficacy over 6–12 weeks of treatment, and modest benefit has been found for the treatment of aggression but not for nonaggressive symptoms of agitation.
- One meta-analysis of RCTs found support for the use of risperidone and aripiprazole but not olanzapine or quetiapine (Schneider et al. 2006).
- In the Clinical Antipsychotic Trials of Intervention Effectiveness—Alzheimer's Disease (CATIE-AD) project (Sultzer et al. 2008), outpatients with AD and psychosis or agitated/aggressive behavior were treated for up to 36 weeks with olanzapine, quetiapine, risperidone, or placebo. Clinical symptoms such as anger, aggression, and paranoid ideas improved somewhat with the atypical antipsychotics, but overall functioning and quality of life did not change. Olanzapine and risperidone were associated with improved Neuropsychiatric Inventory total scores. No significant change occurred with quetiapine, although the dosage was relatively low because of sedation with higher dosages. The mean dosages for olanzapine, quetiapine, and risperidone were 5.5 mg/day, 56.5 mg/day, and 1.0 mg/day, respectively.
- Treatment beyond 6–12 months has generally not been found beneficial, and/or the adverse effects outweigh the advantages (Ballard et al. 2009a).

Adverse effects.

Increased mortality. The FDA's 2005 warning regarding the increased risk of death with atypical antipsychotics was based on a review of RCTs that included risperidone, olanzapine, quetiapine, and aripiprazole. Fifteen of the 17 trials showed a higher mortality rate, with an approximate rate of 1.6–1.7 over 12 weeks (but the absolute risk was small). Cardiac-related events and infection were the most common causes of mortality in these studies. The relationship of antipsychotics and mortality is complex and not yet understood (Kales et al. 2007).

Increased mortality with prolonged treatment. The dementia antipsychotic withdrawal trial showed increased mortality for patients who were randomized to continue antipsychotic treatment than for those allocated to placebo, with marked differences appearing between groups during periods of follow-up longer than 12 months. Survival at 36 months was 30% for patients who continued taking antipsychotics compared with 60% for patients taking placebo (Ballard et al. 2009b). In one study of patients who were very frail and had a mean age of 86 years, antipsychotic use did not increase mortality or hospital admissions at 2-year follow-up, but use of restraints doubled mortality (Raivio et al. 2007).

Cerebrovascular events. Risperidone has been associated with a threefold risk of serious cerebrovascular events, and a similar risk has been demonstrated with olanzapine, although this finding has been debated. If an association exists, it is likely related to the entire class of atypical antipsychotics (Ballard et al. 2009a).

Cognitive decline. Acceleration in the rate of cognitive decline has been demonstrated in patients treated with atypical antipsychotics compared with those taking placebo over 12 weeks (Schneider et al. 2006).

Other adverse effects. Other adverse effects of atypical antipsychotics include sedation, parkinsonism, QTc prolongation, and metabolic syndrome.

Cholinesterase Inhibitors

Cholinesterase inhibitors, if maintained over 6 months, may provide mild improvement in anxiety and apathy, but no changes in agitation (Ballard et al. 2009a).

Antidepressants for the Agitation of Dementia

- In a comparison of citalopram and risperidone in an RCT of patients with dementia but not depression, both medication groups experienced improvement, including decreased psychotic symptoms and agitation (Pollock et al. 2007).
- The evidence does not support use of trazodone for the treatment of agitation in patients with dementia of the Alzheimer's type (Teri et al. 2000).
- Although some data are encouraging, further studies are needed before treatment with antidepressants for agitation of dementia in nondepressed patients is recommended.

Anticonvulsants

- Valproate is not indicated due to sedation with no demonstrated benefit in the treatment of neuropsychiatric symptoms.
- Preliminary results show that carbamazepine can help in managing agitation in patients with AD, but additional data are needed (Ballard et al. 2009a).

References

American Psychiatric Association: Diagnostic and Statistical Manual of Mental Disorders, 4th Edition, Text Revision. Washington DC, American Psychiatric Association, 2000

American Psychiatric Association Work Group on Alzheimer's Disease and Other Dementias, Rabins PV, Blacker D, et al: American Psychiatric Association practice guideline for the treatment of patients with Alzheimer's disease and other dementias, second edition. Am J Psychiatry 164:5–56, 2007

Ayalon L, Gum AM, Feliciano L, et al: Effectiveness of nonpharmacological interventions for the management of neuropsychiatric symptoms in patients with dementia: a systematic review. Arch Intern Med 166:2182–2188, 2006

Ballard CG, Gauthier S, Cummings JL, et al: Management of agitation and aggression associated with Alzheimer disease. Nat Rev Neurol 5:245–255, 2009a

Ballard C, Hanney ML, Theodoulou M, et al: The dementia antipsychotic withdrawal trial (DART-AD): long-term follow-up of a randomised placebo-controlled trial. Lancet Neurol 8:151–157, 2009b

Barnes DE, Covinsky KE, Whitmer RA, et al: Predicting risk of dementia in older adults: the late-life dementia risk index. Neurology 73:173–179, 2009

Chertkow H, Massoud F, Nasreddine Z, et al: Diagnosis and treatment of dementia, III: mild cognitive impairment and cognitive impairment without dementia. CMAJ 178:1273–1285, 2008

Cummings JL: Alzheimer's disease. N Engl J Med 351:56–67, 2004

Feldman HH, Jacova C, Robillard A, et al: Diagnosis and treatment of dementia, II: diagnosis. CMAJ 178:825–836, 2008

Folstein MF, Folstein SE, McHugh PR: Mini-Mental State: a practical method for grading the cognitive state of patients for the clinician. J Psychiatr Res 12:189–198, 1975

Fossey J, Ballard C, Juszczak E, et al: Effect of enhanced psychosocial care on antipsychotic use in nursing home residents with severe dementia: cluster randomised trial. BMJ 332:756–761, 2006

Gill SS, Bronskill SE, Normand SL, et al: Antipsychotic drug use and mortality in older adults with dementia. Ann Intern Med 146:775–786, 2007

Green RC, Cupples LA, Go R, et al: Risk of dementia among white and African American relatives of patients with Alzheimer disease. JAMA 287:329–336, 2002

Hogan DB, Bailey P, Black S, et al: Diagnosis and treatment of dementia, 5: nonpharmacologic and pharmacologic therapy for mild to moderate dementia. CMAJ 179:1019–1026, 2008

Holsinger T, Deveau J, Boustani M, et al: Does this patient have dementia? JAMA 297:2391–2404, 2007

Kales HC, Valenstein M, Kim HM, et al: Mortality risk in patients with dementia treated with antipsychotics versus other psychiatric medications. Am J Psychiatry 164:1568–1576, 2007

Knopman DS, DeKosky ST, Cummings JL, et al: Practice parameter: diagnosis of dementia (an evidence-based review). Report of the Quality Standards Subcommittee of the American Academy of Neurology. Neurology 56:1143–1153, 2001

Knopman DS, Boeve BF, Petersen RC: Essentials of the proper diagnoses of mild cognitive impairment, dementia, and major subtypes of dementia. Mayo Clin Proc 78:1290–1308, 2003

Kokmen E, Smith GE, Petersen RC, et al: The short test of mental status. Correlations with standardized psychometric testing. Arch Neurol 48:725–728, 1991

Li H, Wetten S, Li L, et al: Candidate single-nucleotide polymorphisms from a genome-wide association study of Alzheimer disease. Arch Neurol 65:45–53, 2008

McKeith IG, Galasko D, Kosaka K, et al: Consensus guidelines for the clinical and pathologic diagnosis of dementia with Lewy bodies (DLB): report of the consortium on DLB international workshop. Neurology 47:1113–1124, 1996

Mendez MF, Lauterbach EC, Sampson SM, et al: An evidence-based review of the psychopathology of frontotemporal dementia: a report of the ANPA Committee on Research. J Neuropsychiatry Clin Neurosci 20:130–149, 2008

Nasreddine ZS, Phillips NA, Bédirian V, et al: The Montreal Cognitive Assessment, MoCA: a brief screening tool for mild cognitive impairment. J Am Geriatr Soc 53:695–699, 2005

Neary D, Snowden JS, Gustafson L, et al: Frontotemporal lobar degeneration: a consensus on clinical diagnostic criteria. Neurology 51:1546–1554, 1998

Pollock BG, Mulsant BH, Rosen J, et al: A double-blind comparison of citalopram and risperidone for the treatment of behavioral and psychotic symptoms associated with dementia. Am J Geriatr Psychiatry 15:942–952, 2007

Raivio MM, Laurila JV, Strandberg TE, et al: Neither atypical nor conventional antipsychotics increase mortality or hospital admissions among elderly patients with dementia: a two-year prospective study. Am J Geriatr Psychiatry 15:416–424, 2007

Scherder E, Oosterman J, Swaab D, et al: Recent developments in pain in dementia. BMJ 330:461–464, 2005

Schneider LS, Dagerman K, Insel PS: Efficacy and adverse effects of atypical antipsychotics for dementia: meta-analysis of randomized, placebo-controlled trials. Am J Geriatr Psychiatry 14:191–210, 2006

Silverman JM, Smith CJ, Marin DB, et al: Familial patterns of risk in very late-onset Alzheimer disease. Arch Gen Psychiatry 60:190–197, 2003

Sink KM, Holden KF, Yaffe K: Pharmacological treatment of neuropsychiatric symptoms of dementia: a review of the evidence. JAMA 293:596–608, 2005

Sitzer DI, Twamley EW, Jeste DV: Cognitive training in Alzheimer's disease: a meta-analysis of the literature. Acta Psychiatr Scand 114:75–90, 2006

Sultzer DL, Davis SM, Tariot PN, et al: Clinical symptom responses to atypical antipsychotic medications in Alzheimer's disease: phase 1 outcomes from the CATIE-AD effectiveness trial. Am J Psychiatry 165:844–854, 2008

Tang-Wai DF, Knopman DS, Geda YE, et al: Comparison of the Short Test of Mental Status and the Mini-Mental State Examination in mild cognitive impairment. Arch Neurol 60:1777–1781, 2003

Teng EL, Chui HC: The Modified Mini-Mental State (3MS) examination. J Clin Psychiatry 48:314–318, 1987

Teri L, Logsdon RG, Peskind E, et al: Treatment of agitation in AD: a randomized, placebo-controlled clinical trial. (Erratum in Neurology 56:426, 2001.) Neurology 55:1271–1278, 2000

van Duijn CM, Clayton D, Chandra V, et al; EURODEM Risk Factors Research Group: Familial aggregation of Alzheimer's disease and related disorders: a collaborative re-analysis of case-control studies. Int J Epidemiol 20 (suppl 2):S13–S20, 1991

Viswanathan A, Rocca WA, Tzourio C: Vascular risk factors and dementia: how to move forward? Neurology 72:368–374, 2009

Wang PS, Schneeweiss S, Avorn J, et al: Risk of death in elderly users of conventional vs. atypical antipsychotic medications. N Engl J Med 353:2335–2341, 2005

Zubenko GS, Zubenko WN, McPherson S, et al: A collaborative study of the emergence and clinical features of the major depressive syndrome of Alzheimer's disease. Am J Psychiatry 160:857–866, 2003

9

Eating Disorders

Although eating disorders are infrequently diagnosed in the medical setting, eating disorder symptoms, such as restricted intake, uncontrolled eating, and body image distress, are common in patients (Devlin et al. 2011). Eating disorders are associated with high rates of all-cause mortality and suicide (Crow et al. 2009), and eating disorder symptoms may complicate treatment of medical illness.

Definitions and Clinical Features

Diagnostic Overlap

The course and outcome of eating disorders are associated with a substantial degree of crossover from one eating disorder diagnosis to another. More than half of patients with anorexia nervosa cross over between restricting and binge-eating/purging subtypes, and about one-third cross over to bulimia but are likely to relapse to anorexia. Patients with bulimia most often cross over to eating disorder not otherwise specified (Steinhausen and Weber 2009) and are less likely to develop anorexia nervosa (Eddy et al. 2008).

Definition of Anorexia Nervosa

To be diagnosed with anorexia nervosa, a patient needs to meet four criteria as defined by DSM-IV-TR (American Psychiatric Association 2000):

1. Refusal to maintain weight at or above minimally normal weight for height and age (body weight is more than 15% below ideal weight)
2. Intense fear of weight gain or of becoming fat, despite being underweight
3. Severe body image disturbance in which body image is the predominant measure of self-worth with denial of the seriousness of low body weight
4. In postmenarchal females, amenorrhea (i.e., absence of at least three menstrual cycles)

Restricting or Binge-Eating/Purging Subtypes of Anorexia Nervosa

Patients with the restricting subtype of anorexia nervosa primarily use restriction of intake to reduce their weight, whereas those with the binge-eating/purging subtype regularly engage in binge eating or purging (e.g., vomiting, abuse of laxatives or diuretics) or both to control their weight. A patient with anorexia may induce vomiting yet still be considered anorexic (rather than bulimic) if criteria for anorexia are met (American Psychiatric Association 2000).

Definition of Bulimia Nervosa

DSM-IV-TR criteria for bulimia nervosa include the following (American Psychiatric Association 2000):

1. Episodes of binge eating occur with a sense of loss of control.
2. Binge eating is followed by compensatory behavior of the purging type (e.g., self-induced vomiting, laxative abuse, diuretic abuse) or nonpurging type (e.g., excessive exercise, fasting, strict dieting).
3. Binges and compensatory behavior occur at least two times per week for 3 months.
4. Patient feels dissatisfaction with body shape and weight.

Eating Disorder Not Otherwise Specified

Patients with clearly aberrant eating patterns and weight management habits who do not meet the criteria for anorexia nervosa or bulimia nervosa are diagnosed with eating disorder not otherwise specified (NOS). The treatment literature has been predominantly focused on bulimia nervosa and anorexia nervosa, although eating disorder NOS is the most common eating disorder (Crow and Peterson 2009). One example of eating disorder NOS is binge-eating disorder, which is currently a research diagnosis requiring patients to meet three of the five following criteria (American Psychiatric Association 2000, p. 787):

1. Eating much more rapidly than normal
2. Eating until uncomfortably full
3. Eating large amounts of food when not feeling physically hungry
4. Eating alone because of embarrassment about how much one is eating
5. Feeling disgusted, depressed, or very guilty after overeating

Night Eating Syndrome

Night eating syndrome is characterized by evening hyperphagia (eating more than one-third of total daily calories after the evening meal) and nocturnal awakenings with ingestion of food. It is likely to co-occur with substance use disorders, use of atypical antipsychotics, and obesity (Lundgren et al. 2006).

Epidemiology

Prevalence

Lifetime prevalence estimates of anorexia nervosa, bulimia nervosa, and binge-eating disorder are 1%, 1.5%, and 3.5%, respectively, among women, and 0.3%, 0.5%, and 2.0%, respectively, among men (Hudson et al. 2007).

Chronic Course of Illness

Less than half of patients with bulimia have full recovery, and 25% have a chronic protracted course (Steinhausen and Weber 2009). In one study, two-thirds of women with anorexia nervosa showed clinical recovery by 5 years, with no difference in recovery between cases that had been detected and cases that were undetected in the medical system (Keski-Rahkonen et al. 2007). The mean lifetime duration of binge-eating disorder is 14 years, significantly longer than that of bulimia nervosa or anorexia nervosa, each of which has a mean duration of about 6 years (Pope et al. 2006).

Comorbid Psychiatric Illness With High Rates of Anxiety Disorders

Two-thirds of patients with anorexia and bulimia nervosa have had one or more anxiety disorders in their lifetime, most commonly obsessive-compulsive disorder and social phobia. For the majority of patients, the onset of the anxiety disorder occurs in childhood before development of the eating disorder (Kaye et al. 2004). Comorbid depression and substance use frequently co-occur; alcohol use is more often associated with bulimia nervosa and the binge-eating/purging subtype of anorexia nervosa than with the restricting type of anorexia nervosa (Bulik et al. 2004; Halmi et al. 1991).

Increased Mortality

Mortality rates for anorexia and bulimia nervosa are approximately 4%. Although eating disorder NOS is sometimes viewed as less serious than the other eating disorders, it has a similar mortality rate (Crow et al. 2009).

Pathogenesis

The etiology of eating disorders is multifactorial and includes genetics, central nervous system abnormalities, personality traits, cultural influences, and family environment. Substantial evidence supports the familial aggregation of eating disorders, and twin studies show higher rates among monozygotic twins than among dizygotic twins. Personality traits such as perfectionism, impulsivity, and negative affect are potential risk factors (Yager and Andersen 2005).

Assessment and Differential Diagnosis

Assessment

Assessment of patients in the medical setting is challenging for many reasons, including the difficulty of determining whether behaviors such as vomiting or food restriction are due to somatic illness or psychological factors. Patients with eating disorders are often secretive about their illness and may deny the severity. A thorough history is the most important part of the assessment, and no diagnostic tests are required to make a diagnosis unless the history suggests an organic etiology.

1. *Physical assessment.* The physical examination should focus on evidence of dehydration, lanugo, acrocyanosis, salivary gland enlargement, and scarring on the dorsum of the hand (Russell's sign). The patient should also be checked for orthostatic hypotension and body mass index. Patients who purge need a dental examination.

2. *Laboratory assessment.* The laboratory evaluation is individualized for each patient but typically includes serum electrolytes, blood urea nitrogen and creatinine, liver enzymes, serum albumin, thyroid function, complete blood cell count, and urinalysis. For patients who are severely malnourished, the assessment includes calcium, magnesium, and phosphate levels and an electrocardiogram. Serum amylase may be considered for patients suspected of self-induced vomiting but is not sufficiently sensitive or specific to be a useful routine screening tool.

3. *Other studies to consider.* Dual-energy X-ray absorptiometry of bone may be used for patients who have been chronically underweight. Magnetic resonance imaging (MRI) or computed tomography (CT) of the brain may be needed for patients who have persistent cognitive impairment or other mental status changes despite weight restoration (American Psychiatric Association 2006).

Differential Diagnosis

Preoccupation with body image or the presence of intentional weight manipulation is helpful in differentiating an eating disorder from other medical etiologies. In the absence of these features, the diagnosis of an eating disorder should be considered provisional, and other causes need to be thoroughly evaluated (Devlin et al. 2011). Table 9–1 lists medical conditions to consider in the differential diagnosis.

Medical Complications

Eating disorders have some serious medical complications, as discussed in this section. The medical effects of individual eating disorder symptoms are listed in Table 9–2.

Table 9–1.   Medical differential diagnosis of eating disorders

System	Diagnosis
Endocrine	Diabetes mellitus, hyperthyroidism, Addison's disease, Sheehan's syndrome (postpartum pituitary necrosis), panhypopituitarism
Gastrointestinal	Malabsorption, pancreatitis, inflammatory bowel disease, peptic ulcer disease, dysmotility disorders, superior mesenteric artery syndrome, cystic fibrosis
Neurological	Psychomotor or limbic seizures, neurodegenerative disorders, hypothalamic or diencephalic tumor
Other medical	Malignancies (especially lymphomas and gastrointestinal cancers), collagen vascular disorders, human immunodeficiency virus, parasitic infections, chronic renal failure, drug-induced weight change

Source.   Adapted from Devlin et al. 2011.

Osteopenia

Osteopenia is one of the most severe complications of anorexia nervosa and is difficult to reverse. The risk for fractures later in life is increased (Lucas et al. 1999). Treatment recommendations include weight gain, 1,200–1,500 mg/day of elemental calcium, a multivitamin with vitamin D, and individual assessments for estrogen/progestin replacement.

Cardiac Changes

Congestive heart failure, pericardial effusions, bradycardia, and conduction abnormalities with arrhythmias or prolonged QTc interval can occur in patients who are undernourished (Cooke et al. 1994). Prolongation of the QTc is often associated with hypokalemia, hypomagnesemia, or hypocalcemia and may be exacerbated by medications. Syrup of ipecac used to induce vomiting may cause muscle damage, including cardiotoxicity with manifestations of bradycardia, hypotension, and conduction defects.

Endocrine Changes

Reduced metabolic rate due to starvation results in a change in thyroid hormone synthesis, including normal thyroid-stimulating hormone level, low or normal

Table 9–2. Eating disorder symptoms and medical effects

System	Medical effect
Restrictive eating	Cognitive dysfunction, fatigue, cold intolerance, constipation, dizziness, hypoglycemia, acrocyanosis, orthostatic pulse and blood pressure, edema, amenorrhea
Vomiting	Dehydration, metabolic alkalosis, hypokalemia, arrhythmias, esophagitis/gastritis, esophageal tears, dental caries, parotid/submandibular gland hypertrophy, gastroesophageal reflux disease, pharyngitis
Binge eating/overeating with weight gain	Obesity, dyslipidemia, hypertension, type 2 diabetes mellitus, coronary artery disease, stroke, gallbladder disease, osteoarthritis, sleep apnea, respiratory disorders
Laxative abuse	Cathartic colon, dehydration, hypokalemia, metabolic acidosis or mild metabolic alkalosis
Diuretic abuse	Dehydration, hypokalemia, hypomagnesemia
Appetite-suppressant abuse	Hypertension, tremor, arrhythmias
Compulsive exercise	Bradycardia, overuse syndrome, stress fractures
Water loading	Hyponatremia, headache, nausea, dizziness, seizure

Source. Adapted from Devlin et al. 2011.

thyroxine (T_4) and triiodothyronine (T_3) concentrations, and elevated concentration of reverse T_3 (euthyroid sick syndrome). Other endocrine features that are associated with starvation and that normalize with weight restoration include increased cortisol and growth hormone levels, decreased estrogen, luteinizing hormone, and follicle-stimulating hormone levels in women, and decreased testosterone level in men. In women with anorexia, amenorrhea is due to decreased pulsatile secretion of gonadotropin-releasing hormone, and patients with bulimia may develop amenorrhea without body weight changes (Devlin et al. 2011).

Electrolyte Imbalances and Nutritional Deficiencies

Eating disorder behaviors such as vomiting, diuretic or laxative abuse, and fluid restriction may lead to severe dehydration with decreased potassium, magnesium, phosphate, sodium, and calcium levels. If hypokalemia is chronic, it may lead to nephropathy and renal failure (Devlin et al. 2011). Deficiencies in thiamine among patients with anorexia can be associated with adult beriberi or Wernicke-Korsakoff syndrome.

Concurrent General Medical Conditions

Eating Disorders and Diabetes Mellitus

Data are conflicting about the frequency of eating disorders in patients with insulin-dependent diabetes mellitus, although high rates of intentional insulin omission appear to occur in young women with type 1 diabetes for the purpose of weight control. Blood glucose is elevated in these patients, and the risk of ketoacidosis and other complications is increased (Crow et al. 1998). Patients with binge-eating disorder may have an increased risk of metabolic syndrome independent of the risk of obesity (Hudson et al. 2010). Among individuals with type 2 diabetes who are overweight or obese and are binge eaters, the rate of success with weight loss intervention programs appears to be similar to those who are not binge eaters (Gorin et al. 2008).

Eating Disorders and Pregnancy

Infertility

One study found that 17% of women with infertility have an eating disorder (Stewart et al. 1990). Long-term studies have shown no differences in cumulative pregnancy rates in women with bulimia nervosa compared with those who do not have an eating disorder (Crow et al. 2002), although women with anorexia have more difficulty conceiving (European Society of Human Reproduction and Embryology [ESHRE] Capri Workshop Group 2006).

Pregnancy and Postpartum Period

The data are conflicting, but eating disorder symptoms often improve during pregnancy and return during the postpartum period (Andersen and Ryan 2009). Patients who present with hyperemesis gravidarum should be assessed for potential warning signs of an eating disorder, such as lack of weight gain during the second trimester, abnormal body mass index, unexplained hyperkalemia from laxative use, or dental problems indicative of a long-standing history of frequent emesis. Compared to women without eating disorders, women with eating disorders are more likely to have pregnancies complicated by fetal growth restriction and preterm labor (Bansil et al. 2008). Pregnant women with active eating disorders appear to be at elevated risk for delivery by cesarean section and for postpartum depression (Franko et al. 2001), and those with bulimia have an increased risk of miscarriage and preterm birth (Morgan et al. 2006). Infant feeding may also be affected by eating disorders. For example, infants of women with anorexia nervosa have a higher risk of feeding difficulties between birth and 6 months (Micali et al. 2009). Mealtime interactions have also been described as less positive and less interactive for mothers with an eating disorder than for those without an eating disorder (Waugh and Bulik 1999).

Treatments

Anorexia Nervosa

Inpatient Care

Weight restoration is the first treatment challenge for low-weight patients with anorexia nervosa. The following criteria are suggested for determination of inpatient psychiatric care (American Psychiatric Association 2006):

1. Severe malnutrition—less than 85% of ideal body weight or acute weight decline with refusal to eat
2. Autonomic dysfunction—bradycardia (heart rate <40 beats/minute), hypotension, or temperature dysregulation
3. Electrolyte abnormalities or glucose <60 mg/dL
4. Acute medical complication of malnutrition (e.g., pancreatitis, cardiovascular compromise, delirium, seizures, syncope)

Refeeding Syndrome

When patients who are severely malnourished (i.e., less than 75% of ideal body weight) are re-fed too rapidly, refeeding syndrome may occur. Refeeding syndrome is a potentially lethal condition resulting from rapid shifts in fluids and electrolytes. The risk is particularly high with enteral and parenteral feeding, but it can also occur with aggressive oral refeeding. Patients with chronic malnutrition and those who have rapidly lost a substantial amount of weight are at risk of this development during the first 2–3 weeks of refeeding. The cardinal feature of the syndrome is severe hypophosphatemia with manifestations of heart failure, rhabdomyolysis, seizures, and delirium. Other abnormalities include hypokalemia, hypomagnesemia, low glucose, hypocalcemia, and thiamine deficiency. Prevention of refeeding syndrome begins with identification of high-risk patients. Vitamin supplements, including thiamine, should be started immediately, and refeeding needs to be done slowly (e.g., 20 kcal/kg and increase by 100–200 kcal/day). In addition to monitoring patients' electrolytes (phosphate, magnesium, and potassium), physicians need to observe patients for signs of edema, congestive heart failure, and mental status changes (American Psychiatric Association 2006American Psychiatric Association 2000; Mehanna et al. 2008).

Pharmacological and Behavioral Interventions

Literature on behavioral and pharmacological interventions for anorexia nervosa is scarce, and the results are inconclusive. Cognitive-behavioral therapy (CBT) may decrease the likelihood of relapse for adults after weight restoration, and family therapy is effective for adolescents but not adults (Bulik et al. 2007). Selective serotonin reuptake inhibitors (SSRIs) may be considered for patients with depressive, anxiety, or obsessive-compulsive symptoms, but studies have not shown an advantage in weight restoration. Second-generation antipsychotics, including olanzapine, quetiapine, and risperidone, are used, but limited data are available regarding efficacy, and patient compliance is a limiting factor.

Bulimia

Psychological Treatments

CBT for bulimia nervosa results in better patient outcomes than do minimal treatment, supportive therapy, or purely behavioral interventions. The goal of CBT is to address cognitive disturbances, such as overemphasis on weight and shape, rigid rules about eating, and low self-esteem, in addition to the behaviors of purging and weight regulation. Interpersonal therapy (IPT) has also been shown to result in significant symptom change, although CBT may result in more rapid improvement (Agras et al. 2000).

Pharmacological Treatments

Antidepressants are more effective than placebo in treating bulimia, with the most evidence supporting SSRIs. Fluoxetine at dosages of 60 mg/day or higher has been found to improve outcome and decrease the likelihood of relapse, although pharmacotherapy alone is not sufficient for long-term remission (Romano et al. 2002).

Binge-Eating Disorder

Psychological Treatments

Both CBT and IPT are effective treatments for binge eating, especially for patients with low self-esteem and high eating disorder psychopathology; rather than weight reduction, the primary change is in reducing binge days and improving psychological features. At 2-year follow-up, one study found that guided self-help based on CBT and IPT resulted in greater remission than behavioral weight loss treatment. Findings on whether behavioral weight loss treatment results in significant weight reduction have been inconsistent, although obese individuals with binge-eating disorder appear to lose less weight than obese patients without binge-eating disorder while undergoing behavioral weight loss treatment (Wilfley et al. 2008; Wilson et al. 2010).

Pharmacological Treatments

Sibutramine, a serotonin-norepinephrine reuptake inhibitor, has been approved by the U.S. Food and Drug Administration for the long-term treatment of obesity, and some evidence supports its efficacy in the treatment of obese patients with binge-eating disorder (Appolinario et al. 2003; Wilfley et al. 2008). Topiramate has also been found to be efficacious in the short-term treatment of binge-eating disorder associated with obesity (McElroy et al. 2003).

Bariatric Surgery

Approximately 25% of patients seeking bariatric surgery have binge-eating disorder. (For more information, see Chapter 16, "Bariatric Surgery.")

References

Agras WS, Walsh T, Fairburn CG, et al: A multicenter comparison of cognitive-behavioral therapy and interpersonal psychotherapy for bulimia nervosa. Arch Gen Psychiatry 57:459–466, 2000

American Psychiatric Association: Diagnostic and Statistical Manual of Mental Disorders, 4th Edition, Text Revision. Washington, DC, American Psychiatric Association, 2000

American Psychiatric Association: Treatment of patients with eating disorders, third edition. Am J Psychiatry 163 (suppl):4–54, 2006

Andersen AE, Ryan GL: Eating disorders in the obstetric and gynecologic patient population. Obstet Gynecol 114:1353–1367, 2009

Appolinario JC, Bacaltchuk J, Sichieri R, et al: A randomized, double-blind, placebo-controlled study of sibutramine in the treatment of binge-eating disorder. Arch Gen Psychiatry 60:1109–1116, 2003

Bansil P, Kuklina EV, Whiteman MK, et al: Eating disorders among delivery hospitalizations: prevalence and outcomes. J Womens Health (Larchmt) 17:1523–1528, 2008

Bulik CM, Klump KL, Thornton L, et al: Alcohol use disorder comorbidity in eating disorders: a multicenter study. J Clin Psychiatry 65:1000–1006, 2004

Bulik CM, Berkman ND, Brownley KA, et al: Anorexia nervosa treatment: a systematic review of randomized controlled trials. Int J Eat Disord 40:310–320, 2007

Cooke RA, Chambers JB, Singh R, et al: QT interval in anorexia nervosa. Br Heart J 72:69–73, 1994

Crow S, Peterson CB: Refining treatments for eating disorders (comment). Am J Psychiatry 166:266–267, 2009

Crow SJ, Keel PK, Kendall D: Eating disorders and insulin-dependent diabetes mellitus. Psychosomatics 39:233–243, 1998

Crow SJ, Thuras P, Keel PK, et al: Long-term menstrual and reproductive function in patients with bulimia nervosa. Am J Psychiatry 159:1048–1050, 2002

Crow SJ, Peterson CB, Swanson SA, et al: Increased mortality in bulimia nervosa and other eating disorders. Am J Psychiatry 166:1342–1346, 2009

Devlin MJ, Johraus JP, DiMarco ID: Eating disorders, in The American Psychiatric Publishing Textbook of Psychosomatic Medicine, 2nd Edition. Edited by Levenson JL. Washington, DC, American Psychiatric Publishing, 2011, pp 305–334

Eddy KT, Dorer DJ, Franko DL, et al: Diagnostic crossover in anorexia nervosa and bulimia nervosa: implications for DSM-V. Am J Psychiatry 165:245–250, 2008

European Society of Human Reproduction and Embryology (ESHRE) Capri Workshop Group: Nutrition and reproduction in women. Hum Reprod Update 12:193–207, 2006

Franko DL, Blais MA, Becker AE, et al: Pregnancy complications and neonatal outcomes in women with eating disorders. Am J Psychiatry 158:1461–1466, 2001

Gorin AA, Niemeier HM, Hogan P, et al: Binge eating and weight loss outcomes in overweight and obese individuals with type 2 diabetes: results from the Look AHEAD trial. Arch Gen Psychiatry 65:1447–1455, 2008

Halmi KA, Eckert E, Marchi P, et al: Comorbidity of psychiatric diagnoses in anorexia nervosa. Arch Gen Psychiatry 48:712–718, 1991

Hudson JI, Hiripi E, Pope HG, et al: The prevalence and correlates of eating disorders in the National Comorbidity Survey Replication. Biol Psychiatry 61:348–358, 2007

Hudson JI, Lalonde JK, Coit CE, et al: Longitudinal study of the diagnosis of components of the metabolic syndrome in individuals with binge-eating disorder. Am J Clin Nutr 91:1568–1573, 2010

Kaye WH, Bulik CM, Thornton L, et al: Comorbidity of anxiety disorders with anorexia and bulimia nervosa. Am J Psychiatry 161:2215–2221, 2004

Keski-Rahkonen A, Hoek HW, Susser ES, et al: Epidemiology and course of anorexia nervosa in the community. Am J Psychiatry 164:1259–1265, 2007

Lucas AR, Melton LJ, Crowson CS, et al: Long-term fracture risk among women with anorexia nervosa: a population-based cohort study. Mayo Clin Proc 74:972–977, 1999

Lundgren JD, Allison KC, Crow S, et al: Prevalence of the night eating syndrome in a psychiatric population. Am J Psychiatry 163:156–158, 2006

McElroy SL, Arnold LM, Shapira NA, et al: Topiramate in the treatment of binge eating disorder associated with obesity: a randomized, placebo-controlled trial. (Erratum in Am J Psychiatry 160:612, 2003.) Am J Psychiatry 160:255–261, 2003

Mehanna HM, Moledina J, Travis J: Refeeding syndrome: what it is, and how to prevent and treat it. BMJ 336:1495–1498, 2008

Micali N, Simonoff E, Treasure J: Infant feeding and weight in the first year of life in babies of women with eating disorders. J Pediatr 154:55–60.e1, 2009

Morgan JF, Lacey JH, Chung E: Risk of postnatal depression, miscarriage, and preterm birth in bulimia nervosa: retrospective controlled study. Psychosom Med 68:487–492, 2006

Pope HG, Lalonde JK, Pindyck LJ, et al: Binge eating disorder: a stable syndrome. Am J Psychiatry 163:2181–2183, 2006

Romano SJ, Halmi KA, Sarkar NP, et al: A placebo-controlled study of fluoxetine in continued treatment of bulimia nervosa after successful acute fluoxetine treatment. Am J Psychiatry 159:96–102, 2002

Steinhausen HC, Weber S: The outcome of bulimia nervosa: findings from one-quarter century of research. Am J Psychiatry 166:1331–1341, 2009

Stewart DE, Robinson E, Goldbloom DS, et al: Infertility and eating disorders. Am J Obstet Gynecol 163:1196–1199, 1990

Waugh E, Bulik CM: Offspring of women with eating disorders. Int J Eat Disord 25:123–133, 1999

Wilfley DE, Crow SJ, Hudson JI, et al: Efficacy of sibutramine for the treatment of binge eating disorder: a randomized multicenter placebo-controlled double-blind study. Am J Psychiatry 165:51–58, 2008

Wilson GT, Wilfley DE, Agras WS, et al: Psychological treatments of binge eating disorder. Arch Gen Psych 67:94–101, 2010

Yager J, Andersen AE: Clinical practice: anorexia nervosa. N Engl J Med 353:1481–1488, 2005

10

Mood Disorders

Depression

Epidemiology of Depression

Prevalence

General population.   The lifetime prevalence of major depressive disorder (MDD) in the general U.S. adult population is 16% (Kessler et al. 2003). The point prevalence rates are 2%–3% for men and 5%–9% for women.

Patients with chronic medical illnesses.   Rates of depression are higher in patients with chronic medical illnesses—such as diabetes mellitus, myocardial infarction, HIV–related illness, cancer, stroke, Parkinson's disease, and epilepsy—than in those without medical conditions. The prevalence of depression is estimated to be almost three times as high in patients with chronic disease as in healthy control subjects (Egede 2007). The rates of depression appear to increase progressively from community settings (3%–5%) to primary care settings (5%–10%) to inpatient medical settings (10%–15%) (Katon 2003).

High Rates of Comorbid Psychiatric Disorders

The majority of patients (70%) with lifetime MDD have a comorbid anxiety disorder, substance use disorder, or impulse-control disorder (Kessler et al. 2003).

Worse Depression Outcomes in Medically Ill Patients

The mean duration of MDD in the general population is estimated to be 16 weeks (Kessler et al. 2003). Despite similar rates of treatment for depression, patients with comorbid medical illness have worse depression outcomes, including increased likelihood of depressive symptoms at 6- and 12-month follow-ups (Koike et al. 2002). In a study of medical inpatients, McKenzie et al. (2010) found that depression persisted for at least 3 months after discharge in 35%–50% of patients. Poorer physical and mental functioning during hospitalization and a family history of depression were associated with persistence of depressive symptoms.

Greater Functional Impairment

Nearly 60% of respondents in the National Comorbidity Survey Replication described role impairment from depression as severe or very severe. Among individuals with chronic medical conditions, those with concurrent major depression have higher degrees of functional disability and productivity losses than do those without depression (Egede 2007). Several studies have suggested that depression and anxiety are more predictive of functional impairment over time than is the severity of physical illness (Mayou et al. 2000; Sullivan et al. 1997, 2000). Functional impairment in elderly patients is a predictor of the development of major depression (Katon 2003).

Increased Medical Utilization and Costs

Substantially higher costs are associated with the medical care of patients with depression than of those without depression. The cost is related to all types of care, including primary care, specialty care, emergency department, and mental health visits; pharmacy costs; diagnostic tests; and inpatient fees (Katon 2003). One study showed that total ambulatory and inpatient costs were about 50% higher for depressed than nondepressed patients after adjustment for chronic medical illness costs (Katon 2003; Katon et al. 2003).

Sociodemographic Characteristics

The factors associated with increased risk of major depression are similar in patients with and without chronic illness. These characteristics include female sex, younger age (<65 years), lower income, higher body mass index, smoking, unemployment, and declining health status (Egede 2007). Maladaptive coping styles also increase the risk of developing a mood disorder (Vinberg et al. 2010). Factors that may influence the likelihood of depression in medically ill patients include the physical effects of the illness and treatment, the personal meaning associated with the medical condition, and the level of social support.

Relationship of Depression With Medical Outcomes

Complex Interrelationship

Not only does medical illness increase the likelihood of developing depression, but the reverse is also true: depression may increase risk for medical illness such as cardiovascular disease and stroke. The interplay among depression, risk factors for depression, and chronic medical illness is complex. Genetic vulnerability, childhood adversity, and stressful life events are three known risk factors for the development of major depression (Kendler et al. 2002). Childhood adversity, including neglect and sexual abuse, may lead to maladaptive attachment, which then may contribute to difficulty collaborating with physicians (Ciechanowski et al. 2001). Both childhood adversity and major depression are associated with risk factors for medical illnesses such as smoking, obesity, and sedentary lifestyle. The symptom burden and functional impairment associated with medical illnesses, in addition to the indirect pathophysiological effects that medical illnesses have on the central nervous system (CNS) through increased cytokine levels or other inflammatory factors, may contribute to the development of depression. The negative impact of depression on patients' collaboration with their physician and compliance with treatment, as well as the direct pathophysiological effects of depression, increases morbidity and mortality in patients with major depression and chronic medical illness (Katon 2003).

Higher Likelihood of Noncompliance With Medical Treatment

Compared with nondepressed patients, depressed patients are reported to be three times more likely to be noncompliant with medical treatment. Having positive beliefs and expectations regarding the effectiveness of medical treatment improves compliance, and if a patient is hopeless due to depression, the capacity to be optimistic is diminished. Social support is also important for treatment adherence, and patients who are depressed may withdraw and isolate themselves from their support network. If cognitive functioning is affected by depression, the patient's ability to remember and follow through with treatment may be affected (DiMatteo et al. 2000).

Increased Mortality

The data have been mixed, but growing evidence supports an association between major depression (even subthreshold depression) and increased mortality. The relationship is most strongly established in patients with cardiovascular or cerebrovascular disease (Roose et al. 2001; von Ammon Cavanaugh et al. 2001; Wulsin et al. 1999). In a prospective study of stroke patients, depressed patients were three times more likely than nondepressed patients to die during the 10-year follow-up (Morris et al. 1993). One study found that in-hospital mortality of medical inpatients was predicted by the severity of medical illness, a diagnosis of major depression based on modified criteria, and a past history of depression (von Ammon Cavanaugh et al. 2001).

Higher Number of Unexplained Symptoms

Patients with depression have more medically unexplained symptoms, even when controlling for severity of medical illness. In a study of patients with diabetes, cardiac disease, arthritis, and pulmonary disease, somatic symptoms were as strongly associated with depression and anxiety as were objective physiological measures (Katon et al. 2007).

Diagnosing Depression in Medically Ill Patients

Misinterpreting Depression as "Appropriate" Reaction

A common but misleading and potentially harmful approach is for physicians to consider depression in medically ill patients to be an "appropriate" reaction; this attitude trivializes the importance of depression and leads to undertreatment. Sadness, however, is an expectable response to the many adverse effects associated with medical illness (Cassem 1995).

Challenges of Making a Diagnosis

Historically, the issue of diagnosing major depression in medically ill patients has been fraught with controversy for the following reasons (Li and Rodin 2011):

- At least four of the DSM-IV-TR (American Psychiatric Association 2000) criterion A symptoms of major depressive disorder—fatigue, anorexia or weight loss, impairment in concentration, and sleep disturbance—can also be accounted for by medical illness or medical treatment.

- Patients may present with anhedonia when physical symptoms such as pain interfere with the capacity to experience pleasure in the absence of comorbid depression.
- Patients with advanced medical disease may report suicidal ideation or desire for death in the absence of depressed mood.
- Depressive symptoms may manifest in atypical forms, such as noncompliance with treatment or increased intensity of somatic symptoms.
- A new diagnosis of a medical problem or the progression of medical disease may be associated with intense feelings of loss and grief, and defining the boundary between normal grief and depression can be difficult.

Diagnostic Approaches

Exclusive approach. Specificity is maximized by eliminating anorexia and fatigue from the list of nine DSM-IV-TR criterion A symptoms of major depressive episode (Table 10–1), and then requiring four of the remaining symptoms for a diagnosis. The method is more often used for research than for clinical practice.

Etiological approach. The clinician makes a subjective judgment to determine whether a symptom should be attributed to depression or medical illness.

Substitutive approach. Physical symptoms are replaced by emotional symptoms. For example, low energy is replaced by brooding, self-pity, or pessimism, and difficulty concentrating is replaced by nonreactive mood (Endicott 1984).

Inclusive approach. Symptoms of depression are taken at face value, without exclusion or substitution due to comorbid medical issues. This is the most sensitive approach and, given the generally favorable risk-benefit profile of most antidepressants, is the most commonly applied approach at the clinical bedside.

Demoralization

Demoralization has been described as a syndrome of hopelessness, loss of meaning, and existential distress accompanied by a subjective sense of incompetence. Patients may feel demoralized by disability, bodily disfigurement, dependency,

Table 10–1. DSM-IV-TR diagnostic criteria for major depressive episode

A. Five (or more) of the following symptoms have been present during the same 2-week period and represent a change from previous functioning; at least one of the symptoms is either (1) depressed mood or (2) loss of interest or pleasure. **Note:** Do not include symptoms that are clearly due to a general medical condition, or mood-incongruent delusions or hallucinations.

   (1) depressed mood most of the day, nearly every day, as indicated by either subjective report (e.g., feels sad or empty) or observation made by others (e.g., appears tearful). **Note:** In children and adolescents, can be irritable mood.

   (2) markedly diminished interest or pleasure in all, or almost all, activities most of the day, nearly every day (as indicated by either subjective account or observation made by others)

   (3) significant weight loss when not dieting or weight gain (e.g., a change of more than 5% of body weight in a month), or decrease or increase in appetite nearly every day. **Note:** In children, consider failure to make expected weight gains.

   (4) insomnia or hypersomnia nearly every day

   (5) psychomotor agitation or retardation nearly every day (observable by others, not merely subjective feelings of restlessness or being slowed down)

   (6) fatigue or loss of energy nearly every day

   (7) feelings of worthlessness or excessive or inappropriate guilt (which may be delusional) nearly every day (not merely self-reproach or guilt about being sick)

   (8) diminished ability to think or concentrate, or indecisiveness, nearly every day (either by subjective account or as observed by others)

   (9) recurrent thoughts of death (not just fear of dying), recurrent suicidal ideation without a specific plan, or a suicide attempt or a specific plan for committing suicide

B. The symptoms do not meet criteria for a mixed episode (see DSM-IV-TR, p. 365)

C. The symptoms cause clinically significant distress or impairment in social, occupational, or other important areas of functioning.

Table 10–1. DSM-IV-TR diagnostic criteria for major depressive episode *(continued)*

D. The symptoms are not due to the direct physiological effects of a substance (e.g., a drug of abuse, a medication) or a general medical condition (e.g., hypothyroidism).

E. The symptoms are not better accounted for by bereavement, i.e., after the loss of a loved one, the symptoms persist for longer than 2 months or are characterized by marked functional impairment, morbid preoccupation with worthlessness, suicidal ideation, psychotic symptoms, or psychomotor retardation.

Source. Reprinted from American Psychiatric Association: *Diagnostic and Statistical Manual of Mental Disorders,* 4th Edition, Text Revision. Washington, DC, American Psychiatric Association, 2000, p. 356. Used with permission.

feelings of being a burden on others, and fear of loss of dignity (Cockram et al. 2009; Kissane et al. 2001). Debate is ongoing as to whether demoralization represents a disorder or a normal reaction to overwhelming circumstances. The prevalence of demoralization in medically ill patients has been estimated to be 30% (Mangelli et al. 2005). Jerome Frank (1974) described demoralization as a characteristic of all conditions that respond to psychotherapy. The psychotherapeutic approach with demoralized patients includes helping them mobilize hope, self-agency, and connection with others (Griffith and Gaby 2005). (See Chapter 15, "Psychosocial Management.")

Depression Secondary to General Medical Condition

In the section on other mood disorders, DSM-IV-TR includes mood disorder due to a general medical condition, which refers to mood disorders judged to be the direct physiological consequence of a specific medical illness. Conditions such as pancreatic cancer, Parkinson's disease, multiple sclerosis, and hypothyroidism are known to directly cause depression, but in many cases, a causal relationship is difficult to confirm because other biological, psychological, and social factors may also be contributing to the patient's mood symptoms (Li and Rodin 2011). Table 10–2 lists medical conditions and toxic agents associated with depression.

Table 10–2.   Medical conditions and toxic agents associated with secondary depressive disorders

Endocrine disorders
Addison's disease
Cushing's disease
Hypopituitarism
Hypothyroidism

Infections
Encephalitis
Epstein-Barr virus
Hepatitis
HIV
Pneumonia
Postinfluenza
Tertiary syphilis

Medications
Amphetamine withdrawal
Antihypertensives: methyldopa,
  clonidine, guanethidine, reserpine
Barbiturates
Benzodiazepines
Cocaine withdrawal
Corticosteroids
Opiates
Chemotherapeutic agents: vinblastine,
  vincristine, procarbazine, L-asparaginase,
  interferon alfa
Gonadotropin-releasing hormone
  agonists
Interleukin
Interferon alfa-2
Mefloquine
Metoclopramide
Progesterone-releasing implanted
  contraceptives

Miscellaneous
Alcoholism
Anemia
Heavy metal poisoning
Hypercalcemia
Hypermagnesemia
Hypokalemia
Systemic lupus erythematosus

Neurological disorders
Cerebrovascular disease
Dementia (particularly subcortical)
Epilepsy (particularly with a temporal
  lobe focus)
Huntington's disease
Multiple sclerosis
Parkinson's disease
Postconcussional disorder
Progressive supranuclear palsy
Sleep apnea
Stroke
Subarachnoid hemorrhage

Tumors
Central nervous system
Lung
Pancreas

Cognitive Changes Associated With Depression

Depression as a Neurodegenerative Disorder

A growing body of evidence suggests that depression, at least in some individuals, is a neurodegenerative disorder (MacQueen et al. 2003). Young patients who are depressed show deficits in executive function and memory, and such deficits seem to worsen in older patients who are chronically depressed (Fossati et al. 2002).

Correlation Between Depression Severity and Cognitive Performance

An association between depression severity and cognitive performance has been demonstrated in the domains of episodic memory, executive function, and processing speed, but not for semantic memory or visuospatial memory (McDermott and Ebmeier 2009).

Involvement of Pathological Alterations of Limbic and Cortical Structures in Depression

Decreased volumes of the hippocampus, basal ganglia, and orbitofrontal and subgenual prefrontal cortex are found in patients who have had multiple episodes of MDD or longer illness duration. Gender, medication, stage of illness, and family history all influence the nature of the findings in a regionally specific manner (Lorenzetti et al. 2009).

Differentiating Depression From Dementia

Distinguishing between early dementia and depression is often difficult, and the two illnesses frequently coexist. Clinically helpful considerations are summarized in Table 10–3.

Screening Instruments for Depression

Beck Depression Inventory–II

The Beck Depression Inventory–II (BDI-II) is a 21-item self-report scale that has been well studied and widely used. Although several studies have found the BDI-II to be an accurate measure of depressive symptoms, its utility in assessing medically ill patients has been questioned because of the high proportion of somatic items (Berard et al. 1998; Clarke et al. 1993; Wilhelm et al., 2004).

Table 10–3.   Differentiating depression and dementia

	Depression	Dementia
Insidious onset	Weeks to months	Months to years
Psychological distress present	Yes	Yes
Frequently answers "I don't know"	Yes	No
Higher cortical function deficits (dysphasia, dyspraxia)	No	Yes
Remote memory less impaired than recent memory	No	Yes
Inconsistent mental status examination findings on repeated examinations	Yes	No
Past or family history of mood disorder	Yes	No
Awareness of cognitive deficits	Yes	No
Neuroimaging study results usually abnormal	No	Yes

Note.   Depression and dementia can occur together, especially in subcortical dementias. When a patient with dementia also has comorbid major depression, his or her cognitive deficits are greatly magnified.

Center for Epidemiologic Studies Depression Scale

The Center for Epidemiologic Studies Depression Scale (CES-D) is a valuable instrument in screening for depression in medically ill patients, although some studies have found it to have a low positive predictive value (Pandya et al. 2005; Thomas et al. 2001; van Wilgen et al. 2006). The CES-D is a 20-item self-report measure in which only 4 of the items are somatic.

Hospital Anxiety and Depression Scale

The Hospital Anxiety and Depression Scale (HADS) is a 14-item self-report scale specifically designed for use with medically ill patients (Zigmond and Snaith 1983). It includes separate 7-item subscales for depression and anxiety; the depression subscale does not include somatic items and focuses on anhedonia. Studies have supported the value of the HADS as a screening instrument for many different medical populations (Bambauer et al. 2005; Herrmann 1997; Katz et al. 2004; Stafford et al. 2007; Walker et al. 2007), although it may not be a valid instrument for palliative care patients (Lloyd-Williams et al. 2001).

Patient Health Questionnaire

The Patient Health Questionnaire (PHQ-9) is a self-administered diagnostic instrument for depression. Each of the nine symptom categories in DSM-IV-TR criterion A is scored from 0 (not at all) to 3 (nearly every day). The PHQ-9 is a commonly used instrument for depression screening in primary care clinics and may be able to detect depression outcome and changes over time (Dejesus et al. 2007; Kroenke et al. 2001; Lowe et al. 2004; Williams et al. 2005).

Very Brief Screening Instruments

Some studies suggest that a single-item screening question (e.g., "Are you depressed?") or a two-item subset of the PHQ-9 is as effective as the longer instruments (Chochinov et al. 1997; Lowe et al. 2005).

Pharmacological Management

Selective Serotonin Reuptake Inhibitors

Because of their tolerability and relative safety, selective serotonin reuptake inhibitors (SSRIs) are generally considered first-line treatment for depression in medically ill patients. The success of the SSRIs in displacing the tricyclic antidepressants (TCAs) as first-line treatment is not due to efficacy but rather to fewer anticholinergic and cardiac side effects and to greater safety in overdose.

Benefits. SSRIs may have benefits independent of effects on depression, such as in the treatment of hot flashes in cancer patients (Kimmick et al. 2006) and global cognitive functioning in stroke patients (Jorge et al. 2010).

Adverse effects. Although SSRIs are generally well tolerated in depressed medically ill patients, they do have some adverse effects (see also Chapter 14, "Biological Treatments").

- The most common side effects are gastrointestinal distress, nervousness, sexual dysfunction, and insomnia.
- Anxiety and jitteriness may occur in at least 10% of patients, primarily arising during early treatment and typically improving after the acute phase. Short-term use of benzodiazepines may be helpful in alleviating these symptoms. Nausea also occurs, most frequently in the early phase of treatment. Other adverse effects include excessive sweating, headaches, flushing, dry mouth, and appetite changes.

- Less common side effects of SSRIs, especially when taken with nonsteroidal anti-inflammatory agents or warfarin, include the syndrome of inappropriate antidiuretic hormone, hyponatremia, and increased gastrointestinal bleeding.
- During long-term treatment, weight gain, sleep disturbances, fatigue, apathy, cognitive symptoms, and sexual dysfunction are possible side effects (Smith et al. 2008).

Active metabolites and elimination half-life.   SSRIs differ based on the presence of active metabolites and elimination half-life. For example, fluoxetine, which has an elimination half-life of 1–3 days, is converted to norfluoxetine, a potent SSRI with a half-life of 7–9 days. Therefore, steady-state plasma levels of fluoxetine are not reached for 5–6 weeks; a similar length of time is required to clear norfluoxetine after discontinuation. The longer half-life reduces the effect of missed doses and mitigates the SSRI discontinuation syndrome. In contrast, paroxetine has a short elimination half-life and is often associated with discontinuation symptoms (Mann 2005).

Drug interactions.   SSRIs differ in their risk for interactions with other drugs. Citalopram, escitalopram, and sertraline are least likely to affect the metabolism of other drugs, whereas fluoxetine, paroxetine, and especially fluvoxamine are more likely to do so.

Serotonin-Norepinephrine Reuptake Inhibitors

- *Venlafaxine* blocks reuptake of serotonin at lower dosages and of norepinephrine at higher dosages; its dual action at higher dosages, usually thought to occur in the 150–225+ mg/day range, appears to benefit some patients whose condition has not responded to SSRIs or other antidepressants, and is effective in reducing the pain of diabetic neuropathy (Davis and Smith 1999). Venlafaxine reduces hot flashes in cancer patients (Loprinzi et al. 2000). The side-effect profile is similar to that of the SSRIs, except venlafaxine has the added potential of dose-related high blood pressure.
- *Desvenlafaxine* is the major active metabolite of venlafaxine. The most common side effects are nausea, dizziness, and insomnia (Rickels et al. 2010).
- *Duloxetine,* a newer dual agent, is approved for the treatment of diabetic neuropathy and fibromyalgia in addition to depression. Unlike venlafax-

ine, duloxetine does not appear to be associated with a significant risk of elevated blood pressure.

- *Milnacipran,* the newest dual agent, has been approved by the U.S. Food and Drug Administration (FDA) only for fibromyalgia, but the medication has demonstrated efficacy and is marketed in Europe for the treatment of depression. It is distinguished from the other serotonin-norepinephrine reuptake inhibitors (SNRIs) by its equipotent serotonin and norepinephrine reuptake inhibition (Pae et al. 2009a) and the fact that cytochrome P450 enzymes are not involved in its metabolism. Dosing should be reduced in the presence of renal failure.

Other Novel Antidepressants

- *Bupropion,* a norepinephrine-dopamine reuptake inhibitor, can be stimulating, has minimal cardiac effects, rarely causes sexual dysfunction, and is not associated with weight gain. However, bupropion may produce anxiety, agitation, anxiety, and headache, and its use is avoided in patients with seizures or at risk for seizures (e.g., patients with brain tumors).
- *Mirtazapine,* an α_2-adrenergic receptor antagonist, is moderately anticholinergic and very antihistaminic; therefore, it promotes appetite, weight gain, and sedation. Mirtazapine is well suited for certain patients (e.g., a patient with advanced cancer who is depressed, cannot sleep, and has decreased appetite). Due to its serotonin type 3 receptor–blocking antiemetic effects, it may also be useful in patients who have nausea.
- *Trazodone* acts mainly postsynaptically as a serotonin type 2 receptor antagonist. Its sedating properties and lack of anticholinergic side effects contribute to its common use in lower dosages as a sleep aid. However, its association with orthostatic hypotension, sedation, and priapism limits its use in antidepressant dosages. Trazodone lacks the quinidine-like properties of the cyclic antidepressants but in rare cases has been associated with cardiac arrhythmias.

Tricyclic Antidepressants

TCAs are still used in the hospital and clinic. They are effective for treating chronic neuropathic pain, fibromyalgia, headache, insomnia, anxiety, and depression.

Altered dosages. Lower dosages of TCAs are sometimes required for patients with liver disease, patients who are elderly or malnourished, and patients taking medications (e.g., paroxetine, fluoxetine) that can inhibit metabolism of TCAs. Higher TCA dosages may be needed for patients taking medications (e.g., carbamazepine, phenytoin, barbiturates) that induce hepatic enzymes.

Precautions. Prior to starting a TCA, a medical history should be performed to determine whether the patient has cardiac conduction system disease. An electrocardiogram (ECG) should be obtained if the patient has had cardiac disease or cardiac symptoms, and should be considered for patients ages 40 years and older.

Adverse effects. At therapeutic levels, TCAs may produce sedation, orthostatic hypotension, and anticholinergic effects, and may decrease the seizure threshold. Like type Ia antiarrhythmic drugs (e.g., quinidine), TCAs may prolong ventricular depolarization and actually improve ventricular dysrhythmias. However, a patient who has preexisting bundle branch disease is at risk for second- or third-degree heart block. Conduction delay will appear on the ECG as increased duration of the QTc, QRS, or PR intervals. When blood levels are in the therapeutic range, TCAs have little if any effect on left ventricular performance, even in patients with low ejection fractions. For patients with a history of angina, an important consideration is that anticholinergic effects may increase the heart rate and slightly increase cardiac workload (Glassman and Bigger 1981).

Monoamine Oxidase Inhibitors

Indications and adverse effects. Despite their side-effect profile, dietary restrictions, and drug-drug interactions, monoamine oxidase inhibitors (MAOIs) can be particularly useful agents for the treatment of anxiety and "atypical" depression (e.g., depression with hyperphagia, hypersomnia, psychomotor slowing, and rejection sensitivity) and can be effective in patients with treatment-resistant depression (Pae et al. 2009b). MAOIs have potent hypotensive effects, a fact that is particularly important when treating elderly patients, who may be both more sensitive to orthostasis and more likely to fall and sustain fractures. Other common side effects are dry mouth, gastrointestinal upset, urinary hesitancy, sexual dysfunction, weight gain, myoclonic jerks, and headache.

Mechanism of action. MAOIs irreversibly block monoamine oxidase (MAO), the enzyme responsible for the oxidative deamination of neurotransmitters such as serotonin, norepinephrine, and dopamine. The enzyme MAO comes in two forms, MAO-A and MAO-B. The blockade of MAO-A in the gastrointestinal tract is responsible for the severe hypertensive crisis that can occur if patients ingest foods containing the sympathomimetic tyramine. Tyramine is usually metabolized in the gastrointestinal tract, but the blockade of MAO-A allows it to flow into the general circulation.

Oral and transdermal forms available. Phenelzine (45–90 mg/day) and tranylcypromine (30–50 mg/day) irreversibly inhibit both MAO-A and MAO-B. Selegiline at lower dosages is a selective irreversible inhibitor of MAO-B and is indicated for the treatment of Parkinson's disease. At higher dosages, it is a nonselective inhibitor of MAO and functions as a traditional MAOI with antidepressant properties. A transdermal patch form of selegiline was approved by the FDA in 2006 for use in the treatment of depression. No dietary restrictions are necessary with transdermal selegiline when it is used at 6 mg/day because direct inhibition of MAO-A in the gastrointestinal tract is bypassed. MAOI dietary restrictions *are* required if the 9-mg/day or 12-mg/day patch is used, because of limited clinical and experimental experience with higher dosages (Patkar et al. 2006). Caution must be exercised when switching from an MAOI to another antidepressant: a 2-week drug-free period is recommended to allow time for MAO to regenerate. Fluoxetine, due to its longer half-life, requires a 5-week drug-free interval.

Psychostimulants

Indications and administration. Psychostimulant medications, such as methylphenidate (plasma half-life = 1–2 hours) and dextroamphetamine (plasma half-life = 6–8 hours), are an important treatment option in some situations (Table 10–4). Psychostimulants are fast acting, well tolerated, and reasonably safe among elderly and medically ill patients (Masand et al. 1991). Usual dosage ranges are 5–20 mg/day for both methylphenidate and dextroamphetamine. Administration is typically divided into two doses per day, in the morning and at noon or early afternoon, because of the short half-lives. Doses later than 3:00 P.M. should be avoided so that sleep is not disturbed. When effective, the onset of action is usually within 2–3 days.

Table 10–4.   Clinical situations in which psychostimulants are an important treatment option

When neurovegetative features of depression threaten health or life and a rapid response is needed

In terminally ill patients with profound psychomotor retardation

For treatment-resistant depression

For adult attention-deficit disorder

For late-stage HIV disease (AIDS)–associated secondary mood disorders

For poststroke depression

For depression associated with subcortical dementias (e.g., dementia associated with Parkinson's disease)

Adverse effects.   Adverse effects are relatively few but may include sinus tachycardia, dysrhythmias, blood pressure elevation, psychosis, insomnia, anorexia, and exacerbation of spasticity in patients with upper motor neuron disease. These side effects usually occur at dosages much higher than those recommended. Stimulants are contraindicated in patients with structural heart disease or tachyarrhythmia. Although some physicians are reluctant to prescribe psychostimulants because of their abuse potential, the risk is low in patients without a substance abuse history at the dosages recommended for use in the medical setting.

Commonly Used Augmentation Strategies

Commonly used augmentation strategies that have proved effective for depression include bupropion, buspirone, lithium, mirtazapine, and thyroid supplementation with triiodothyronine or liothyronine (T_3). Evidence is accumulating that atypical antipsychotics can also be useful adjunctive treatments for treatment-resistant depression, although data are lacking regarding the efficacy of atypical antipsychotics compared with other augmenting agents. Although aripiprazole was approved in 2007 and an olanzapine/fluoxetine combination in 2009 for treatment-resistant depression, the risk of the long-term side effects of atypical antipsychotics must be weighed against the benefits (DeBattista and Hawkins 2009).

Treatment Strategies and Outcomes

Remission Versus Response

The current standard goal of treatment is remission, or the absence of depressive symptoms, often defined as a score of ≤7 on the 17-item Hamilton Rating Scale for Depression (Ham-D17) or a score of ≤5 on the Quick Inventory of Depressive Symptomatology Self-Report (QIDS-SR). With a response to treatment, usually defined as a 50% or greater reduction in baseline symptoms, a patient may subjectively feel better, but residual depressive symptoms result in a higher risk of relapse, continued impairments, and increased use of medical services (Doraiswamy et al. 2001).

Sequenced Treatment Alternatives to Relieve Depression (STAR*D) Study

Study goal.   Remission was the goal in the STAR*D study.

Study design.   The multicenter, prospective, sequentially randomized controlled trial of outpatients with nonpsychotic unipolar depression was designed to mimic real-world clinical decision making. The protocol allowed patients to be randomized to available treatment options (switching agents, augmentation, and cognitive therapy) based on patient preference.

- For all treatments, a move to the next step could occur whenever intolerable adverse affects were encountered or when the maximally tolerated dosage did not result in meaningful symptom reduction in 6–8 weeks.
- Patients with significant comorbid medical problems were not excluded unless the conditions contraindicated the use of the study's medications (average number of general medical conditions=3).
- More than 75% of the participants had recurrent depression, with a 15-year average duration of illness (Rush et al. 2009).

Remission rates and dosages.   Remission rates and dosages were similar in the primary care and psychiatry settings.

First-step treatment: citalopram.   One-third of patients remitted in first-step treatment with citalopram.

- Among the patients who remitted, 50% achieved remission within 6 weeks, and a substantial number responded or remitted at or after 8 weeks.

- Greater medical comorbidity was associated with lower remission rates.
- Other factors associated with poor outcomes included minority status, lower socioeconomic status, concurrent psychiatric disorders (especially substance use and anxiety disorders), lower function and quality of life, and longer index episodes.
- Higher remission rates occurred among participants who had higher levels of education or income and who were Caucasian, female, and employed (Trivedi et al. 2006).

Second-step treatment. Switching to within-class, out-of-class, or dual-action agents led to similar remission rates. About one-fourth of patients remitted when switched from citalopram to sertraline, bupropion sustained release (SR), or venlafaxine extended release (ER).

- Augmentation of citalopram had similar remission rates between bupropion SR (39%) and buspirone (33%), although bupropion had greater symptom reduction and tolerability.
- Augmentation of citalopram with cognitive therapy or switching to cognitive therapy had similar remission rates (Trivedi et al. 2006).

Third-step treatment. No differences in remission were found between patients switched to mirtazapine (8%) and those switched to nortriptyline (12%) (Fava et al. 2006). Likewise, no differences in remission were found for augmentation with lithium (13%) or T_3 (25%), although more participants discontinued lithium due to adverse effects (Nierenberg et al. 2006).

Fourth-step treatment. Remission rates were similar for patients switched to the MAOI tranylcypromine (14%) and those switched to venlafaxine ER plus mirtazapine (16%). More adverse effects occurred with tranylcypromine. The dropout rate was higher with tranylcypromine, and the symptom reduction was greater with venlafaxine ER plus mirtazapine (McGrath et al. 2006).

Implications for clinical practice. The STAR*D results indicate that in treating patients with depression, clinicians should do the following (Rush et al. 2009):

1. Aim for remission rather than response (i.e., 50% reduction in symptoms) to minimize the risk of relapse.
2. Encourage patients to stay in treatment. Of participants who remained for up to four treatment steps, 67% achieved remission.
3. Dose aggressively to maximize the chances of remission.
4. Because average time to remission was 5–6 weeks, wait 6–8 weeks before determining that a treatment is ineffective.
5. If the patient is tolerating first-step monotherapy and is beginning to experience improvement, consider augmentation as a second step.
6. Prepare the patient for the possibility of two or more treatment attempts. The number of steps necessary will likely increase with greater comorbidity and chronicity.
7. Consider aggressive treatments, such as combination or augmentation strategies, early during therapy to achieve remission as quickly as possible.

Comparative Efficacy and Tolerability Among New-Generation Antidepressants

Many studies have compared the new-generation antidepressants (i.e., SSRIs, SNRIs, bupropion, and mirtazapine). Generally, the efficacy is similar, and if a difference has been found, it has been modest (Hansen et al. 2005; Papakostas et al. 2007). One meta-analysis suggested that mirtazapine, escitalopram, venlafaxine, and sertraline were more efficacious than duloxetine, fluoxetine, fluvoxamine, and paroxetine, and that sertraline and escitalopram had the best tolerability (Cipriani et al. 2009). When balancing efficacy, acceptability, and drug cost, Cipriani and colleagues suggested that sertraline may be the most appropriate first-line agent. These findings were based on only 8 weeks of treatment, which is a significant limitation of the meta-analysis (Cipriani et al. 2009).

Depression Severity Associated With Antidepressant Drug Effects

A recent meta-analysis found that the benefit of antidepressant therapy over placebo increases with severity of depression symptoms and, on average, may be minimal for patients with mild to moderate symptoms. The benefit of medications over placebo was substantial for patients with very severe depression (Fournier et al. 2010).

Electroconvulsive Therapy

Electroconvulsive therapy (ECT) is a highly effective treatment for severe depression with functional impairment, psychotic depression, and catatonia. (See Chapter 14, "Biological Treatments," for information on ECT and two other brain stimulation techniques: vagal nerve and deep brain stimulation.)

Psychological Interventions

General Issues

The psychiatric examination is not complete without an attempt by the psychiatric consultant to understand the meaning of the illness to the patient, including the ways in which past experiences are affecting the patient's current approach to his or her illness. The value to the patient of "just talking" is often underestimated. Because most hospital stays are short, brief therapies are used. For patients seen in outpatient consultation, cognitive therapy, psychodynamic psychotherapy, and supportive psychotherapy are available treatment options. Group psychotherapy promotes support, improves interpersonal relationships, models adaptive coping mechanisms, decreases loneliness, and helps the patient develop a sense of meaning in life. Cognitive therapy is particularly useful for patients with false assumptions or beliefs about their illness, such as patients who believe that illness represents punishment or weakness, who have unrealistic or distorted fears and expectations, and who have exaggerated or inappropriate responses to loss (Fava et al. 1988).

Efficacy of Psychological Interventions

Evidence indicates that cognitive therapy may be as effective as medication for treating mild and moderate depression (DeRubeis et al. 1999). When psychological treatment is combined with antidepressant therapy, patients experience higher rates of improvement than with drug treatment alone (Pampallona et al. 2004). In primary care clinics, psychological interventions are more effective for treating depression than usual care alone in both the short term and the long term (Bortolotti et al. 2008). (See also Chapter 15, "Psychosocial Management.")

Bipolar Disorder and Secondary Mania

Epidemiology of Bipolar Disorder

The incidence and prevalence of mania due to a general medical condition are unknown. Lifetime prevalence estimates for bipolar disorder are 1% for bipolar I, 1% for bipolar II, and 2% for subthreshold bipolar disorder (Merikangas et al. 2007). Lifetime recurrence is frequent, and residual mood symptoms early in recovery appear to be a powerful predictor of recurrence (Perlis et al. 2006b). Patients with residual affective symptoms develop a subsequent major affective episode three times faster than patients who have an asymptomatic initial recovery (Judd et al. 2008).

Effects of Comorbid Bipolar Disorder and Medical Disease on Medical and Psychiatric Outcomes

Studies suggest that medical comorbidity is associated with worse bipolar outcomes (Pirraglia et al. 2009). The reverse relationship is also true: bipolar disorder predicts worse medical outcomes. Bipolar spectrum disorders are associated with premature mortality due to general medical illness; compared with the general population, patients with bipolar disorder have twice the risk of cardiovascular mortality (Murray et al. 2009). Potential causes of premature mortality include adverse pharmacological effects, biological factors, health care disparities, and poor lifestyle choices (Roshanaei-Moghaddam and Katon 2009). Modifiable risk factors, such as dyslipidemia, hyperglycemia, hypertension, smoking, and obesity, are common in this population and contribute to illnesses such as diabetes and coronary heart disease. Many psychotropic agents used in the treatment of bipolar disorder have similar efficacy, but some are associated with more metabolic side effects, a potentially important factor that deserves consideration when choosing among these medications (Newcomer 2009).

Diagnosis

General Issues

Bipolar disorder is frequently unrecognized in patients who present with depression, especially in the primary care setting; efforts to screen for both depression and manic episodes can improve diagnosis and treatment (Das et al. 2005). In medically ill patients, mania can be confused with delirium because abrupt onset, agitation, sleep disturbance, inattention, and psychosis can occur in both illnesses (Arora and Daughton 2007). Compared with patients with MDD, patients with bipolar depression are more likely to have a family history of bipolar disorder, an earlier age at onset, and a greater number of previous depressive episodes (Perlis et al. 2006a).

Diagnostic Criteria for Mania

The diagnostic criteria for manic episode (American Psychiatric Association 2000, p. 362) include the following:

1. The patient has had a distinct period of abnormally and persistently elevated, expansive, or irritable mood, lasting at least 1 week (or any duration if hospitalization is necessary).
2. During the period of mood disturbance, at least three of the following symptoms are present: inflated self-esteem or grandiosity, decreased need for sleep, more talkative than usual, racing thoughts or flight of ideas, distractibility, increase in goal-directed activity, and excessive involvement in pleasurable activities that have a high potential for painful consequences (e.g., spending money, sexual indiscretion).
3. The mood disturbance leads to significant impairment in social or occupational functioning.

Secondary Mania

According to DSM-IV-TR, secondary mania is diagnosed either as mood disorder due to general medical condition with manic features or as substance-induced mood disorder with manic features. Secondary mania requires a prominent and persistent elevated, expansive, or irritable mood, as well as evidence from the history, physical examination, or laboratory findings that the disturbance is the direct physiological consequence of a general medical condition (American Psychiatric Association 2000). Secondary mania is not diagnosed if the mood disturbance occurs in the course of delirium.

Differentiation of Primary and Secondary Mania

A temporal correlation of the onset of mania and an organic factor helps to differentiate primary from secondary mania. Secondary mania usually begins hours or days after the physiological or toxic insult. Before mania can be assumed to be due to an organic etiology, a careful history and examination are necessary to determine whether a patient has had prior mood episodes (Arora and Daughton 2007). Secondary mania can occur at any age, whereas primary mania is more likely to occur in the first three decades of life. A family history of bipolar disorder suggests but does not prove that mania is primary.

Table 10–5. Selected causes of secondary mania

Neurological conditions	Medications and substances
Frontotemporal dementia	Alcohol
HIV encephalopathy	Amantadine
Huntington's disease	Amphetamines
Multiple sclerosis	Anabolic steroids
Psychomotor seizures	Antidepressants
Stroke (temporal, right hemispheric)	Cocaine
Traumatic brain injury	Corticosteroids/corticosteroid withdrawal
Tumors	Cyclobenzaprine
Viral encephalitis	Dextromethorphan
Wilson's disease	Dopamine agonists (levodopa, pramipexole)
Other systemic conditions	*Hypericum perforatum* (St. John's wort)
Carcinoid	Isoniazid
Cushing's syndrome	Methylphenidate and other stimulants
Hyperthyroidism	Modafinil
Niacin deficiency	Phencyclidine
Postoperative delirium	Procarbazine
Puerperal postpartum psychosis	Propafenone
Vitamin B_{12} deficiency	Sympathomimetic amines (e.g., ephedrine)
	Thyroid preparations
	Zidovudine

Etiology of Secondary Mania

Table 10–5 lists potential causes of secondary mania. (For additional information, see McDaniel and Sharma 2002.)

Neurological disorders.   The presence of a neurological disorder is a significant risk factor for secondary mania, particularly in patients who are elderly (Shulman et al. 1992). Manic symptoms are associated with many neurological disorders, such as some movement disorders, multiple sclerosis, head trauma, stroke, CNS HIV infection, and epilepsy (Rundell and Wise 1989). The prevalence of mania in HIV-infected patients is estimated to be 4%–8% (Kilbourne et al. 2001). Evidence suggests that compared with HIV patients with primary mania, HIV-infected patients with secondary mania are older, have more severe cognitive impairment, and are more likely to have CD4 cell counts below 350 cells/mm^3. Manic symptoms in the secondary mania group are more severe, with increased aggressiveness, paranoid delusions, auditory hallucinations, and visual hallucinations (Nakimuli-Mpungu et al. 2006). Secondary mania is more likely to occur in patients with traumatic brain injury (~10%) than in patients with other brain injuries, such as stroke (Jorge et al. 1993). Some studies have suggested an association with right-sided lesions in patients with brain injury who develop secondary mania (Robinson et al. 1988; Starkstein et al. 1988).

Substance-induced mania.　Corticosteroids and dopaminergic agonists are frequent causes of medication-induced mania. Hypomania and mania are the most common acute mood changes related to corticosteroid therapy (symptoms usually develop within 1 week), whereas depression occurs more often with long-term corticosteroid therapy. Dosage is the most significant risk factor for the development of mood symptoms, and symptoms typically resolve with dose reduction or discontinuation of corticosteroids. For patients with psychosis or agitation, therefore, antipsychotics are considered the first-line treatment (Warrington and Bostwick 2006).

Treatment of Bipolar Mania

General Considerations

The treatments for secondary and primary mania are similar, with two exceptions. First, in secondary mania, the etiological agent is identified and removed, whenever possible. Patients might require surgical procedures to remove tumors, medications to correct metabolic abnormalities, or removal of toxic agents associated with secondary mania. Second, lithium is not usually a first-line treatment for secondary mania because of increased side effects in patients who are medically ill, elderly, or both. However, there are exceptions: lithium has been used successfully in treating mania secondary to corticosteroids and brain tumors without seizures (McDaniel and Sharma 2002). Medication choice depends on the acuity of presentation, underlying medical condition, route of administration, potential drug-drug interactions, and side-effect profile.

Lithium

Decreased suicide and all-cause mortality.　According to findings from a meta-analysis, lithium is effective in the prevention of suicide, deliberate self-harm, and death from all causes in patients with mood disorders (unipolar depression, bipolar, schizoaffective disorder, and dysthymia) (Cipriani et al. 2005). For patients with bipolar disorder, lithium reduces the risk of relapse, at least of manic episodes (Geddes et al. 2004).

Dosage and monitoring.   Lithium is titrated within a rather narrow therapeutic range. Toxic effects occur at dosages only moderately higher than those needed for therapeutic effects. Therefore, the clinician must monitor serum lithium levels carefully; the levels are typically drawn 12 hours after the last dose. Dosages should generally begin at 300 mg/day and be increased gradually to achieve serum lithium concentrations within the generally accepted therapeutic range (0.6–1.2 mEq/L). Patients in an acute manic phase are best treated with lithium dosages that achieve serum concentrations at the upper end of this therapeutic range (0.8–1.2 mEq/L). However, for severely ill medical patients, elderly patients, or patients with renal disease, lower dosages are typically used. Steady-state serum levels typically take 5–8 days to achieve, and clinical effects usually begin around 10–14 days. For this reason, concomitant use of an antipsychotic or benzodiazepine (e.g., clonazepam) is often necessary for acute control of agitation and psychosis. Evidence suggests that lithium combined with risperidone or haloperidol is more effective than lithium alone for treatment of acute mania (Sachs et al. 2002).

Adverse effects.   In healthy individuals, the side effects of lithium are usually mild, generally well tolerated, and often transient. The most common side effects are tremor, nausea, vomiting, diarrhea, polyuria, and polydipsia. Hypothyroidism, rashes, nephrogenic diabetes insipidus, interstitial nephritis, and weight gain are less frequent. Nonspecific ST segment and T-wave changes are commonly seen on the ECG; conduction defects and arrhythmias are rare. Approximately 50% of patients taking lithium will have benign and reversible T-wave flattenings (Cassem 2004). Before patients start taking lithium, the following should be considered: ECG, electrolyte measurements, thyroid function tests, weight measurements, and renal function tests, as well as pregnancy tests in women of childbearing age. The concomitant use of nonsteroidal antiinflammatory drugs, thiazide diuretics, angiotensin-converting enzyme inhibitors, and cyclooxygenase-2 inhibitors may result in increased lithium levels. Lithium toxicity markedly affects the CNS and can be a life-threatening emergency. Symptoms of lithium-induced CNS toxicity include ataxia, slurred speech, and nystagmus and can proceed to convulsions, coma, and death if lithium levels are greater than 2.5 mEq/L. The threshold for more serious side effects is lower in predisposed or medically ill patients. Dialysis is the treatment of choice in cases of life-threatening lithium toxicity.

Anticonvulsant Mood Stabilizers

- *Valproate* has demonstrated efficacy for treatment of mania; there is also increasing but limited evidence for an antidepressant effect in bipolar depression. The onset of antimanic activity generally occurs within several days to 2 weeks of achieving a serum valproate concentration of ≥50 mg/L (Malhi et al. 2009). When valproate is prescribed for medically ill patients, the clinician should be alert to gastrointestinal side effects, hepatotoxicity, coagulation effects, and possible drug-drug interactions. Although hepatic toxicity is a concern when prescribing valproate, it is relatively rare. Hepatic necrosis, a major risk factor for children younger than 2 years, is an uncommon complication in adults taking valproate, occurring in 1 in 10,000 patients (Eadie et al. 1988).

- *Carbamazepine* has shown effectiveness in treating acute mania and may also be effective for maintenance (Ceron-Litvoc et al. 2009), but its side-effect profile has made it a less popular choice than valproic acid. When prescribing carbamazepine to medically ill patients, a clinician must consider its potential hematological toxicity, quinidine-like effects on cardiac conduction, antidiuretic actions, and enzyme induction that can alter the effects of other drugs. Toxic carbamazepine levels may occur when it is given to a patient also taking the calcium channel blockers diltiazem and verapamil (Stoudemire et al. 1993). Because carbamazepine is a potent inducer of cytochrome P450 3A4, it influences the metabolism of many drugs that rely on this enzyme; the blood levels of some drugs may decrease if carbamazepine is added to a patient's medication regimen. Carbamazepine induces its own metabolism, necessitating gradual increases in dosage over the first few weeks of treatment to maintain a steady blood level.

- *Lamotrigine* has been shown in controlled studies to be effective for the recurrence of bipolar depression, but it does not prevent mania (Bowden et al. 2003; Calabrese et al. 2003). Although rash occurs in 10% of patients, the incidence of Stevens-Johnson syndrome is 0.08%, and the risk appears to be minimized by a slow dose titration. The dosage of lamotrigine is generally doubled when combined with carbamazepine because of enzyme induction; however, it is halved when used with valproate because of inhibition of metabolism. Other side effects include headache, blurred vision, nausea, and vomiting.

- Despite their clinical use, *gabapentin* and *topiramate* have been found to be no more effective than placebo (Malhi et al. 2009).

Antipsychotics

Antipsychotics are effective for acute mania, and several second-generation antipsychotics have FDA approval for bipolar depression. The second-generation antipsychotics have efficacy similar to haloperidol for mania and are comparable to treatment with a mood stabilizer. If an antipsychotic is required for long-term therapy, the second-generation antipsychotics are most often used due to decreased risk of extrapyramidal symptoms, although evidence is emerging regarding the development of extrapyramidal symptoms associated with these agents in patients with bipolar disorder. The addition of a second-generation antipsychotic to a mood stabilizer appears to be better than treatment with a mood stabilizer alone (Scherk et al. 2007).

Treatment of Bipolar Depression

Pharmacological Management

Treatment of bipolar depression is especially challenging. The use of antidepressants has been controversial, and increasing data support the lack of efficacy of antidepressants. In a large randomized controlled trial, the Systematic Treatment Enhancement Program for Bipolar Disorder (STEP-BD), an antidepressant (paroxetine or bupropion) or placebo was added to lithium or anticonvulsant treatment for patients with bipolar I or II disorder; neither antidepressant was more effective than placebo (Sachs et al. 2007). TCAs and venlafaxine are particularly associated with mood switching into mania, and bupropion is the least likely to cause mood switch; the risk is reduced when antidepressants are given in combination with a mood stabilizer (Leverich et al. 2006; Salvi et al. 2008). Randomized controlled trials of quetiapine and olanzapine (olanzapine monotherapy and combination olanzapine/fluoxetine therapy) have demonstrated efficacy for bipolar depression, with an onset of action in 1 week (Cruz et al. 2010). One study showed improvement in depressive symptoms with adjunctive modafinil (Frye et al. 2007).

Psychological Interventions

In a group of patients with bipolar depression who did not receive benefit from adjunctive antidepressant therapy in the STEP-BD study, cognitive-behavioral therapy, interpersonal and social rhythms therapy, and family-focused therapy were found to increase the likelihood of recovery, enhance interpersonal functioning, and improve recovery speed (Miklowitz et al. 2007). For long-term treatment, adjunctive psychotherapy improves symptomatic and functional outcomes over 2-year periods (Miklowitz 2008).

References

American Psychiatric Association: Diagnostic and Statistical Manual of Mental Disorders, 4th Edition, Text Revision. Washington, DC, American Psychiatric Association, 2000

Arora M, Daughton J: Mania in the medically ill. Curr Psychiatry Rep 9:232–235, 2007

Bambauer KZ, Locke SE, Aupont O, et al: Using the Hospital Anxiety and Depression Scale to screen for depression in cardiac patients. Gen Hosp Psychiatry 27:275–284, 2005

Berard RM, Boermeester F, Viljoen G: Depressive disorders in an out-patient oncology setting: prevalence, assessment, and management. Psychooncology 7:112–120, 1998

Bortolotti B, Menchetti M, Bellini F, et al: Psychological interventions for major depression in primary care: a meta-analytic review of randomized controlled trials. Gen Hosp Psychiatry 30:293–302, 2008

Bowden CL, Calabrese JR, Sachs G, et al: A placebo-controlled 18-month trial of lamotrigine and lithium maintenance treatment in recently manic or hypomanic patients with bipolar I disorder. (Erratum in Arch Gen Psychiatry 61:680, 2004.) Arch Gen Psychiatry 60:392–400, 2003

Calabrese JR, Bowden CL, Sachs G, et al: A placebo-controlled 18-month trial of lamotrigine and lithium maintenance treatment in recently depressed patients with bipolar I disorder. J Clin Psychiatry 64:1013–1024, 2003

Cassem EH: Depressive disorders in the medically ill: an overview. Psychosomatics 36:S2–S10, 1995

Cassem NH: Mood-disordered patients, in Massachusetts General Hospital Handbook of General Hospital Psychiatry. Edited by Stern TA, Cassem NH, Jellinek MS, et al. St. Louis, MO, CV Mosby, 2004, pp 69–92

Ceron-Litvoc D, Soares BG, Geddes J, et al: Comparison of carbamazepine and lithium in treatment of bipolar disorder: a systematic review of randomized controlled trials. Hum Psychopharmacol 24:19–28, 2009

Chochinov HM, Wilson KG, Enns M, et al: "Are you depressed?" Screening for depression in the terminally ill. Am J Psychiatry 154:674–676, 1997

Ciechanowski PS, Katon WJ, Russo JE, et al: The patient-provider relationship: attachment theory and adherence to treatment in diabetes. Am J Psychiatry 158:29–35, 2001

Cipriani A, Pretty H, Hawton K, et al: Lithium in the prevention of suicidal behavior and all-cause mortality in patients with mood disorders: a systematic review of randomized trials. Am J Psychiatry 162:1805–1819, 2005

Cipriani A, Furukawa TA, Salanti G, et al: Comparative efficacy and acceptability of 12 new-generation antidepressants: a multiple-treatments meta-analysis. Lancet 373:746–758, 2009

Clarke DM, Smith GC, Herrman HE: A comparative study of screening instruments for mental disorders in general hospital patients. Int J Psychiatry Med 23:323–337, 1993

Cockram CA, Doros G, de Figueiredo JM: Diagnosis and measurement of subjective incompetence: the clinical hallmark of demoralization. Psychother Psychosom 78:342–345, 2009

Cruz N, Sanchez-Moreno J, Torres F, et al: Efficacy of modern antipsychotics in placebo-controlled trials in bipolar depression: a meta-analysis. Int J Neuropsychopharmacol 13:5–14, 2010

Das AK, Olfson M, Gameroff MJ, et al: Screening for bipolar disorder in a primary care practice. JAMA 293:956–963, 2005

Davis JL, Smith RL: Painful peripheral diabetic neuropathy treated with venlafaxine HCl extended release capsules. Diabetes Care 22:1909–1910, 1999

DeBattista C, Hawkins J: Utility of atypical antipsychotics in the treatment of resistant unipolar depression. CNS Drugs 23:369–377, 2009

Dejesus RS, Vickers KS, Melin GJ, et al: A system-based approach to depression management in primary care using the Patient Health Questionnaire–9. Mayo Clin Proc 82:1395–1402, 2007

DeRubeis RJ, Gelfand LA, Tang TZ, et al: Medications versus cognitive behavior therapy for severely depressed outpatients: mega-analysis of four randomized comparisons. Am J Psychiatry 156:1007–1013, 1999

DiMatteo MR, Lepper HS, Croghan TW: Depression is a risk factor for noncompliance with medical treatment: meta-analysis of the effects of anxiety and depression on patient adherence. Arch Intern Med 160:2101–2107, 2000

Doraiswamy PM, Khan ZM, Donahue RM, et al: Quality of life in geriatric depression: a comparison of remitters, partial responders, and nonresponders. Am J Geriatr Psychiatry 9:423–428, 2001

Eadie MJ, Hooper WD, Dickinson RG: Valproate-associated hepatotoxicity and its biochemical mechanisms. Med Toxicol Adverse Drug Exp 3:85–106, 1988

Egede LE: Major depression in individuals with chronic medical disorders: prevalence, correlates and association with health resource utilization, lost productivity and functional disability. Gen Hosp Psychiatry 29:409–416, 2007

Endicott J: Measurement of depression in patients with cancer. Cancer 53:2243–2249, 1984

Fava GA, Sonino N, Wise TN: Management of depression in medical patients. Psychother Psychosom 49:81–102, 1988

Fava M, Rush AJ, Wisniewski SR, et al: A comparison of mirtazapine and nortriptyline following two consecutive failed medication treatments for depressed outpatients: a STAR*D report. Am J Psychiatry 163:1161–1172, 2006

Fossati P, Coyette F, Ergis AM, et al: Influence of age and executive functioning on verbal memory of inpatients with depression. J Affect Disord 68:261–271, 2002

Fournier JC, DeRubeis RJ, Hollon SD, et al: Antidepressant drug effects and depression severity: a patient-level meta-analysis. JAMA 303:47–53, 2010

Frank JD: Psychotherapy: the restoration of morale. Am J Psychiatry 131:271–274, 1974

Frye MA, Grunze H, Suppes T, et al: A placebo-controlled evaluation of adjunctive modafinil in the treatment of bipolar depression. Am J Psychiatry 164:1242–1249, 2007

Geddes JR, Burgess S, Hawton K, et al: Long-term lithium therapy for bipolar disorder: systematic review and meta-analysis of randomized controlled trials. Am J Psychiatry 161:217–222, 2004

Glassman AH, Bigger JT Jr: Cardiovascular effects of therapeutic doses of tricyclic antidepressants: a review. Arch Gen Psychiatry 38:815–820, 1981

Griffith JL, Gaby L: Brief psychotherapy at the bedside: countering demoralization from medical illness. Psychosomatics 46:109–116, 2005

Hansen RA, Gartlehner G, Lohr KN, et al: Efficacy and safety of second-generation antidepressants in the treatment of major depressive disorder. Ann Intern Med 143:415–426, 2005

Herrmann C: International experiences with the Hospital Anxiety and Depression Scale: a review of validation data and clinical results. J Psychosom Res 42:17–41, 1997

Jorge RE, Robinson RG, Starkstein SE, et al: Secondary mania following traumatic brain injury. Am J Psychiatry 150:916–921, 1993

Jorge RE, Acion L, Moser D, et al: Escitalopram and enhancement of cognitive recovery following stroke. Arch Gen Psychiatry 67:187–196, 2010

Judd LL, Schettler PJ, Akiskal HS, et al: Residual symptom recovery from major affective episodes in bipolar disorders and rapid episode relapse/recurrence. Arch Gen Psychiatry 65:386–394, 2008

Katon WJ: Clinical and health services relationships between major depression, depressive symptoms, and general medical illness. Biol Psychiatry 54:216–226, 2003

Katon WJ, Lin E, Russo J, et al: Increased medical costs of a population-based sample of depressed elderly patients. Arch Gen Psychiatry 60:897–903, 2003

Katon W, Lin EHB, Kroenke K: The association of depression and anxiety with medical symptom burden in patients with chronic medical illness. Gen Hosp Psychiatry 29:147–155, 2007

Katz MR, Kopek N, Waldron J, et al: Screening for depression in head and neck cancer. Psychooncology 13:269–280, 2004

Kendler KS, Gardner CO, Prescott CA: Toward a comprehensive developmental model for major depression in women. Am J Psychiatry 159:1133–1145, 2002

Kessler RC, Berglund P, Demler O, et al: The epidemiology of major depressive disorder: results from the National Comorbidity Survey Replication (NCS-R). JAMA 289:3095–3105, 2003

Kilbourne AM, Justice AC, Rabeneck L, et al: General medical and psychiatric comorbidity among HIV-infected veterans in the post-HAART era. J Clin Epidemiol 54 (suppl 1):S22–S28, 2001

Kimmick GG, Lovato J, McQuellon R, et al: Randomized, double-blind, placebo-controlled, crossover study of sertraline (Zoloft) for the treatment of hot flashes in women with early stage breast cancer taking tamoxifen. Breast J 12:114–122, 2006

Kissane DW, Clarke DM, Street AF: Demoralization syndrome: a relevant psychiatric diagnosis for palliative care. J Palliat Care 17:12–21, 2001

Koike AK, Unutzer J, Wells KB: Improving the care for depression in patients with comorbid medical illness. (Erratum in Am J Psychiatry 160:204, 2003.) Am J Psychiatry 159:1738–1745, 2002

Kroenke K, Spitzer RL, Williams JB: The PHQ-9: validity of a brief depression severity measure. J Gen Intern Med 16:606–613, 2001

Leverich GS, Altshuler LL, Frye MA, et al: Risk of switch in mood polarity to hypomania or mania in patients with bipolar depression during acute and continuation trials of venlafaxine, sertraline, and bupropion as adjuncts to mood stabilizers. Am J Psychiatry 163:232–239, 2006

Li M, Rodin G: Depression, in The American Psychiatric Publishing Textbook of Psychosomatic Medicine, 2nd Edition. Edited by Levenson JL. Washington, DC, American Psychiatric Publishing, 2011, pp 175–198

Lloyd-Williams M, Friedman T, Rudd N: An analysis of the validity of the Hospital Anxiety and Depression scale as a screening tool in patients with advanced metastatic cancer. J Pain Symptom Manage 22:990–996, 2001

Loprinzi CL, Kugler JW, Sloan JA, et al: Venlafaxine in management of hot flashes in survivors of breast cancer: a randomised controlled trial. Lancet 356:2059–2063, 2000

Lorenzetti V, Allen NB, Fornito A, et al: Structural brain abnormalities in major depressive disorder: a selective review of recent MRI studies. J Affect Disord 117:1–17, 2009

Lowe B, Kroenke K, Herzog W, et al: Measuring depression outcome with a brief self-report instrument: sensitivity to change of the Patient Health Questionnaire (PHQ-9). J Affect Disord 81:61–66, 2004

Lowe B, Kroenke K, Grafe K: Detecting and monitoring depression with a two-item questionnaire (PHQ-2). J Psychosom Res 58:163–171, 2005

MacQueen GM, Campbell S, McEwen BS, et al: Course of illness, hippocampal function, and hippocampal volume in major depression. Proc Natl Acad Sci USA 100:1387–1392, 2003

Malhi GS, Adams D, Cahill CM, et al: The management of individuals with bipolar disorder: a review of the evidence and its integration into clinical practice. Drugs 69:2063–2101, 2009

Mangelli L, Fava GA, Grandi S, et al: Assessing demoralization and depression in the setting of medical disease. J Clin Psychiatry 66:391–394, 2005

Mann JJ: The medical management of depression. N Engl J Med 353:1819–1834, 2005

Masand P, Pickett P, Murray GB: Psychostimulants for secondary depression in medical illness. Psychosomatics 32:203–208, 1991

Mayou RA, Gill D, Thompson DR, et al: Depression and anxiety as predictors of outcome after myocardial infarction. Psychosom Med 62:212–219, 2000

McDaniel JS, Sharma SM: Mania, in The American Psychiatric Publishing Textbook of Consultation-Liaison Psychiatry, 2nd Edition. Edited by Wise MG, Rundell JR. Washington, DC, American Psychiatric Publishing, 2002, pp 339–359

McDermott LM, Ebmeier KP: A meta-analysis of depression severity and cognitive function. J Affect Disord 119:1–8, 2009

McGrath PJ, Stewart JW, Fava M, et al: Tranylcypromine versus venlafaxine plus mirtazapine following three failed antidepressant medication trials for depression: a STAR*D report. Am J Psychiatry 163:1531–1541; quiz 1666, 2006

McKenzie M, Clarke DM, McKenzie DP, et al: Which factors predict the persistence of DSM-IV depression, anxiety, and somatoform disorders in the medically ill three months post hospital discharge? J Psychosom Res 68:21–28, 2010

Merikangas KR, Akiskal HS, Angst J, et al: Lifetime and 12-month prevalence of bipolar spectrum disorder in the National Comorbidity Survey replication. (Erratum in Arch Gen Psychiatry 64:1039, 2007.) Arch Gen Psychiatry 64:543–552, 2007

Miklowitz DJ: Adjunctive psychotherapy for bipolar disorder: state of the evidence. Am J Psychiatry 165:1408–1419, 2008

Miklowitz DJ, Otto MW, Frank E, et al: Psychosocial treatments for bipolar depression: a 1-year randomized trial from the Systematic Treatment Enhancement Program. Arch Gen Psychiatry 64:419–426, 2007

Morris PL, Robinson RG, Andrzejewski P, et al: Association of depression with 10-year poststroke mortality. Am J Psychiatry 150:124–129, 1993

Murray DP, Weiner M, Prabhakar M, et al: Mania and mortality: why the excess cardiovascular risk in bipolar disorder? Curr Psychiatry Rep 11:475–480, 2009

Nakimuli-Mpungu E, Musisi S, Mpungu SK, et al: Primary mania versus HIV-related secondary mania in Uganda. Am J Psychiatry 163:1349–1354; quiz 1480, 2006

Newcomer JW: Comparing the safety and efficacy of atypical antipsychotics in psychiatric patients with comorbid medical illnesses. J Clin Psychiatry 70 (suppl 3):30–36, 2009

Nierenberg AA, Fava M, Trivedi MH, et al: A comparison of lithium and T(3) augmentation following two failed medication treatments for depression: a STAR*D report. Am J Psychiatry 163:1519–1530, 2006

Pae CU, Marks DM, Shah M, et al: Milnacipran: beyond a role of antidepressant. Clin Neuropharmacol 32:355–363, 2009a

Pae CU, Tharwani H, Marks DM, et al: Atypical depression: a comprehensive review. CNS Drugs 23:1023–1037, 2009b

Pampallona S, Bollini P, Tibaldi G, et al: Combined pharmacotherapy and psychological treatment for depression: a systematic review. Arch Gen Psychiatry 61:714–719, 2004

Pandya R, Metz L, Patten SB: Predictive value of the CES-D in detecting depression among candidates for disease-modifying multiple sclerosis treatment. Psychosomatics 46:131–134, 2005

Papakostas GI, Thase ME, Fava M, et al: Are antidepressant drugs that combine serotonergic and noradrenergic mechanisms of action more effective than the selective serotonin reuptake inhibitors in treating major depressive disorder? A meta-analysis of studies of newer agents. Biol Psychiatry 62:1217–1227, 2007

Patkar AA, Pae CU, Masand PS: Transdermal selegiline: the new generation of monoamine oxidase inhibitors. CNS Spectr 11:363–375, 2006

Perlis RH, Brown E, Baker RW, et al: Clinical features of bipolar depression versus major depressive disorder in large multicenter trials. Am J Psychiatry 163:225–231, 2006a

Perlis RH, Ostacher MJ, Patel JK, et al: Predictors of recurrence in bipolar disorder: primary outcomes from the Systematic Treatment Enhancement Program for Bipolar Disorder (STEP-BD). Am J Psychiatry 163:217–224, 2006b

Pirraglia PA, Biswas K, Kilbourne AM, et al: A prospective study of the impact of comorbid medical disease on bipolar disorder outcomes. J Affect Disord 115:355–359, 2009

Rickels K, Montgomery SA, Tourian KA, et al: Desvenlafaxine for the prevention of relapse in major depressive disorder: results of a randomized trial. J Clin Psychopharmacol 30:18–24, 2010

Robinson RG, Boston JD, Starkstein SE, et al: Comparison of mania and depression after brain injury: causal factors. Am J Psychiatry 145:172–178, 1988

Roose SP, Glassman AH, Seidman SN: Relationship between depression and other medical illnesses. JAMA 286:1687–1690, 2001

Roshanaei-Moghaddam B, Katon W: Premature mortality from general medical illnesses among persons with bipolar disorder: a review. Psychiatr Serv 60:147–156, 2009

Rundell JR, Wise MG: Causes of organic mood disorder. J Neuropsychiatry Clin Neurosci 1:398–400, 1989

Rush AJ, Warden D, Wisniewski SR, et al: STAR*D: revising conventional wisdom. CNS Drugs 23:627–647, 2009

Sachs GS, Grossman F, Ghaemi SN, et al: Combination of a mood stabilizer with risperidone or haloperidol for treatment of acute mania: a double-blind, placebo-controlled comparison of efficacy and safety. Am J Psychiatry 159:1146–1154, 2002

Sachs GS, Nierenberg AA, Calabrese JR, et al: Effectiveness of adjunctive antidepressant treatment for bipolar depression. N Engl J Med 356:1711–1722, 2007

Salvi V, Fagiolini A, Swartz HA, et al: The use of antidepressants in bipolar disorder. J Clin Psychiatry 69:1307–1318, 2008

Scherk H, Pajonk FG, Leucht S: Second-generation antipsychotic agents in the treatment of acute mania: a systematic review and meta-analysis of randomized controlled trials. Arch Gen Psychiatry 64:442–455, 2007

Shulman KI, Tohen M, Satlin A, et al: Mania compared with unipolar depression in old age. Am J Psychiatry 149:341–345, 1992

Smith FA, Wittmann CW, Stern TA: Medical complications of psychiatric treatment. Crit Care Clin 24:635–656, 2008

Stafford L, Berk M, Jackson HJ: Validity of the Hospital Anxiety and Depression Scale and Patient Health Questionnaire–9 to screen for depression in patients with coronary artery disease. Gen Hosp Psychiatry 29:417–424, 2007

Starkstein SE, Boston JD, Robinson RG: Mechanisms of mania after brain injury: 12 case reports and review of the literature. J Nerv Ment Dis 176:87–100, 1988

Stoudemire A, Fogel BS, Gulley LR, et al: Psychopharmacology in the medical patient, in Psychiatric Care of the Medical Patient. Edited by Stoudemire A, Fogel BS. New York, Oxford University Press, 1993, pp 155–206

Sullivan MD, LaCroix AZ, Baum C, et al: Functional status in coronary artery disease: a one-year prospective study of the role of anxiety and depression. Am J Med 103:348–356, 1997

Sullivan MD, LaCroix AZ, Spertus JA, et al: Five-year prospective study of the effects of anxiety and depression in patients with coronary artery disease. Am J Cardiol 86:1135–1138, 2000

Thomas JL, Jones GN, Scarinci IC, et al: The utility of the CES-D as a depression screening measure among low-income women attending primary care clinics. The Center for Epidemiologic Studies-Depression. Int J Psychiatry Med 31:25–40, 2001

Trivedi MH, Rush AJ, Wisniewski SR, et al: Evaluation of outcomes with citalopram for depression using measurement-based care in STAR*D: implications for clinical practice. Am J Psychiatry 163:28–40, 2006

van Wilgen CP, Dijkstra PU, Stewart RE, et al: Measuring somatic symptoms with the CES-D to assess depression in cancer patients after treatment: comparison among patients with oral/oropharyngeal, gynecological, colorectal, and breast cancer. Psychosomatics 47:465–470, 2006

Vinberg M, Froekjaer VG, Kessing LV: Coping styles in healthy individuals at risk of affective disorder. J Nerv Ment Dis 198:39–44, 2010 von Ammon Cavanaugh S, Furlanetto LM, Creech SD, et al: Medical illness, past depression, and present depression: a predictive triad for in-hospital mortality. Am J Psychiatry 158:43–48, 2001

Walker J, Postma K, McHugh GS, et al: Performance of the Hospital Anxiety and Depression Scale as a screening tool for major depressive disorder in cancer patients. J Psychosom Res 63:83–91, 2007

Warrington TP, Bostwick JM: Psychiatric adverse effects of corticosteroids. Mayo Clin Proc 81:1361–1367, 2006

Wilhelm K, Kotze B, Waterhouse M, et al: Screening for Depression in the Medically Ill: a comparison of self-report measures, clinician judgment, and DSM-IV diagnoses. Psychosomatics 45:461–469, 2004

Williams LS, Brizendine EJ, Plue L, et al: Performance of the PHQ-9 as a screening tool for depression after stroke. Stroke 36:635–638, 2005

Wulsin LR, Vaillant GE, Wells VE: A systematic review of the mortality of depression. Psychosom Med 61:6–17, 1999

Zigmond AS, Snaith RP: The hospital anxiety and depression scale. Acta Psychiatr Scand 67:361–370, 1983

11

Sleep Disorders

Insufficient sleep can result in fatigue, sleepiness, inattention, depressed mood, and cognitive changes. Sleep disturbance may be an independent risk factor for depression in older adults (Cho et al. 2008). Common medical problems are associated with sleep abnormalities, and disruption of sleep may worsen the subjective symptoms of the medical illness (Parish 2009). Sleep disorders are categorized as sleep-related breathing disorders, hypersomnias of central origin, circadian rhythm sleep disorders, parasomnias, and sleep-related movement disorders.

Sleep Stages in Healthy Adults

Sleep can be subdivided into two general states: rapid eye movement sleep (REM) and non–rapid eye movement sleep (NREM). The three main features of REM sleep include increased electroencephalographic (EEG) frequency, muscle atonia, and presence of rapid eye movements. NREM sleep includes four stages; most time is spent in stage 2. Stages 3 and 4 are the deeper stages of sleep known as delta-wave sleep, deep sleep, and slow-wave sleep. Patients with disrupted sleep often have decreased slow-wave and REM sleep and spend more time than normal in stages 1 and 2 (Krahn 2011).

Sleep-Related Difficulties Associated With Medical Problems

Sleep-related difficulties are frequently associated with common medical problems. Patients with heart failure or chronic lung disease often have sleep problems due to oxygen desaturation, paroxysmal nocturnal dyspnea, orthopnea, and coughing. Some patients with coronary artery disease experience nocturnal angina. Poor sleep quality is associated with both obstructive and restrictive lung diseases. Gastroesophageal reflux disease may result in difficulty initiating and maintaining sleep, as well as increased nocturnal awakenings (Parish 2009). Patients with renal disease have a high prevalence of sleep disorders, including insomnia, restless legs, excessive daytime sleepiness, and obstructive sleep apnea. About half of patients with end-stage renal disease report excessive daytime sleepiness, and 20% of patients undergoing dialysis have restless legs (Hanly 2004). Diabetes is associated with sleep-related complaints, especially insomnia and excessive daytime sleepiness. In patients with HIV infection, the severity of sleep problems appears to be correlated with the stage of the disease (Darko et al. 1992). Disrupted sleep occurs in most patients with fibromyalgia, and the perception of pain is increased in patients with poor sleep quality (Affleck et al. 1996). The prevalence of chronic insomnia in menopausal patients approaches 60%; vasomotor instability is a primary cause (Ohayon 2006). Cancer patients undergoing treatment are likely to have sleep problems, including excessive fatigue, insomnia, and daytime somnolence. Even in healthy older adults with no subjective sleep complaints, specific EEG sleep characteristics may predict increased risk of all-cause mortality (Dew et al. 2003).

Evaluation of Sleep

History and Physical Examination

A detailed diagnostic history and a physical examination are necessary to differentiate whether the patient's symptoms are related primarily to a medical, neurological, or psychiatric disorder; the patient's environment; or both. Because patients may minimize the level of their daytime sleepiness, other informants such as family members are important in providing additional history. Obtaining history from a bed partner is helpful, especially for information regarding sleep-related breathing and movement disorders. The Epworth Sleepiness Scale and the Stanford Sleepiness Scale are brief questionnaires that subjectively quantify sleepiness. Areas of the physical examination that warrant particular attention include the patient's level of alertness, neck circumference, body mass index, nasopharyngeal abnormalities, thyroid size, pulmonary and cardiac findings, and cognitive changes. Screening laboratory tests to consider include thyroid-stimulating hormone, ferritin, vitamin B_{12}, folate, and complete blood count (Krahn 2011).

Diagnostic Tests

Although polysomnography provides the best diagnostic accuracy in the evaluation of sleep disorders, it is not necessary when patients have certain disorders, such as restless legs syndrome, or when the symptoms clearly represent a specific disorder. Portable devices are available in some tertiary care hospitals. Overnight pulse oximetry has limitations, including false negatives, but can be beneficial in the medical setting in the initial evaluation of obstructive sleep apnea. Used for the assessment of excessive daytime sleepiness, including narcolepsy, the Multiple Sleep Latency Test (MSLT) objectively measures a patient's tendency to fall asleep (Krahn 2011). The Maintenance of Wakefulness Test (MWT) is used to determine the outcome of treatment by measuring the patient's ability to stay awake.

Insomnia

Definition

Insomnia is present when all three of the following criteria are met (American Academy of Sleep Medicine 2005):

1. The patient complains of difficulty initiating sleep, difficulty maintaining sleep, or waking up too early. Alternatively, the patient complains that sleep is chronically nonrestorative or poor in quality.

2. The difficulty occurs despite adequate opportunity and circumstances for sleep.
3. The impaired sleep produces deficits in daytime function.

Epidemiology

Insomnia is one of the most common medical complaints. Each year, approximately 30% of adults develop symptoms of insomnia and 7% develop an insomnia syndrome (LeBlanc et al. 2009). Prevalence is higher among elderly people and occurs more often in women than men. More than half of elderly people likely have at least one sleep complaint (Foley et al. 1995).

Causes of Insomnia

Medical, neurological, psychiatric, and environmental factors should be considered in the assessment of insomnia (Table 11–1). Medications that commonly contribute to insomnia, especially for elderly patients, include acetylcholinesterase inhibitors, carbidopa-levodopa, corticosteroids, diuretics (which cause nocturia), phenytoin, selective serotonin reuptake inhibitors, theophylline, and beta-blockers. Caffeine can have a stimulant effect for 8–14 hours, and caffeine clearance is reduced in patients with hepatic dysfunction. Alcohol is often used by patients as a sleep aid but results in disrupted slow-wave sleep, intense dreaming, and nocturnal awakenings (Wolkove et al. 2007).

Treatment of Insomnia

Factors that may cause or exacerbate insomnia should be addressed first, but insomnia is often a primary rather than a secondary problem. Treatment approaches include improvement of sleep hygiene (Table 11–2), relaxation training, stimulus control, sleep restriction therapy, cognitive-behavioral therapy (CBT), and medications.

Nonpharmacological Strategies

Nonpharmacological strategies are effective in treating insomnia. Stimulus control therapy targets the associations patients have with their bed and bedroom, and their fears about not falling asleep. Patients often try to compensate for lost sleep by staying in bed longer, which results in a circadian shift; sleep restriction therapy increases the drive to sleep by decreasing the total time

Table 11-1.   Selected causes of insomnia

Primarily medical
Obstructive sleep apnea
Angina
Chronic obstructive pulmonary
  disease
Hypoglycemia
Asthma
Congestive heart failure
Gastroesophageal reflux
Hyperthyroidism
Acute and chronic pain
Medication induced

Primarily neurological
Central sleep apnea
Dementia
Restless legs syndrome

Primarily environmental
Community noise (traffic, alarms,
  neighbors)
Hospital factors (blood draws, medication
  administration, alarms, hospital staff)
Altered temperature

Primarily psychiatric
Psychophysiological insomnia
Anxiety disorders
Altered sleep-wake schedule
Sleep state misperception
Mood disorders (mania, depression)
Withdrawal related

Source.   Adapted from Krahn LE: "Sleep Disorders," in *The American Psychiatric Publishing Textbook of Psychosomatic Medicine,* 2nd Edition. Edited by Levenson JL. Washington, DC, American Psychiatric Publishing, 2011, p. 338. Used with permission.

Table 11-2.   Strategies for sleep hygiene

Sleep only as much as needed to feel rested

Avoid daytime naps

Exercise regularly, preferably at least 4 hours before bedtime

Avoid forcing sleep and go to bed when sleepy

Keep a regular sleep-wake cycle

Minimize caffeine

Avoid alcohol

Avoid nicotine especially prior to bedtime

Do not use the bedroom for activities other than sleep and sexual activity

Manage stress and avoid worrying in bed

spent in bed. CBT combines the previously described therapies and has been found to be effective if used alone or in combination with pharmacotherapy (Morin et al. 2009; Sivertsen et al. 2006). One study found CBT alone to be superior to zopiclone alone in the treatment of acute and chronic insomnia in older adults (Sivertsen et al. 2006). Combined CBT and pharmacotherapy for the initial 6 weeks of treatment followed by CBT alone has been shown to have the best long-term outcome (Morin et al. 2009). The medications most commonly used include benzodiazepines, nonbenzodiazepine hypnotics, and melatonin agonists (Table 11–3).

Benzodiazepines

Meta-analyses of randomized, placebo-controlled trials suggest that benzodiazepines and nonbenzodiazepine hypnotics decrease sleep latency and the number of awakenings, thereby improving the quality and duration of sleep (Buscemi et al. 2007). The primary difference between the benzodiazepines is the duration of action, as outlined in Table 11–3. Their use is limited by adverse effects, which include impaired memory, motor incoordination, sedation, respiratory suppression, and dependence. Complex sleep-related behaviors may also occur, including driving, making telephone calls, and eating while not fully awake. Elderly patients are at particular risk for delirium, agitation, night wandering, and falls.

Nonbenzodiazepine Hypnotics

The nonbenzodiazepine hypnotics differ from the benzodiazepines in that they have more selective effects on one γ-aminobutyric acid (GABA) type A receptor. The selectivity also results in fewer anxiolytic and anticonvulsant effects. The adverse effects are similar to those of benzodiazepines but possibly are less severe and less frequent.

Melatonin Agonists

Ramelteon, a melatonin agonist, provides most benefit for patients with sleep-onset insomnia. It should be avoided in patients with hepatic dysfunction. Rare side effects include headache, somnolence, and sore throat, but it is not associated with dependence, withdrawal, or rebound insomnia (Griffiths and Johnson 2005).

Table 11–3. Medications for treatment of insomnia

Drug	Half-life (hours)	Usual adult dose (mg)
Benzodiazepines		
Triazolam	2–5	0.125–0.25
Oxazepam	5–10	15–30
Temazepam	8–12	15
Lorazepam	10–14	0.5–1
Clonazepam	18–50	0.25–0.5
Nonbenzodiazepines		
Zaleplon	1	5–10
Zolpidem	1–3	5–10
Eszopiclone	6–9	1–3
Melatonin agonist		
Ramelteon	1–5	8

Other Medications

Medications and over-the-counter products that have sedative properties but have not been approved by the U.S. Food and Drug Administration for insomnia are frequently used for their sleep-promoting effects; these medications include antidepressants, antipsychotics, diphenhydramine, herbal products, and melatonin. Trazodone is frequently used, but limited evidence is available to support its use (Mendelson 2005). Doxepin and amitriptyline are the most sedating tricyclic antidepressants and may be helpful for patients with comorbid insomnia and neuropathic pain, but they are associated with adverse effects, especially for patients who are medically ill. One study showed that in the treatment of insomnia alone, low-dose doxepin was effective in elderly patients (Scharf et al. 2008). Low-dose mirtazapine has antihistaminergic effects, but other side effects including weight gain need to be considered. Quetiapine is commonly used as a sleep aid; however, limited data support its use (Sateia 2009), and it is expensive. Some studies have shown quetiapine to be efficacious in patients with comorbid mood disorders or posttraumatic stress disorder (PTSD) (Endicott et al. 2007; Robert et al. 2005; Todder et al. 2006). Diphenhydramine is generally not recommended because it may rapidly lose its effectiveness, and anticholinergic side effects are problematic in patients who are medically ill. Melatonin has not been found to be effective for primary insomnia, but it may be beneficial for delayed sleep phase syndrome (Buscemi et al. 2005).

Sleep-Related Breathing Disorders

Sleep-related breathing disorders are characterized by abnormal respiratory patterns (e.g., apneas, hypopneas, or respiratory effort–related arousals) or abnormal reductions in gas exchange (e.g., hypoventilation) during sleep. These disorders are associated with significant morbidity and impairment, including cardiovascular disease, impaired daytime functioning, and depression (Peppard et al. 2006). Sleep-related breathing disorders include central sleep apnea, obstructive sleep apnea, and sleep-related hypoventilation/hypoxemic syndromes.

Central Sleep Apnea

Central sleep apnea is differentiated from obstructive sleep apnea by the absence of snoring. Patients are often older, have cerebrovascular and cardiovascular disease, and present with insomnia rather than excessive daytime sleepiness. Treatment can include hypnotics to decrease arousals, or supplemental oxygen (Krahn 2011).

Hypoventilation Syndromes

Patients with hypoventilation syndromes due to obesity or congenital abnormalities have mild hypercarbia and elevated serum bicarbonate while awake and which worsen during sleep. Hypnotics should not be given to these patients.

Obstructive Sleep Apnea

Obstructive sleep apnea is the most common sleep-related breathing disorder; mild symptoms occur in 20% of adults and moderate to severe symptoms in approximately 7%. Medical sequelae include systemic hypertension, mild pulmonary hypertension, cardiovascular morbidity, and cognitive impairment. Obstructed breathing during sleep and excessive daytime sleepiness are the cardinal features of the disorder. Signs of obstructed breathing include snoring, restlessness, and resuscitative snorts. The diagnosis, which is confirmed by polysomnography, requires more than five episodes of apnea an hour in addition to frequent arousals, oxygen desaturation due to apnea, or bradytachycardia. Risk factors include obesity, craniofacial abnormalities, upper airway soft tissue abnormalities, and possibly heredity, smoking, diabetes, and nasal congestion (Young et al. 2004). Positive airway pressure therapy is first-line treatment, and other treatments include oral appliances or surgery.

Hypersomnias of Central Origin

Hypersomnias of central origin include narcolepsy (with or without cataplexy), idiopathic hypersomnia, and behaviorally induced insufficient sleep. Narcolepsy is a condition that is often unrecognized, with an estimated prevalence of 0.06% (Silber et al. 2002). Elements of REM sleep intrude into wakefulness, and the overall effect is excessive daytime sleepiness. Additional features of narcolepsy include hypnagogic hallucinations, sleep paralysis, and cataplexy. Questioning a patient's history of emotionally triggered transient weakness is helpful diagnostically, because cataplexy is unique to narcolepsy. The etiology of narcolepsy includes the absence of the neuropeptide orexin, genetic factors, and rare brain lesions. Behavioral modifications such as a regular sleep schedule, daytime naps, and avoidance of medications that disrupt sleep can be beneficial. The mainstays of pharmacological treatment include modafinil, methylphenidate, and amphetamines. Cataplexy is treated with REM sleep–suppressing agents, such as venlafaxine, atomoxetine, fluoxetine, and γ-hydroxybutyrate.

Circadian Rhythm Sleep Disorders

Circadian rhythm sleep disorders consist of jet lag type, shift work type, delayed sleep phase pattern, advanced sleep phase pattern, and irregular sleep-wake pattern. Patients with prolonged stays in an intensive care unit are prone to developing circadian rhythm disorders. Patients with delayed sleep phase pattern have difficulty falling asleep at night and waking in the morning, as well as associated daytime sleepiness that interferes with functioning. Advanced sleep phase pattern is less common and is characterized by habitually early sleep and wake times that are at least several hours earlier than desired times. Treatment approaches include chronotherapy, light therapy, and melatonin (Lu and Zee 2006).

Parasomnias

Parasomnias are undesirable motor events or experiences (emotions, perceptions, dreams) that occur during entry to sleep, within sleep, or during arousals from sleep. The patient has no conscious awareness of the movements or behaviors, but they can appear purposeful.

Non–Rapid Eye Movement–Related Parasomnias

NREM-related parasomnias include disorders of arousal such as sleepwalking, sleep terrors, and confusional states.

Rapid Eye Movement–Related Parasomnias

Patients with REM sleep behavior disorder appear to be acting out their dreams because they lack normal muscle atonia during REM sleep. REM sleep behavior disorder is associated with Parkinson's disease, multiple system atrophy, and dementia with Lewy bodies, and most commonly occurs in elderly males. Initial treatment involves modification of the environment to reduce the likelihood of injury, and clonazepam is considered the first-line pharmacotherapy. For patients who are unable to tolerate clonazepam, melatonin is an alternative (Gagnon et al. 2006).

A common REM disorder associated with psychiatric illness is nightmare disorder, particularly in patients with PTSD. Prazosin has been shown to decrease PTSD-related nightmares (Dierks et al. 2007). Nonpharmacological treatments, particularly imagery rehearsal therapy, reduce chronic nightmares and improve sleep quality (Krakow et al. 2001).

Miscellaneous Parasomnias

Miscellaneous parasomnias not involving a specific stage of sleep can occur from medication or substance use. The use of zolpidem has been associated with complex behaviors such as sleepwalking, sleep-related eating, and sleep-driving (Dolder and Nelson 2008).

Sleep-Related Movement Disorders

Restless legs syndrome (RLS) is characterized by an urge to move the legs, usually accompanied by uncomfortable sensations that occur during rest and are relieved by movement. The sensation may be described by patients as creeping, crawling, or pulling, and it is localized to deep structures rather than the skin. The prevalence of clinically significant RLS is estimated to be 2.7%, and RLS occurs more commonly in females (Allen et al. 2005). The cause of primary RLS is unknown, but studies suggest a genetic basis for the disorder (Montplaisir et al. 1997). Secondary RLS can occur with iron deficiency, end-stage renal disease, diabetes mellitus, multiple sclerosis, Parkinson's disease, pregnancy, and venous insufficiency. The majority of patients with RLS also have periodic limb movement disorder (PLMD), which involves involuntary jerking movements that occur during sleep and result in daytime sleepiness. Medications and other substances, such as caffeine, nicotine, alcohol, dopamine-blocking antiemetics, antidepressants, and antipsychotics, may exacerbate the symptoms. If a patient requires an antidepressant, bupropion has been shown to reduce periodic limb movements in patients with depression (Nofzinger et al. 2000). First-line treatment options for patients with periodic limb movements include pramipexole, ropinirole, and carbidopa-levodopa preparations. Benzodiazepines and gabapentin are alternatives, and low dosages of low-potency opioids may also be effective (Silber et al. 2004).

References

Affleck G, Urrows S, Tennen H, et al: Sequential daily relations of sleep, pain intensity, and attention to pain among women with fibromyalgia. Pain 68:363–368, 1996

Allen RP, Walters AS, Montplaisir J, et al: Restless legs syndrome prevalence and impact: REST general population study. Arch Intern Med 165:1286–1292, 2005

American Academy of Sleep Medicine: International Classification of Sleep Disorders: Diagnostic and Coding Manual, 2nd Edition. Westchester, IL, American Academy of Sleep Medicine, 2005

Buscemi N, Vandermeer B, Hooton N, et al: The efficacy and safety of exogenous melatonin for primary sleep disorders: a meta-analysis. J Gen Intern Med 20:1151–1158, 2005

Buscemi N, Vandermeer B, Friesen C, et al: The efficacy and safety of drug treatments for chronic insomnia in adults: a meta-analysis of RCTs. J Gen Intern Med 22:1335–1350, 2007

Cho HJ, Lavretsky H, Olmstead R, et al: Sleep disturbance and depression recurrence in community-dwelling older adults: a prospective study [see comment]. Am J Psychiatry 165:1543–1550, 2008

Darko DF, McCutchan JA, Kripke DF, et al: Fatigue, sleep disturbance, disability, and indices of progression of HIV infection. Am J Psychiatry 149:514–520, 1992

Dew MA, Hoch CC, Buysse DJ, et al: Healthy older adults' sleep predicts all-cause mortality at 4 to 19 years of follow-up [see comment]. (Erratum in Psychosom Med 65:210, 2003.) Psychosom Med 65:63–73, 2003

Dierks MR, Jordan JK, Sheehan AH: Prazosin treatment of nightmares related to post-traumatic stress disorder. Ann Pharmacother 41:1013–1017, 2007

Dolder CR, Nelson MH: Hypnosedative-induced complex behaviours: incidence, mechanisms and management. CNS Drugs 22:1021–1036, 2008

Endicott J, Rajagopalan K, Minkwitz M, et al: A randomized, double-blind, placebo-controlled study of quetiapine in the treatment of bipolar I and II depression: improvements in quality of life. Int Clin Psychopharmacol 22:29–37, 2007

Foley DJ, Monjan AA, Brown SL, et al: Sleep complaints among elderly persons: an epidemiologic study of three communities. Sleep 18:425–432, 1995

Gagnon JF, Postuma RB, Montplaisir J: Update on the pharmacology of REM sleep behavior disorder. Neurology 67:742–747, 2006

Griffiths RR, Johnson MW: Relative abuse liability of hypnotic drugs: a conceptual framework and algorithm for differentiating among compounds. J Clin Psychiatry 66 (suppl 9):31–41, 2005

Hanly P: Sleep apnea and daytime sleepiness in end-stage renal disease. Semin Dial 17:109–114, 2004

Krahn LE. Sleep disorders, in The American Psychiatric Publishing Textbook of Psychosomatic Medicine, 2nd Edition. Edited by Levenson JL. Washington, DC, American Psychiatric Publishing, 2011, pp 335–360

Krakow B, Hollifield M, Johnston L, et al: Imagery rehearsal therapy for chronic nightmares in sexual assault survivors with posttraumatic stress disorder: a randomized controlled trial. JAMA 286:537–545, 2001

LeBlanc M, Mérette C, Savard J, et al: Incidence and risk factors of insomnia in a population-based sample. Sleep 32:1027–1037, 2009

Lu BS, Zee PC: Circadian rhythm sleep disorders. Chest 130:1915–1923, 2006

Mendelson WB: A review of the evidence for the efficacy and safety of trazodone in insomnia. J Clin Psychiatry 66:469–476, 2005

Montplaisir J, Boucher S, Poirier G, et al: Clinical, polysomnographic, and genetic characteristics of restless legs syndrome: a study of 133 patients diagnosed with new standard criteria. Mov Disord 12:61–65, 1997

Morin CM, Vallieres A, Guay B, et al: Cognitive behavioral therapy, singly and combined with medication, for persistent insomnia: a randomized controlled trial. JAMA 301:2005–2015, 2009

Nofzinger EA, Fasiczka A, Berman S, et al: Bupropion SR reduces periodic limb movements associated with arousals from sleep in depressed patients with periodic limb movement disorder. J Clin Psychiatry 61:858–862, 2000

Ohayon MM: Severe hot flashes are associated with chronic insomnia. Arch Intern Med 166:1262–1268, 2006

Parish JM: Sleep-related problems in common medical conditions. Chest 135:563–572, 2009

Peppard PE, Szklo-Coxe M, Hla KM, et al: Longitudinal association of sleep-related breathing disorder and depression. Arch Intern Med 166:1709–1715, 2006

Robert S, Hamner MB, Kose S, et al: Quetiapine improves sleep disturbances in combat veterans with PTSD: sleep data from a prospective, open-label study. J Clin Psychopharmacol 25:387–388, 2005

Sateia MJ: Update on sleep and psychiatric disorders. Chest 135:1370–1379, 2009

Scharf M, Rogowski R, Hull S, et al: Efficacy and safety of doxepin 1 mg, 3 mg, and 6 mg in elderly patients with primary insomnia: a randomized, double-blind, placebo-controlled crossover study. J Clin Psychiatry 69:1557–1564, 2008

Silber MH, Krahn LE, Olson EJ, et al: The epidemiology of narcolepsy in Olmsted County, Minnesota: a population-based study. Sleep 25:197–202, 2002

Silber MH, Ehrenberg BL, Allen RP, et al: An algorithm for the management of restless legs syndrome. (Erratum in Mayo Clin Proc 79:1341, 2004.) Mayo Clin Proc 79:916–922, 2004

Sivertsen B, Omvik S, Pallesen S, et al: Cognitive behavioral therapy vs. zopiclone for treatment of chronic primary insomnia in older adults: a randomized controlled trial. JAMA 295:2851–2858, 2006

Todder D, Caliskan S, Baune BT: Night locomotor activity and quality of sleep in quetiapine-treated patients with depression. J Clin Psychopharmacol 26:638–642, 2006

Wolkove N, Elkholy O, Baltzan M, et al: Sleep and aging, 2: management of sleep disorders in older people. CMAJ 176:1449–1454, 2007

Young T, Skatrud J, Peppard PE: Risk factors for obstructive sleep apnea in adults. JAMA 291:2013–2016, 2004

12

Somatoform and Related Disorders

Patients have expectations of their physicians. They think they can tell the physician what is not right, and the physician can identify the problem, treat it, and relieve any dysfunction, pain, or suffering. Physicians, in turn, harbor their own expectations for patients who have physical complaints: "A patient should complain in reasonable proportion to demonstrative pathology, report physical distress in bodily terms and emotional distress in psychological terms, and accept a doctor's opinion and advice compliantly" (Lipowski 1988, p. 1361). These expectations may align agreeably when patient and physician are faced with a fractured radius, but they often diverge when the patient has chronic or cryptic abdominal pain. More than 50% of the general population experiences somatic complaints during any given week; however, physicians cannot find a definitive medical cause in a comparable proportion of patients with physical symptoms who present for medical care (Kellner 1985). These patients commonly use medical resources frequently, are often dissatisfied with the outcome, and may engender additional medical complications.

A Challenging Arena

Physicians are well trained to detect, measure, and manage pathology of the body—that is, those anatomical and physiological perturbations that are exposed to the five senses (e.g., wheezing, a thready pulse, icteric sclerae, the fruity fragrance of ketosis) or to the technology of the laboratory. However, pathology of emotion and behavior, or the mind and soul, often eludes objective metrics. Physicians are familiar with coronary artery occlusion that sets the stage for oxygen demand to exceed supply, resulting in myocardial ischemia reflected in chest or jaw pain; if there is poor collateral flow and no prompt lysis of the clot, myocardial infarction follows and congestive failure may develop. In contrast, physicians do not typically think of medical illness or interpersonal stressors as setting the stage for coping demands to exceed resources, resulting in emotional ischemia reflected in dysphoria or heartache; nor can physicians anticipate that if no emotional oxygen is forthcoming, the patient may develop an infarction of identity followed by congestive despondency.

Disease and Illness

Distinguishing between disease and illness is useful for consultation psychiatrists (Eisenberg 1977). *Disease* involves objectively measurable anatomical deformations and pathophysiological states. *Illness* involves those experiences, behaviors, and functional changes associated with disease (or the patient's perception of disease), including the personal suffering, alienation, and debilitation that shape a patient's quality of life (Folks et al. 2000). In other words, disease is a pathophysiological process that is often but not always associated with documentable lesions, whereas illness also encompasses the patient's response to the disease. A patient can have a disease without illness or could have illness behavior without known disease. Mismatches are common and are at the root of many management problems. For example, a patient with hypertension may experience no symptoms and therefore deny that he or she is ill; nonadherence to treatment soon follows. In contrast, the patient with a somatoform spectrum disorder experiences illness without evidence of a disease, or if evidence is present, the patient's reaction extends beyond conventional expectations.

Hybrid Pathology

When a physiological cause cannot be found for a symptom or when the physician thinks that a significant disparity exists between the patient's subjective complaints and the objective findings, psychiatric consultation may be requested to confirm or exclude a so-called functional, psychogenic, or psychosomatic etiology. The amplification or magnification of somatic sensations varies widely among patients. Moreover, patients with hypervigilant sensitivity who amplify somatic symptoms (i.e., somatizers) are a heterogeneous group and defy simple categorization or explanation. Not all somatizers have a somatoform disorder. This amplification process has both trait and state characteristics and is influenced by multiple factors (Barsky et al. 1992), which include the following:

- The patient's cognition (information, beliefs, opinions, and attribution)
- Developmental history
- Context of the symptom (feedback from others and expectations)
- Cultural setting
- Amount of attention to the symptom (when attention is increased, the symptom is amplified; when decreased, the symptom is diminished)
- Comorbid conditions (anxiety and depression commonly amplify symptoms)

Clues to Somatoform Spectrum Illness

Brodsky (1984) listed clues that suggest that a patient has a somatoform spectrum illness:

- Developmental associations may have included prominent somatic emphases.
- Somatoform language is used in the family of origin.
- Parents are demanding or unrewarding except when child is ill.
- Parental figure has suffered a significant illness.
- Coping mechanisms apart from illness behavior are absent or unacceptable.
- Disengagement from anger, aggression, or usual responsibilities is accomplished through somatic reactions.

Common Presentations

Patients with somatoform spectrum illness have the tendency to experience, amplify, and communicate psychological and interpersonal distress in the form of somatic suffering and medically unexplained symptoms (Abbey 2002). Most cases can be grouped into one of these categories:

- *Medically unexplained symptoms*—Somatic symptoms are not explained after appropriate medical and psychiatric assessment. This absence of explanation argues that *idiopathic symptoms* is a more accurate descriptor and may portend a shift in future taxonomy.
- *Somatic presentation of psychiatric disorder*—Patients with psychiatric disorders, especially depression and anxiety disorders, often present to primary care physicians with somatic symptoms as a prominent part of the clinical picture.
- *Somatoform disorders*—Patients present with physical symptoms that suggest a medical disorder, worry excessively about contracting a disease, or both; however, no medical disorder exists, or if one exists, it cannot fully explain the complaint(s). Despite medical evaluation and reassurance, the patient's bodily preoccupation and worry about medical illness continue. For many patients with somatoform disorders, illness is a "way of life" (Ford 1983).
- *Conversion disorders*—Patients exhibit signs and/or symptoms of disease and/or disability as an expression of internal conflict—that is, their psychological dilemma is converted into somatic dysfunction. Both the conflict and the conversion are unconsciously driven and are therefore beyond voluntary control.
- *Factitious disorders*—Patients are understood to deliberately induce signs and/or symptoms of disease so as to elicit medical care, thereby answering an unconscious longing to engage in the role of patient for whatever purposes it may serve.

Inadequacy of Conventional Treatment

Conventional treatment of somatoform and related disorders falls short. Fourteen common physical symptoms are responsible for almost half of all primary care visits; over a 1-year follow-up period, many of these symptoms prove to be benign and only 10%–15% are found to be caused by a persisting organic illness (Katon and Walker 1998). Somatizing patients have higher average health care costs than do other patients: total charges are 9 times greater, hospital charges 6 times greater, and physician services 14 times greater. Somatizing patients spend up to 7 days per month sick in bed, compared with the general population average of half a day (G. R. Smith et al. 1986).

High Viscosity Between Societal Mores and Somatic Symptoms

Disability, formal or informal, attributed to a specific somatic complaint is generally respected more readily than an emotional complaint. Children learn that a stomachache is more likely to earn reprieve from school than is anxiety over a bully; employees know that colleagues will be more forgiving of an absence occasioned by a migraine headache than by dysphoria over a romantic loss; and patients understand that physicians attend to somatic symptoms and respond with action but may grow weary of, or even put off, patients who complain of vague malaise.

Current Nosology Deliberations

The diagnoses presently classified as somatoform or related disorders have earned close scrutiny by researchers and work groups, inside and outside psychiatry (Dimsdale and Creed 2009; R. C. Smith and Dwamena 2007; Voigt et al. 2010). DSM-5, scheduled for publication in 2013, is likely to introduce substantial changes in nomenclature (American Psychiatric Association 2010). The research cited in this volume is based on existing categories and directs consideration along conventional, topical lines, avoiding the proposals currently unfolding in the construction of DSM-5.

Comorbidities and Differential Diagnosis

Somatic complaints may be the foremost concern of patients presenting with a wide range of psychiatric conditions. A psychiatric referral requesting confirmation of a somatoform spectrum diagnosis requires careful consideration of alternate explanations and frequent comorbidities, as discussed in the following subsections.

Medical Disorders

The consultant's first task is to remain alert for medical disorders. The patient's personality or exaggerated behavior may have decreased the primary physician's index of suspicion for a medical diagnosis and attenuated the preconsultation workup. Thorough review of the medical record is a time-consuming but imperative task.

Cognitive Disorders

Patients with dementia, delirium, or other cognitive disorders may present with increased physical complaints, particularly when anxious.

Adjustment Disorders

If the symptom occurs as a reaction to significant acute stress, it is often self-limited. Identification of the stressor and its significance to the individual is the first and most important step in planning treatment.

Anxiety Disorders

A high correlation exists between anxiety and the development of somatic symptoms (Simon and VonKorff 1991). Patients with an anxiety disorder, particularly panic disorder, are especially aware of bodily sensations.

Mood Disorders

Depressed patients often have multiple somatic concerns, including the neurovegetative signs of depression, and other physical complaints. Hypochondriacal preoccupation during depressive episodes increases with age (Cassem and Barsky 1991).

Substance-Related Disorders

Patients with substance abuse, dependence, withdrawal, and the medical sequelae of chronic substance use are seen commonly in the general hospital. These patients commonly report physical symptoms.

Psychotic Disorders

Patients who are actively psychotic may report bizarre physical symptoms. The consultant must ensure that physical symptoms are not ignored simply because the patient has a chronic psychotic disorder. On the other hand, pursuit of bizarre physical symptoms that are clearly secondary to psychosis is unnecessary.

Delusional Disorders

The following are the most common somatic delusions (sometimes called monosymptomatic hypochondriacal psychosis):

- Delusions of infestation (e.g., complaints of insects or foreign bodies on or under the skin)
- Olfactory delusions (e.g., a complaint of a foul odor from skin, mouth, rectum, or vagina)
- Body dysmorphia (i.e., the belief that one's body or a body part is ugly or misshapen; however, the majority of patients with body dysmorphic disorder are not delusional, as discussed in "Body Dysmorphic Disorder" later in this chapter)

Personality Disorders

Histrionic and dependent personality disorders are more common among women presenting with prominent somatic concerns. In men, antisocial personality disorder is more common among those who emphasize somatic complaints without discernible medical or surgical pathology.

General Principles of Approach

The common feature shared by the somatoform spectrum disorders is the presence of physical symptoms that suggest a medical condition but are not fully explained by a medical condition or by the direct effects of a substance or another mental disorder. Somatoform illness behavior involves an individual's conscious or unconscious use of the body or bodily symptoms for psychological purposes or personal benefit. Nonetheless, somatoform illness is almost never an ordinal either/or (i.e., all one or all the other) phenomenon and therefore requires a methodical, comprehensive assessment (Folks et al. 2000).

Evaluation

Although the patient identified by primary care physicians or specialists as a potential somatizer may not have a somatoform or other psychiatric disorder, data gathering is similar to that in a typical psychiatric consultation. The consultant should do the following:

1. Establish the medical context (Abbey 2002):
   - Collaborate with referral sources to better understand the reason for referral.
   - Review the medical records before the interview.
2. Understand the patient. In addition to the patient's historical account of his or her symptoms, the psychiatrist is attentive to the following questions:
   - What is the extent of the patient's disease?
   - What is the magnitude of his or her suffering?
   - Are disease and illness proportional?
   - Does the illness serve to resolve particular issues?
   - How do collateral observers (e.g., family) perceive the patient?
3. Consider potential functions served unconsciously by the somatic symptoms. For example, the patient might be unconsciously doing any of the following:
   - Removing himself or herself from an overwhelming situation
   - Gaining the sick role and meeting dependency needs
   - Moderating systems problems (e.g., diverting family attention)
   - Punishing himself or herself for perceived wrongdoing
   - Masking expression of an unacceptable wish or impulse
   - Identifying with an important figure in his or her life
   - Communicating with the only vocabulary patient knows
4. Use suggested interview tips. Many evaluations for somatoform disorders are single encounters. The interview necessarily becomes an important diagnostic and therapeutic instrument: the psychiatrist's approach to clarifying a diagnosis can build an alliance and become a stepping-stone to constructive intervention. "Acknowledging and witnessing the awfulness of someone's experience can be a powerful counter to both isolation and confusion; task is inquiry, not exhortation" (Griffith and Gaby 2005).
   - Address patient's ambivalence about seeing a psychiatrist early.
   - Take the patient's symptoms seriously.
   - Pay particular attention to the range and depth of emotional response to issues raised during the examination, level of denial, meaning of

symptoms and normal test results to the patient, and evidence of unwarranted hostility toward physicians.

- When appropriate, conduct limited, relevant portions of a physical and neurological examination, which may improve patient alliance (Abbey 2002).
- Reframe and educate when asked, "Is this physical or psychological?"
- Pay close attention to symptoms, but listen also for the unspoken (i.e., consider whether anything is conspicuous by its absence).
- Be respectfully curious about the patient's life, looking for relational gaps and/or a current dilemma.
- Sniff for a silver lining (e.g., say to the patient, "From what you have described, I imagine you wouldn't wish this on your worst enemy. Even so, do you ever look back and see that it has somehow helped you become a better person?").
- Interview questions that often shed light include the following:
  - How has this illness affected your life?" or "How would you have been different if I had met you before these symptoms began?"
  - "Who truly understands what you're experiencing?"
  - "Is there anyone in your family with similar struggles?"
  - "How is your partner managing?"
  - "Do you feel that your symptoms drive him away, or is he someone who is inspired to go the extra mile for you?"
  - "Can he tell if you're having a bad day just by looking at you?"
  - If the patient identifies herself as religious, ask, "Does God have some purpose in this suffering for you? Do you have any ideas what that may be?"

5. Use collateral tools. The Minnesota Multiphasic Personality Inventory (MMPI) is particularly useful for patients who may be malingering and/or who have severe characterological problems.

6. Distinguish "normal" from "abnormal." Illness behavior refers to the manner in which individuals interpret their symptoms, take remedial action, and use sources of help (Mechanic 1986). Abnormal illness behavior is indicated by amplified, inappropriate, or maladaptive perception, evaluation, and reaction to one's symptoms, particularly when this behavior

pattern persists despite a physician's offering an accurate explanation of the symptoms and an appropriate course of management. The following clues often indicate an overvaluation of somatic symptoms:

- Symptom multiplicity, severity, and chronicity
- Difficulty coping: degree of role impairment
- Disease conviction: resistance to benign findings and reassurance
- Illness as a way of life: invalidism
- Maladaptive response to medical care
- Refractoriness to palliative, symptomatic treatment

Management

In managing patients with somatoform spectrum disorders, the consulting psychiatrist should do the following:

1. Support a thorough workup and maintain humility.
2. Align yourself with the patient and invite him or her to join you in collaborative curiosity about the symptoms—their history, patterns, meaning, and consequences.
3. Use analogies or stories to teach interaction of mind and body. After hearing, for example, about some individuals with performance anxiety who encounter increased gastrointestinal motility before a public presentation, most patients will understand the connection and even smile when the psychiatrist shares the vignette and ends by asking, "Now is that diarrhea a physical problem or a psychological problem?"
4. Encourage a formulation that honors the unconscious and respects the patient's perseverance despite adversity. For example, when explaining conversion symptoms, the consultant might comment, "I admire the creativity of your unconscious mind to find a way to balance these competing loyalties in a very difficult situation."
5. Adopt care and palliation, rather than "cure," as a goal.
6. Recognize and control one's own negative reactions and countertransference. Somatizing patients commonly evoke strong negative emotional responses in physicians that may interfere with optimal clinical care.
7. Insofar as possible, consolidate medical contact—that is, have as much care as possible under the oversight of a single primary physician.

8. Regular appointments, irrespective of a patient's symptoms, will decrease the use of other health care services. Without this proactive arrangement, illness behavior is reinforced because symptoms become the necessary prerequisite for attention; the patient also learns that if symptoms abate, the physician's attention is turned elsewhere. By scheduling regular appointments, the physician uncouples the linkage between symptoms and attention.

9. Assiduously evaluate and treat comorbid psychiatric conditions, particularly mood and anxiety disorders because these tend to exacerbate somatic amplification.

10. Be alert for new medical problems, but use diagnostic tests for objective changes only.

11. Maintain awareness of psychosocial context. The health care system may be the organizing hub for the patient's life. If possible, educate and persuade significant others in the patient's life regarding the value of rewarding non-illness-related behaviors.

12. Anticipate the risk for prescription or over-the-counter drug abuse because these patients often seek the opinions of multiple physicians.

13. Minimize polypharmacy to reduce the risk of iatrogenic complications. The process of tapering unnecessary medications (whose meaning is likely far different for the patient) can be long and difficult, so taking small, realistic steps increases the chance for success.

14. Gradually shift emphasis from listening to somatic language to encouraging translation to psychosocial stressors.

15. Anticipate extending time and patience in caring for the patient.

16. Understand that getting better and saying "Thank you" would threaten the patient's new relationship with the physician (this dynamic is similar to the description in item 8 in this list).

Collateral Management Tools

Physical Reactivation and Physical Therapy

Although engaging patients with somatoform disorders in exercise is often difficult, once they become more active, they often find the activity pleasurable and report feelings of accomplishment, reduced stress, and greater confidence in their body. Physical therapy is helpful for patients with conversion disorder and may be the only treatment required.

Relaxation Therapies, Biofeedback, Meditation, and Hypnotherapy

Patients with somatoform disorders may be helped by relaxation therapies, biofeedback, meditation, and hypnotherapy. Relaxation therapies aim to modulate somatic sensations and give patients a sense of self-empowerment.

Cognitive Therapy

Cognitive therapy is effective for some patients with somatization (Kronke and Swindle 2000) and hypochondriasis (Barsky and Ahern 2004; Hiller et al. 2002) and can reduce health care use (Hiller et al. 2003). It is used in both individual and group formats. A cognitive model directs attention to factors maintaining preoccupation with worries about health, including attentional factors, avoidant behaviors, beliefs, and misinterpretation of symptoms, signs, and medical communications (Salkovskis 1989). Cognitive therapy is a valuable adjunctive management tool for pain disorders, helping the patient to identify and replace distorted, negative attributions with more constructive coping strategies.

Group Psychotherapy

Group psychotherapy can provide gratification of social yearning, and the need to somatize to establish or maintain relationships may be reduced (Ford 1984). A patient usually accepts confrontation regarding primary or secondary gain more easily from group members than from the individual's therapist (Abbey 2002). Dependency needs and anger at physicians or family are more easily tolerated in the group setting, which tends to diffuse intense affects. Many somatizers, however, will not attend group therapy.

Potential Consequences of Failure to Engage the Patient

When a psychiatrist fails to engage the patient constructively, the following consequences are possible:

- Physician-patient conflict
- "Doctor shopping"
- Unnecessary diagnostic testing and treatment
- Iatrogenic side effects
- Excessive health care utilization
- Overlooking of new medical conditions
- Continued suffering because primary issues remain unrecognized

Somatization Disorder

Epidemiology

The general population lifetime prevalence of somatization disorder is estimated at 0.1%–1.1%, depending on the criteria used (Karvonen et al. 2004; Regier et al. 1988). The prevalence in medical settings is higher, up to 5% in some outpatient primary care clinics (deGruy et al. 1987). Somatization disorder is more common in lower socioeconomic strata and is perhaps 10 times more common in women than in men. Symptom onset is usually during the teen years, often at the time of menarche. Sexual or physical abuse, if not other markers of parental neglect, is common among women with somatization (Waldinger et al. 2006).

Clinical Features

The typical patient with somatization disorder is a woman who began to experience medically unexplained symptoms in early adolescence and has, over the years, continued to have repeated unexplained physical complaints involving multiple organ systems. According to DSM-IV-TR (American Psychiatric Association 2000), the patient requires a history over several years of at least four pain symptoms, two gastrointestinal symptoms, one sexual symptom, and one pseudoneurological symptom, all unexplained medically and sufficient to either impair function or warrant medical attention. Much more common than those who meet full DSM criteria for the disorder are individuals with multiple symptoms but not the minimum of eight necessary for diagnosis.

Associated Features

As high as 75% of patients with somatization disorder have comorbid Axis I diagnoses (Katon et al. 1991), most commonly major depressive disorder, dysthymic disorder, panic disorder, simple phobia, or substance abuse. Up to 65% of patients with somatization disorder meet criteria for one or more personality disorders (Rost et al. 1992), most frequently avoidant, paranoid, obsessive-compulsive, or histrionic.

Differential Diagnosis

Patients with uncommon medical syndromes, mysterious medical illnesses, atypical presentations of common diseases, factitious disorder, or malingering may all elicit consideration of somatization disorder. A detailed review of all past medical records is key. Presence of the following raises the likelihood of a somatization diagnosis:

1. A medical record best measured in pounds, or the electronic equivalent, rather than pages
2. A lifelong history of medically unexplained symptoms
3. A long list of medication "allergies" and unusual reactions
4. Recurring stories of possible conversion symptoms
5. Vague, impressionistic, and often inconsistent or contradictory details
6. Like a greased pig at a county fair, a narrative that becomes more elusive the more firmly a methodical physician attempts to lay hold of it
7. Despite prominent, prolonged complaints, a relative paucity of medical comorbidity

Clinical Course and Prognosis

The psychiatric consultant first must ensure that patients receive an appropriate diagnosis. Somatization disorder is a chronic but fluctuating disorder that rarely remits completely; once established, this diagnosis influences how physicians and the medical system respond to a patient. These patients are at risk for iatrogenic complications from numerous repetitive tests, procedures, and medications; the cost of the disorder is staggering.

Management of Somatization Disorder

Appropriate management of somatization disorder is difficult to implement. Most patients resist psychiatric consultation. The consultant must identify and treat comorbid psychiatric conditions. Additional management recommendations are largely identical to those discussed previously for the approach to patients with somatoform spectrum disorders in general (see "General Principles of Approach" earlier in chapter).

Undifferentiated Somatoform Disorder

Epidemiology

In the general population, 4%–11% of people have multiple medically unexplained symptoms consistent with a subsyndromal form of somatization disorder (Escobar et al. 1989). Further support for this diagnosis comes from the study of distressed high utilizers of medical care, which has shown significantly increased health care use by patients with functional somatic symptoms who have too few symptoms to meet DSM-IV (American Psychiatric Association 1994) criteria for somatization (e.g., Katon et al. 1991). These patients far outnumber those who meet criteria for somatization disorder.

Clinical Features

Undifferentiated somatoform disorder is a residual diagnostic category for patients whose symptoms do not meet criteria for another somatoform disorder but who nevertheless have significant dysfunction caused by unexplained medical symptoms.

Differential Diagnosis

When a detailed review of a patient's history and past medical records reveals the characteristics of somatization disorder but the symptoms fall short of the full criteria, undifferentiated somatoform disorder is a likely diagnosis. If one or only a few medically unexplained symptoms have occurred, and especially if the time course is brief, the consultant should look for an alternative diagnosis. The absence of a general medical diagnosis (by itself) is not sufficient evidence for a psychiatric diagnosis.

Clinical Course and Prognosis

Individuals with undifferentiated somatoform disorder are probably a heterogeneous group and include those for whom an eventual diagnosis of a general medical condition may explain their initial symptoms.

Management

Management of undifferentiated somatoform disorder is usually best served by the same principles enumerated for somatoform patients in the earlier section "General Principles of Approach." For the consultation psychiatrist who hopes to alleviate the intrusion of medically unexplained symptoms, it is useful to remember the following (Maldonado 1999):

- The role or meaning of a symptom for a particular patient must be respected.
- A symptom whose psychological value or purpose has not been understood will not be easily extinguished.

- The psychiatrist should beware of seeking to excise a symptom before providing the patient with a better defense.
- Patients will not give up a symptom until they believe they are strong enough to do without it.
- Patients always do better when they have a powerful incentive for a symptom-free state.
- The purpose of therapy is to enable patients to experience a healthy relationship that survives without reliance on somatic symptoms alone.

Hypochondriasis

Epidemiology

The prevalence of hypochondriasis depends on the diagnostic criteria used (Barsky et al. 1986). A narrow definition estimates a 1%–3% rate of hypochondriasis among various ethnic groups. Hypochondriasis is equally common in men and women. Onset typical occurs during early adulthood.

Clinical Features

The core feature of hypochondriasis is fear of disease or conviction that one has a serious disease based on the misinterpretation of bodily symptoms, despite normal physical examination findings and physician reassurance. Bodily preoccupation (i.e., increased observation of and vigilance toward bodily sensations) is common and lasts for 6 months or more. Patients with hypochondriasis believe that good health is a symptom-free state, and they are more likely than control patients to believe that symptoms mean disease (Barsky et al. 1992). "Concern about the feared illness often becomes a central feature of the individual's self-image, a topic of social discourse, and a response to life stresses" (American Psychiatric Association 2000, p. 504). Central clinical features of hypochondriasis are summed up by the four Ds:

- Disease conviction
- Disease fear
- Disease preoccupation
- Disability

Associated Features

Nearly 90% of the hypochondriacal patients in a general medical outpatient clinic had one or more concurrent Axis I diagnoses; the most common were generalized anxiety disorder (>70%), dysthymia and major depression (each >40%), and somatization disorder (>20%) (Barsky et al. 1992). In keeping with the prevalence of comorbid anxiety, individuals with hypochondriasis are often obsessive in style, whereas somatizers are commonly highly expressive and histrionic. Patients with hypochondriasis are high utilizers of medical services and have the potential for iatrogenic complications from repeated investigations (Abbey 2002).

Differential Diagnosis

Hypochondriasis in a general medical setting is most often secondary to a mood or anxiety disorder. The salient distinction between hypochondriasis and a delusional disorder is that patients with hypochondriasis typically describe a perceived symptom that fuels their conviction or fear of a disease, and the conviction is more pliable than in a delusional disorder.

Clinical Course and Prognosis

Hypochondriasis is typically a chronic condition that benefits little from hospitalization, adding to the suggestion that it is better understood as a personality style or an anxiety disorder (Barsky et al. 1992). Symptoms may improve with resolution of underlying stressors, interpersonal conflicts, or mood and anxiety disorders.

Treatment and Management

The psychiatric consultant should reassure patients regularly—even though reassurance usually does not change their behavior—and should protect them from iatrogenic harm, especially nonindicated surgical procedures. Educating family and significant others about the nature of hypochondriasis may help decrease anxiety and stress at home. Pharmacotherapy with a selective serotonin reuptake inhibitor (SSRI) may be a useful adjunct for patients whose symptoms are especially obsessional (Fallon 2004). Compared with usual medical care, brief cognitive-behavioral therapy has demonstrated clinically significant improvement at 6- and 12-month follow-ups (Barsky and Ahern 2004).

Conversion Disorder

Epidemiology

The estimated prevalence of conversion disorder varies: 0.3% in the general population, 1%–3% in medical outpatient settings, and 1%–4.5% in inpatient neurological and medical settings (Toone 1990). Women outnumber men with the disorder by a ratio varying from 2:1 to 10:1 (Murphy 1990). Onset typically occurs during adolescence or early adulthood, although cases can begin throughout the life cycle.

Clinical Features

Conversion disorder is a loss of or alteration in function that suggests a physical disease (usually neurological), although none can be established by usual diagnostic means. The following are common presentations of conversion:

- Motor symptoms (e.g., paralysis, disturbances in coordination or balance, localized weakness, akinesia, dyskinesia, aphonia, urinary retention)
- Sensory symptoms (e.g., blindness, double vision, anesthesia, paresthesia)
- Combined motor and sensory components, as with some epileptiform events

The initiation or exacerbation of the symptom is associated with a stress that is perceived as extreme by the patient, although this psychological threat or dilemma is characteristically not consciously grasped. *Conversion* refers to the unconscious transformation of intrapsychic conflict to a physical symptom; this process is sometimes referred to as primary gain. Persons with a conversion symptom frequently have a psychological "bind" as in the case that follows.

> **Case example:** A devoted father and Army Airborne paratrooper has developed paralysis of his right arm 2 weeks after a close buddy was killed in a training jump and 3 weeks before his second child is due. The conscientious paratrooper is in a no-win bind: he is immobilized between the push of loyalty

to his comrades, duty to country, and machismo of his unit, and the conflicting pull of his wife, his child(ren), and the fresh reminder that his work is dangerous. Paralysis provides an honorable resolution, if temporary: his buddies and commander are concerned for his medical welfare, and his wife is relieved that he will not be sent to Central America for drug interdiction training as had been planned.

Caveats

In considering whether a patient has conversion disorder, the consultant should keep in mind the following caveats (Stone 2009, p. 181), which in fact apply to the evaluation of all functional symptoms:

- Don't believe all the physical diagnoses in the medical notes.
- Don't wade in early with blunt questions about "depression" or "anxiety."
- Don't make a diagnosis of functional symptoms because someone has an obvious psychiatric problem/personality disorder.
- Don't avoid a diagnosis of a functional problem because someone seems too "normal."
- Don't misinterpret "exaggeration to convince" as "exaggeration to deceive."

Associated Features

Protracted conversion reactions are sometimes associated with secondary physical changes (e.g., disuse atrophy). Patients frequently have a model for the symptom in a family member or close friend. Individuals with psychogenic nonepileptic seizures (described in "Clinical Course and Prognosis" below) have a comorbid seizure disorder in 10%–30% of cases; the range reflects the stringency of diagnostic criteria for establishing a current seizure disorder (Jones et al. 2010).

Differential Diagnosis

The pitfall in making a diagnosis of conversion disorder is the potential for a later appearance of a medical disorder that, in retrospect, explains the so-called conversion symptom. It is therefore imperative that positive presumptive evidence for conversion—that is, intrapsychic conflict or another stressor associated with initiation or exacerbation of the symptom—exists prior to the diagnosis. In follow-up studies, subsequent evidence of a disease process that retrospectively explained the so-called conversion symptom was found in about 5%–30% of cases, with the most recent studies suggesting that 5% is the more accurate figure (Lazare 1981; Stone et al. 2003). The unconscious nature of conversion helps distinguish it from the consciously planned manipulative behaviors associated with malingering and factitious disorders.

Clinical Course and Prognosis

Individual episodes of conversion typically have a sudden onset, are brief in duration, and resolve when the associated psychosocial stressor (bind) remits (American Psychiatric Association 2000; Murphy 1990). However, one follow-up study found that >80% of the patients reported weakness and sensory symptoms at intervals of 9–16 years after the initial occurrence (Stone et al. 2003).

Predisposing Factors for Conversion Disorder

The following factors have been reported as predisposing to conversion disorder (Toone 1990):

- Prior neurological disorders in the individual or in a close contact who provides a model for the conversion symptoms
- Severe social stressors, including bereavement, rape, incest, warfare, and other forms of psychosocial trauma

Improved Prognosis

A better prognosis for conversion disorder is linked to the following (Lazare 1981):

- Acute and recent onset
- Traumatic or stressful life event at onset
- Good premorbid health
- Absence of other major medical or psychiatric disorders

Psychogenic Nonepileptic Seizures

Jones et al. (2010) described the following long-term outcomes of patients with psychogenic nonepileptic seizures:

- 90% reported continuing psychogenic nonepileptic seizure episodes
- 50% reported "current mental health problems" at 10-year follow-up
- 40% continued taking an antiepileptic drug
- Poor quality of life and poor overall levels of functioning

Treatment and Management

Many patients with conversion disorder are suggestible and will likely take to heart a physician's conclusion that gradual improvement can be expected. Many patients show a rapid response to treatment, but some do not (Stone et al. 2003). When a clear relationship between a conflict and a conversion symptom is identified, short-term focused or supportive therapy is indicated. Direct confrontation usually does not help and may worsen the symptom. Multidisciplinary inpatient behavioral treatment was successful in 8 of 9 "acute" cases but failed in 27 of 28 "chronic" cases; strategic-behavioral treatment (i.e., the patient and patient's family were told that full recovery constituted proof of an organic etiology and that failure was proof of a psychiatric etiology) worked in 13 of 21 patients with chronic motor conversion disorder who had failed the initial behavioral therapy (Shapiro and Teasell 2004). Pseudoseizures, tremor, and amnesia are less likely to have a rapid, good outcome (Toone 1990).

Helpful Explanations for Patients With Functional Symptoms

Stone (2009) suggested that a clinician can do the following to help patients with functional symptoms:

1. Explain what the patient does have: "You have functional weakness."
2. Emphasize the mechanism rather than the cause: "Your nervous system is not damaged but it is not functioning properly."
3. Explain what the patient does not have: "You do not have [a stroke, multiple sclerosis, epilepsy, etc.]."
4. Express belief in the patient: "I do not think you are making up your symptoms."
5. Emphasize that the symptoms are common: "I have seen many patients with similar symptoms."
6. Emphasize reversibility: "Because there is no damage, you have the potential to get better."

7. Support expectation of resolution: "In my experience, many individuals with symptoms like yours gradually improve."
8. Emphasize that self-help is important: "These symptoms are not your fault, but there are things you can do to help yourself get better."
9. Use metaphors: "Think of your body as being a piano that is out of tune."
10. Use written information: Provide a copy of the consult or other educational literature that the patient can read and digest on his or her own schedule.

Adjunctive Tools

- Referral to a behaviorally based cognitive-behavioral program
- Physical therapy for reconditioning
- Medication, such as an antidepressant or an anxiolytic
- Continued education (e.g., referral of patient to www.neurosymptoms.org)

Body Dysmorphic Disorder

Epidemiology

Onset of body dysmorphic disorder (BDD) is typically during adolescence (Phillips et al. 1993), although many years may pass before diagnosis because of the patients' reluctance to disclose symptoms. Prevalence rates vary from 1.8% in a population-based survey (Buhlmann et al. 2010) to 3.2% of psychiatric patients (Zimmerman and Mattia 1998) and 10% of patients seeking cosmetic surgery (Jakubietz et al. 2007).

Clinical Features

The hallmark of BDD is an obsession or preoccupation with an imagined defect in appearance (or excessive concern with a slight physical anomaly) that is accompanied by significant distress or impairment in social or occupational functioning. The most common complaints involve facial appearance (e.g., wrinkles, nose, mouth), and less common complaints are about hair, breasts, genitalia, or other body parts. Determining whether the patient's complaint is an overvalued idea or a somatic delusion is sometimes difficult (Hollander et al. 1992).

Associated Features

Most patients with BDD have at least one comorbid Axis I psychiatric disorder (Gunstad and Phillips 2003). Common comorbidities include the following (Grant et al. 2002, 2005; Phillips and Stout 2006):

- Mood disorders
- Substance use disorders
- Social phobia
- Obsessive-compulsive disorder
- Eating disorders

Psychosocial dysfunction due to shame over the imagined defect may be profound. Patients may experience the following:

- Social withdrawal (up to 30% of patients with BDD are homebound for periods of time)
- Broken relationships and lower likelihood of being married
- Impaired occupational capacity
- Referential thinking (i.e., attributing scrutinizing behavior to surrounding people)

Common idiosyncratic and often secretive behaviors include these:

- Fastidious grooming behavior
- Attempts to disguise or camouflage the perceived defect
- Avoidance of mirrors or frequent mirror checking
- Repetitive seeking of reassurance about appearance

Differential Diagnosis

Several Axis I disorders may share features with BDD. Salient distinctions include the following (Buhlmann et al. 2008):

- *Major depression.* Patients with comorbid major depression express depressive symptoms that extend beyond the intense dysphoria that is primarily associated with times when a patient is focused on appearance.

- *Social phobia.* Patients with social phobia fear negative evaluation by others that is not limited to concerns about physical appearance and are less likely to adopt ritualistic behaviors surrounding appearance in preparation for venturing out.
- *Obsessive-compulsive disorder.* Patients with obsessive-compulsive disorder are less likely to experience obsessions and associated compulsive rituals that are exclusively centered on physical appearance.
- *Eating disorders.* Patients with eating disorders experience disturbance of body image, with frequent intrusive preoccupation and consequent rituals, but these revolve around weight and shape concerns, whereas patients with BDD typically have several areas of concern (e.g., hair, nose, skin).

Clinical Course and Prognosis

BDD is usually chronic, with few symptom-free intervals, although the intensity of the symptoms often varies over time. Patients often suffer in isolation, are unwilling to present for clinical attention due to embarrassment and shame, and are unlikely to disclose their symptoms unless asked with a specificity that is informed by physician awareness of the disorder.

Serious sequelae are not rare (Buhlmann et al. 2008):

- Suicidal ideation—10 times higher rate than in general population (31% vs. 3.5%)
- Suicide attempts—10 times higher rate than in general population (22% vs. 2.1%)
- Cosmetic surgery—5 times higher rate than in general population (16% vs. 3.0%)

Several factors are associated with lower likelihood of symptom remission (Phillips et al. 2005):

- Severity of BDD (at intake for prospective study)
- Longer duration of BDD at intake
- Comorbid personality disorder

Factors that are not associated with symptom remission include the following (Phillips et al. 2005):

- Gender, ethnicity, socioeconomic status
- Age at onset
- Delusionality of BDD symptoms
- Comorbid Axis I disorder

Treatment and Management

Surgical alteration of the perceived defect almost always offers only fleeting relief and commonly becomes a source of dissatisfaction, new perceived defects, and psychological destabilization; hostility and even violence against the surgeon may follow (Jakubietz et al. 2007). In contrast, SSRIs and cognitive-behavioral therapy have proved efficacious (Bjornsson et al. 2010; Pavan et al. 2008).

Pain Disorder

Epidemiology

The prevalence of pain disorder is unknown, but the frequency with which patients present at a consultation service with chronic pain, either in isolation or associated with opiate dependence, is no surprise considering that it affects over 50 million Americans (Turk and Wilson 2010).

Clinical Features

Psychological factors are important in the onset, exacerbation, or maintenance of the pain, which is sufficiently severe to warrant medical attention or interfere with function. Pain is neither intentionally produced nor contrived. If a medical disorder is also present, psychological factors amplify the patient's experience of pain far beyond objective expectations based on known anatomy and physiology. Patients who qualified for the DSM forerunners (i.e., psychogenic or somatoform pain disorder) were described as having "the disease of the *D*s" (Brena and Chapman 1983):

- Disability
- Disuse and degeneration of functional capacity secondary to pain behavior
- Drug misuse
- Doctor shopping

- Dependency (emotional)
- Demoralization
- Depression
- Dramatic accounts of illness

Associated Features

Depression, posttraumatic stress disorder, and panic disorder are diagnosed frequently in patients with chronic pain syndromes (Sharp and Keefe 2005). Up to 50% of individuals with chronic pain have depressive symptoms, and 25% meet criteria for major depression or an anxiety disorder. Several findings regarding nonmalignant chronic pain and suicidal behavior are relevant for the consultation psychiatrist (M. T. Smith et al. 2004):

1. Family history of suicide is strongly associated.
2. Pain in the abdomen versus other bodily locations is associated with a fivefold increased risk of suicide.
3. Increased risk of suicide has no association with pain severity, pain duration, or comorbid depression.
4. Neuropathic pain is statistically protective against suicidality.

Differential Diagnosis

As with diagnosing conversion disorder, the most common pitfall in making a diagnosis of pain disorder is the later appearance of a medical disorder that explains the pain. Therefore, the consultant should look for positive evidence of somatoform contributions to the patient's perception of pain (e.g., a relevant conflict or stressor associated with initiation or exacerbation of pain).

Clinical Course and Prognosis

Long-term studies on outcomes of patients with pain disorder do not exist, but the estimated cost in the United States of $100 billion annually in lost income and productivity coupled with medical expense provides evidence of the substantial morbidity of chronic pain (Stewart et al. 2003). Central nervous system plasticity may contribute to further morbidity as neural pathways change, leading to heightened pain sensitivity and a lowered pain threshold (Scholz and Woolf 2002). Iatrogenic complications are common and include opiate and benzodiazepine dependence as well as unnecessary surgical interventions (Abbey 2002).

Treatment and Management

Treatment and management of pain syndromes are complex. When pain has not yet become firmly entrenched in the patient's experience, and particularly if sensitive interviewing establishes a plausible functional role for the pain, the patient may respond to an approach that parallels that described for conversion disorder. When the pain is chronic and has become an organizing force in the patient's life, the following are the most effective strategies (Fishbain et al. 2004; Maizels and McCarberg 2005; Sharp and Keefe 2005):

1. Identify and aggressively treat psychiatric comorbidity.
2. Prescribe serotonin-norepinephrine reuptake inhibitors or tricyclic antidepressants.
3. Carefully weigh risks and benefits of adjunctive antiepileptics and atypical antipsychotics.
4. Avoid narcotic analgesics if at all possible.
5. Refer the patient early to a multidisciplinary behaviorally based treatment program.

Factitious Disorders

Epidemiology

Demographic analyses of patients with factitious disorders suggest two general patterns. Patients with chronic factitious disorder (Munchausen syndrome) are usually middle-aged men who are typically unmarried and estranged from their families. Patients with more acute forms of factitious disorder are usually women, ages 20–40, who have work experience in medical occupations such as nursing and medical technology (Ford and Feldman 2002). Classically, Munchausen syndrome included not only chronicity of symptoms but also pseudologia fantastica (telling tall tales) and peregrination (wandering to multiple medical centers).

Clinical Features

Patients with factitious disorders intentionally feign, exaggerate, exacerbate, or induce symptoms. These individuals are aware of their behaviors, although their underlying motivations are understood to be unconscious. Factitious disorder may occur with predominantly physical symptoms, predominantly psychological symptoms, or combined physical and psychological symptoms. In chronic factitious disorder, self-production of sometimes dramatic, often cryptic, and potentially life-threatening illnesses allows the patient to achieve the goal of assuming the sick role. In factitious disorder by proxy, signs and symptoms are created in another person, usually a child or an elderly relative. Although they have overlap, five levels of factitious disorder have been suggested (Folks et al. 2000):

1. Fictitious history
2. Simulation
3. Exaggeration
4. Aggravation
5. Self-induced pathology

An alternative hierarchy, wherein each level tends to include the prior activities, is as follows:

1. Fictitious history
2. Feigned physical signs
3. Manipulation of diagnostic tests
4. Self-induced pathology

Differential Diagnosis

The diagnosis of factitious disorder with physical symptoms is difficult to make, unless direct evidence is found (e.g., a syringe and insulin are found hidden in the room of a hospitalized patient with unexplained episodes of hypoglycemia). The diagnosis of factitious disorder with psychological symptoms is even more difficult to make, because no corresponding definitive laboratory or other objective tests are available. Indirect evidence, such as no medical diagnosis and a dramatic presentation, may cause frustrated medical staff to request psychiatric consultation because they suspect factitious illness or malingering. The psychiatric consultant must see past the staff's countertransference and look for positive evidence of a diagnosis. Some psychiatrists use "unlikely," "possible," "probable," or "definite" to indicate the likelihood of the diagnosis.

Clinical Course and Prognosis

Factitious disorders are associated with considerable morbidity and mortality. Few patients accept treatment, and even fewer achieve freedom from symptoms. If confronted, some patients may deny but stop behavior, very few may acknowledge behavior and enter treatment, and most will seek medical care elsewhere and continue factitious behavior (Krahn et al. 2003; Wise and Ford 1999).

Treatment and Management

Recent changes in medical practice in the United States emphasize patients' rights and informed consent. As a result, practices such as clandestine searches of personal articles, although once commonplace, are now controversial. When a patient is suspected of having a factitious disorder, involvement of hospital administration and advice from the hospital legal office may be necessary. Whatever steps prove necessary, patient confidentiality must be maintained.

Malingering

Epidemiology

Malingering occurs when illness brings tangible gains. Malingering is most often encountered in prisons, courtrooms, and military settings (when disability evaluations are performed) and among persons with addiction.

Clinical Features

Malingering is grossly exaggerating, lying, or faking physical or psychological symptoms for the sole purpose of a concrete, recognizable gain (i.e., secondary gain), as distinct from the unconscious benefit (i.e., primary gain) achieved by conversion and factitious symptoms. Malingerers are motivated by specific external incentives, such as deferment from military service, avoidance of hazardous work assignments, financial rewards such as disability payments, escape from incarceration, or procurement of controlled substances (Ford and Feldman 2002). Vigilance for malingering is prudent if more than one of the following factors is present (McDermott and Feldman 2007; Slick et al. 2004):

- Antisocial personality disorder
- Lack of cooperation with psychiatric or medical evaluation and treatment

- Marked disparity between the claimed disability and objective findings
- Medicolegal presentation
- Notable psychosocial adversity without an apparent viable solution (e.g., homelessness and an estranged family, squandered friendships, and no shelter vacancies)
- Opportunity for inflating compensation

Differential Diagnosis

Malingering is difficult to prove, unless direct evidence is found. The following five conditions often require careful deliberation to distinguish them from malingering (McDermott and Feldman 2007):

1. *Undetected or underestimated physical illness.* Malingering deserves serious consideration before undertaking high-risk diagnostic procedures.
2. *Pain disorder.* The subjective nature of pain underscores the value of inconspicuous observation of the patient.
3. *Somatization disorder.* The range of complaints and involved systems may be broader with somatization.
4. *Hypochondriasis.* These patients welcome diagnostic evaluations and are, at least briefly, relieved by negative results.
5. *Factitious disorder.* Even noxious procedures may be welcomed because they reinforce the sick role.

Course and Prognosis

Anxiety and depression may tilt a patient's perception of his or her circumstances in life and contribute to an impulsive decision to malinger; such a patient may no longer need the benefits of malingering when the underlying condition is treated. On the other hand, individuals with intrinsically poor coping skills or those who stand to gain significant sums of money or other compensation may prove disinterested in any effort to ameliorate their reported symptoms.

Treatment and Management

Occasionally, when malingering is in the context of a hardy antisocial personality disorder, confrontation may be appropriate. More commonly, downstream turbulence will be decreased by allowing the malingerer to save face and by explaining that testing has not revealed a serious condition and that further deterioration is not anticipated. Malingering may emerge as a legal rather than a medical or psychiatric issue. With this in mind, the clinician does well to substitute circumspection for frustration in his or her approach to the patient. Each note should be written with the awareness that it could become a courtroom exhibit (Ford and Feldman 2002).

References

Abbey SE: Somatization and somatoform disorders, in The American Psychiatric Publishing Textbook of Consultation-Liaison Psychiatry: Psychiatry in the Medically Ill, Second Edition. Edited by Wise MG, Rundell JR. Washington, DC, American Psychiatric Publishing, 2002, pp 361–392

American Psychiatric Association: Diagnostic and Statistical Manual of Mental Disorders, 4th Edition. Washington, DC, American Psychiatric Association, 1994

American Psychiatric Association: Diagnostic and Statistical Manual of Mental Disorders, 4th Edition, Text Revision. Washington, DC, American Psychiatric Association, 2000

American Psychiatric Association: DSM-5 Development: Proposed draft revisions to DSM disorders and criteria. 2010. Available at: www.dsm5.org/Pages/Default.aspx. Accessed January 1, 2011.

Barsky AJ, Ahern DK: Cognitive behavior therapy for hypochondriasis: a randomized controlled trial. JAMA 291:1464–1470, 2004

Barsky AJ, Wyshak G, Klerman GL: Medical and psychiatric determinants of outpatient medical utilization. Med Care 24:548–560, 1986

Barsky AJ, Wyshak G, Klerman GL: Psychiatric comorbidity in DSM-III-R hypochondriasis. Arch Gen Psychiatry 49:101–108, 1992

Bjornsson AS, Didie ER, Phillips KA: Body dysmorphic disorder. Dialogues Clin Neurosci 12:221–232, 2010

Brena SF, Chapman SL (eds): Management of Patients With Chronic Pain. New York, Spectrum, 1983

Brodsky CM: Sociocultural and interactional influences on somatization. Psychosomatics 25:673–680, 1984

Buhlmann U, Reese HE, Renaud S, et al: Clinical considerations for the treatment of body dysmorphic disorder with cognitive-behavioral therapy. Body Image 5:39–49, 2008

Buhlmann U, Glaesmer H, Mewes R, et al: Updates on the prevalence of body dysmorphic disorder: a population-based survey. Psychiatry Res 178:171–175, 2010

Cassem NH, Barsky AJ: Functional somatic symptoms and somatoform disorders, in Massachusetts General Hospital Handbook of General Hospital Psychiatry, 3rd Edition. Edited by Cassem NH. St Louis, MO, Mosby–Year Book, 1991, pp 131–157

deGruy F, Columbia L, Dickinson P: Somatization disorder in a family practice. J Fam Pract 25:45–51, 1987

Dimsdale J, Creed F: The proposed diagnosis of somatic symptom disorders in DSM-V to replace somatoform disorders in DSM-IV: a preliminary report. J Psychosom Res 66:473–476, 2009

Eisenberg L: Disease and illness: distinctions between professional and popular ideas of sickness. Cult Med Psychiatry 1:9–23, 1977

Escobar JI, Manu P, Matthews D, et al: Medically unexplained physical symptoms, somatization disorder and abridged somatization: studies with the Diagnostic Interview Schedule. Psychiatr Dev 7:235–245, 1989

Fallon BA: Pharmacotherapy of somatoform disorders. J Psychosom Res 56:455–460, 2004

Fishbain DA, Cutler RB, Lewis J, et al: Do the second-generation "atypical neuroleptics" have analgesic properties? A structured evidence-based review. Pain Med 5:359–365, 2004

Folks DG, Feldman MD, Ford CV: Somatoform disorders, factitious disorders, and malingering, in Psychiatric Care of the Medical Patient, 2nd Edition. Edited by Stoudemire A, Fogel BS, Greenberg DB. New York, Oxford University Press, 2000, pp 459–475

Ford CV: The Somatizing Disorders: Illness as a Way of Life. New York, Elsevier, 1983

Ford CV: Somatizing disorders, in Helping Patients and Their Families Cope With Medical Problems. Edited by Roback HB. Washington, DC, Jossey-Bass, 1984, pp 39–59

Ford CV, Feldman MD: Factitious disorders and malingering, in The American Psychiatric Publishing Textbook of Consultation-Liaison Psychiatry: Psychiatry in the Medically Ill, 2nd Edition. Edited by Wise MG, Rundell JR. Washington, DC, American Psychiatric Publishing, 2002, pp 519–531

Grant JE, Kim SW, Eckert ED: Body dysmorphic disorder in patients with anorexia nervosa: prevalence, clinical features and delusionality of body image. Int J Eat Disord 32:291–300, 2002

Grant JE, Menard W, Pagano ME, et al: Substance use disorders in individuals with body dysmorphic disorder. J Clin Psychiatry 66:309–316, 2005

Griffith JL, Gaby L: Brief psychotherapy at the bedside: countering demoralization from medical illness. Psychosomatics 46:109–116, 2005

Gunstad J, Phillips KA: Axis I comorbidity in body dysmorphic disorder. Compr Psychiatry 44:270–276, 2003

Hiller W, Leibbrand R, Rief W, et al: Predictors of course and outcome in hypochondriasis after cognitive-behavioral treatment. Psychother Psychosom 71:318–325, 2002

Hiller W, Fichter MM, Rief W: A controlled treatment study of somatoform disorders including analysis of healthcare utilization and cost-effectiveness. J Psychosom Res 54:369–380, 2003

Hollander E, Neville D, Frenkel M, et al: Body dysmorphic disorder: diagnostic issues and related disorders. Psychosomatics 33:156–165, 1992

Jakubietz M, Jakubietz RJ, Kloss DF, et al: Body dysmorphic disorder: diagnosis and approach. Plast Reconstr Surg 119–124, 2007

Jones SG, O'Brien TJ, Adams SJ, et al: Clinical characteristics and outcome in patients with psychogenic nonepileptic seizures. Psychosom Med 72:487–497, 2010

Karvonen JT, Veijola J, Jokelainen J, et al: Somatization disorder in young adult population. Gen Hosp Psychiatry 26:9–12, 2004

Katon WJ, Walker EA: Medically unexplained symptoms in primary care. J Clin Psychiatry 59 (suppl 20):15–21, 1998

Katon W, Lin E, Von Korff M et al: Somatization: a spectrum of severity. Am J Psychiatry 148:34–40, 1991

Kellner R: Functional somatic symptoms and hypochondriasis. Arch Gen Psychiatry 42:821–833, 1985

Krahn LE, Hongzhe L, O'Connor MK: Patients who strive to be ill: factitious disorder with physical symptoms. Am J Psychiatry 160:1163–1168, 2003

Kronke K, Swindle R: Cognitive-behavioral therapy for somatization and symptom syndromes: a critical review of controlled clinical trials. Psychother Psychosom 69:205–215, 2000

Lazare A: Current concepts in psychiatry: conversion symptoms. N Engl J Med 305:745–748, 1981

Lipowski ZJ: Somatization: the concept and its clinical application. Am J Psychiatry 145:1358–1368, 1988

Maizels M, McCarberg B: Antidepressants and antiepileptic drugs for chronic noncancer pain. Am Fam Physician 71:483–490, 2005

Maldonado JR: Somatoform disorders. Paper presented at the 12th United States Psychiatric and Mental Health Congress, Atlanta, GA, November 1999

McDermott BE, Feldman MD: Malingering in the medical setting. Psychiatr Clin N Am 30:645–662, 2007

Mechanic D: The concept of illness behaviour: culture, situation and personal predisposition. Psychol Med 16:1–7, 1986

Murphy MR: Classification of the somatoform disorders, in Somatization: Physical Symptoms and Psychological Illness. Edited by Bass C. Oxford, UK, Blackwell Scientific, 1990, pp 10–39

Pavan C, Simonato P, Marini M, et al: Psychopathologic aspects of body dysmorphic disorder: a literature review. Aesthetic Plast Surg 32:473–484, 2008

Phillips KA, Stout RL: Associations in the longitudinal course of body dysmorphic disorder with major depression, obsessive-compulsive disorder, and social phobia. J Psychiatr Res 40:360–369, 2006

Phillips KA, McElroy SL, Keck PE, et al: Body dysmorphic disorder: 30 cases of imagined ugliness. Am J Psychiatry 150:302–308, 1993

Phillips KA, Pagano ME, Menard W, et al: Predictors of remission from body dysmorphic disorder: a prospective study. J Nerv Ment Dis 193:564–567, 2005

Regier DA, Boyd JH, Burke JD, et al: One-month prevalence of mental disorders in the United States based on five Epidemiologic Catchment Area sites. Arch Gen Psychiatry 45:977–986, 1988

Rost KM, Akins RN, Brown FW, et al: The comorbidity of DSM-III-R personality disorders in somatization disorder. Gen Hosp Psychiatry 14:322–326, 1992

Salkovskis PM: Somatic problems, in Cognitive Behaviour Therapy for Psychiatric Problems. Edited by Hawton K, Salkovskis PM, Kirk J, et al. Oxford, UK, Oxford University Press, 1989, pp 235–276

Scholz J, Woolf CJ: Can we conquer pain? Nat Neurosi 5 (suppl):1062–1067, 2002

Shapiro AP, Teasell RW: Behavioural interventions in the rehabilitation of acute versus chronic non-organic (conversion/factitious) motor disorders. Br J Psychiatry 185:140–146, 2004

Sharp J, Keefe B: Psychiatry in chronic pain: a review and update. Curr Psychiatry Rep 7:213–219, 2005

Simon GE, VonKorff M: Somatization and psychiatric disorder in the NIMH Epidemiologic Catchment Area study. Am J Psychiatry 148:1494–1500, 1991

Slick DJ, Tan JE, Strauss EH, et al: Detecting malingering: a survey of experts' practices. Arch Clin Neuropsychol 19:465–473, 2004

Smith GR, Monson RA, Ray DC: Psychiatric consultation in somatization disorder: a randomized controlled study. N Engl J Med 314:1407–1413, 1986

Smith MT, Edwards RR, Robinson RC, et al: Suicidal ideation, plans, and attempts in chronic pain patients: factors associated with increased risk. Pain 111:201–208, 2004

Smith RC, Dwamena FC: Classification and diagnosis of patients with medically unexplained symptoms. J Gen Intern Med 22:685–691, 2007

Stewart WF, Ricci JA, Chee E, et al: Lost productive time and cost due to common pain conditions in the U.S. workforce. JAMA 290:2443–2454, 2003

Stone J: Functional symptoms in neurology. Pract Neurol 9:179–189, 2009

Stone J, Sharpe M, Rothwell PM, et al: The 12-year prognosis of unilateral functional weakness and sensory disturbance. J Neurol Neurosurg Psychiatry 74:591–596, 2003

Toone BK: Disorders of hysterical conversion, in Somatization: Physical Symptoms and Psychological Illness. Edited by Bass C. Oxford, UK, Blackwell Scientific, 1990, pp 207–234

Turk DC, Wilson HD: Fear of pain as a prognostic factor in chronic pain: conceptual models, assessment, and treatment implications. Curr Pain Heachache Rep 14:88–95, 2010

Voigt K, Nagel A, Meyer B, et al: Towards positive diagnostic criteria: a systematic review of somatoform diagnoses and suggestions for future classification. J Psychosom Res 68:403–414, 2010

Waldinger RJ, Schulz MS, Barsky AJ, et al: Mapping the road from childhood trauma to adult somatization: the role of attachment. Psychosom Med 68:129–135, 2006

Wise MG, Ford CV: Factitious disorders. Prim Care 26:315–326, 1999

Zimmerman M, Mattia JI: Body dysmorphic disorder in psychiatric outpatients: recognition, prevalence, comorbidity, demographics, and clinical correlates. Compr Psychiatry 39:265–270, 1998

13

Substance-Related Disorders

Consultation psychiatrists are in a unique position to identify and intervene in substance-related disorders in medically ill patients. Current alcohol abuse or dependence is present in up to 25% of general hospital patients (Curtis et al. 1989; Gerke et al. 1997; Katz et al. 2008), and 20% of medical outpatients drink alcohol at unhealthy levels (Saitz 2005). Only 25% of individuals who develop substance use disorders seek any addiction treatment during their lifetime; of these, fewer than half receive treatment from mental health professionals, whereas most receive treatment from general medical providers (Schuckit 2009). A window of opportunity may open for treating substance-related disorders in medical-surgical patients, because the patients' resistance to treatment may weaken during acute illness. The care of these patients benefits from collaboration between the consultant and the referring physician. Often, the health care team has strong feelings toward the substance-abusing patient, especially when intoxication or overdose prompted the admission and when the team has cared for the patient for substance-related medical problems in previous admissions. The consulting team can support the primary team in the face of frustration with recidivist patients. Both teams must communicate to the patient the medical, psychological, and social consequences of continued alcohol or drug use.

DSM Criteria

In DSM-IV-TR (American Psychiatric Association 2000), substance-related disorders are divided into substance use disorders and substance-induced disorders. Substance use disorders include alcohol and drug abuse and dependence. Substance-induced disorders include intoxication; withdrawal; delirium; dementia; sexual dysfunction; and amnestic, psychotic, mood, anxiety, and sleep disorders. The loss of control over substance use has both neurobiological and behavioral bases, both of which are modified over time as a result of substance-induced changes in the brain (Self 2004).

Substance Abuse

Substance abuse is demonstrated by "a maladaptive pattern of substance use leading to clinically significant impairment or distress, as manifested by one (or more) of the following, occurring within a 12-month period" (American Psychiatric Association 2000, p. 199):

1. Recurrent use resulting in failure to meet major obligations at work, school, or home
2. Recurrent use in situations in which it is physically hazardous
3. Recurrent substance-related legal problems
4. Continued use despite recurrent social or interpersonal problems caused or exacerbated by the effects of the substance

Substance Dependence

Dependence is demonstrated by "a maladaptive pattern of substance use, leading to clinically significant impairment or distress, as manifested by three (or more) of the following, occurring at any time in the same 12-month period" (American Psychiatric Association 2000, p. 197):

1. Tolerance
2. Withdrawal
3. Greater amounts or more prolonged use than initially intended
4. Persistent desire or unsuccessful efforts to cut down or control use
5. Considerable time spent obtaining, using, or recovering from use of substance

6. Sacrifice of important social, occupational, or recreational activities
7. Continued use despite awareness of adverse consequences

Alcohol

Alcohol is the most frequently abused substance. Two-thirds of Americans drink; nearly 15% of men and 5% of women are heavy drinkers. About 25% of men and women admitted to the hospital are heavy drinkers and are likely to have an alcohol-related disorder (Seppa and Makela 1993; Yates 2002). Lifetime prevalence of alcohol abuse among men is 15%, and alcohol dependence is 10%; the rate is lower in women, but a higher percentage of women than men seek help (Hasin et al. 2007). Alcohol-related problems usually begin between ages 16 and 30; children of alcoholic parents have alcoholism four to five times more often than do children of nonalcoholic parents.

Intoxication

Although multiple factors influence both the rate of absorption and eventual blood alcohol concentration, a reasonable generalization is that 1 drink equivalent (12 oz beer, 5 oz wine, 1.5 oz 80-proof whiskey) will yield a blood alcohol concentration of 20 mg/dL, or 0.02%. In turn, the body metabolizes alcohol at an approximate rate of 1–1.5 drink equivalents/hour once it has been absorbed. Unless the person is alcohol tolerant, mild euphoria occurs at blood levels of 30–50 mg/dL, driving impairment is demonstrable at a level of 50 mg/dL, and significant ataxia is present at 100 mg/dL. Disorientation and stupor can occur at 200 mg/dL, and coma and death may occur in the alcohol-naïve person at 400 mg/dL. In contrast, a chronic heavy drinker may develop sufficient tolerance to allow a concentration of 500 mg/dL without the loss of ability to converse or appear grossly alert to the casual observer.

Recognition
Symptoms and signs of alcohol intoxication include the following:

- Alcohol odor (5% of alcohol is metabolized by the lungs)
- Disinhibition
- Mood lability
- Impaired judgment

- Ataxia
- Dysarthria
- Nystagmus

Management

1. Reduce stimulation by providing a quiet environment.
2. Impede absorption by offering food.
3. Alert security if the patient escalates in behavior.
4. If patient is severely agitated, sedate with lorazepam 1–2 mg intravenously (iv) or intramuscularly (im) every hour as needed.
5. If lorazepam is insufficient, administer haloperidol 1–5 mg iv every hour until calm.
6. Administer thiamine 100 mg im before dextrose-containing intravenous fluids (many centers administer combined thiamine, folate, multivitamins, magnesium, and phosphates intravenously in a variously named "goodie bag").
7. Thereafter, administer thiamine 100 mg daily and folate 1 mg daily.
8. Obtain a blood alcohol level and screen for other drug use.

Withdrawal

Withdrawal symptoms may appear within 6–48 hours after significant reduction in or cessation of prolonged alcohol use. Tremors typically peak 24–48 hours after the last drink and subside after 3–5 days of abstinence. However, about 50% of alcohol-dependent individuals do not develop significant symptoms of withdrawal (Schuckit 2006).

Recognition

Symptoms and signs of alcohol withdrawal include the following:

- Tremulousness
- Insomnia
- Irritability
- Nausea and diminished appetite
- Autonomic hyperactivity
- Anxiety

- Hypervigilance
- Mild transient illusions or hallucinations (even in the absence of other stigmata of delirium)

Management

No single regimen will serve all patients equally well. Multiple protocols exist, but the following fundamental elements are shared.

Medical support. Staff should monitor the patient's vital signs; watch especially for hypertension and fever; and maintain hydration, but watch for fluid and electrolyte imbalances, particularly hypoglycemia, hyponatremia, hypokalemia, hypomagnesemia, and hypophosphatemia.

Pharmacological options. Pharmacological options serve the common goals of patient safety by reducing agitation, averting autonomic hyperactivity and seizures, and avoiding exacerbation of concurrent medical issues. Benzodiazepines (BZDs) are the mainstay of alcohol withdrawal protocols (McKeon et al. 2008). One structured detoxification regimen is chlordiazepoxide 50 mg orally every 6 hours for four doses, then 25 mg every 6 hours for eight doses (Franklin et al. 2002); this approach takes advantage of the long half-life of chlordiazepoxide to create an autotapering effect. For the same reason, some clinicians prefer phenobarbital because its very long half-life provides some protection against withdrawal symptoms even if the patient leaves the hospital before withdrawal has been completed. Alternate regimens utilize BZDs that are metabolized by glucuronidation (e.g., lorazepam 2–4 mg every 6 hours or oxazepam 15–45 mg every 6 hours), especially for patients with alcoholic liver disease, because these medications present less risk of excessive buildup of blood levels.

Inpatient versus outpatient treatment. Depending on the severity of symptoms, stage of withdrawal, medical and psychiatric complications, comorbid polysubstance abuse, patient cooperation, ability to follow instructions, social support systems, and patient history, some patients can be safely detoxified in outpatient settings with limited medical supervision (Blondell 2005).

Symptom-triggered BZD administration. Symptom-triggered BZD administration is frequent in withdrawal protocols (Jaeger et al. 2001). The revised

Clinical Institute Withdrawal Assessment for Alcohol (CIWA-Ar) scale is the most commonly used instrument to gauge the severity of alcohol withdrawal (Sullivan et al. 1989; Williams et al. 2001). Ten domains (nausea, diaphoresis, anxiety, agitation, headache, tremor, clouding of sensorium, and auditory, visual, and tactile disturbances) are scored hourly, and the BZD dose administered is proportional to the severity rating; when the rating falls to a mild level, the intervals between assessments are lengthened and patients receive lower BZD doses.

Potential Complications

Medical Complications

Medical complications of chronic alcohol abuse include anemia, esophageal disorders, gastritis, alcoholic hepatitis, cirrhosis, pancreatitis, cardiomyopathy, insomnia, male feminization and impotence, myopathy, peripheral neuropathy, falls and traumatic accidents (leading to fractures, brain injury, subdural hematoma, etc.), Wernicke-Korsakoff syndrome, and dementia. Physical examination may identify bruises, spider angiomata, ascites, muscle wasting, nystagmus, and ataxia.

Management.   Advising a medically ill alcoholic patient to drink in moderation is foolish. After the patient is stabilized, the clinician should encourage the patient to become involved in community resources, especially Alcoholics Anonymous (AA). Although various life circumstances motivate 20%–30% of patients to achieve long-term remission without structured assistance (Rumpf et al. 2006), of the patients who seriously commit to treatment, 50%–60% achieve substantial functional improvement in the following year (Moos and Moos 2006). Both inpatient and outpatient programs should be considered.

Pharmacological aids to relapse prevention.   For a patient without significant hepatic compromise who has realistic access to regular follow-up, and especially if his or her history includes abstinence that gave way to impulsive drinking, the consultation psychiatrist should urge prompt follow-up with a primary care physician to consider an antidipsogenic medication. Current options include the following:

- *Disulfiram*—precipitates accumulation of acetaldehyde, a metabolite of ethanol, by enzyme inhibition, resulting in distinctly noxious flushing,

nausea, diaphoresis, and tachycardia if any alcohol is consumed—even small amounts from over-the-counter liquid medications
- *Naltrexone*—an opioid antagonist that inhibits the expected rise in endorphins after alcohol consumption, thereby reducing craving by decreasing the reinforcing pleasure obtained by a drink following a period of abstinence
- *Acamprosate*—a glutamatergic blocker and γ-aminobutyric acid (GABA) agonist with an uncertain mechanism of action, although it may successfully attenuate destabilizing effects of alcoholism on the balance between excitatory and inhibitory neurotransmission in the brain

These agents are typically not initiated on the consultation service because they best serve patients when integrated with ongoing assistance, whether in formal treatment programs, self-help programs, or consistent primary care follow-up.

Special considerations in medically ill patients.   Although disulfiram is the oldest of the three pharmacological aids to relapse prevention, it has the least support for outcome effectiveness, whereas acamprosate has garnered fair evidence of benefit, and naltrexone has a strong evidence base for its effectiveness. Disulfiram can have serious side effects that include hepatotoxicity and depression, further limiting its use in medically ill patients. Although the decision is controversial, the U.S. Food and Drug Administration has determined that due to potential hepatotoxicity, naltrexone is contraindicated for patients with severe hepatic disease; this is not an absolute contraindication, but naltrexone requires careful monitoring when used in the context of existing hepatic compromise. In contrast, acamprosate has no known risk of hepatotoxicity or significant drug interactions, making it a good choice in patients who are medically ill. However, the dosage should be reduced in patients with impaired renal function, and acamprosate should be avoided completely in the presence of renal failure.

Alcohol Overdose

The lethal level of alcohol does not increase as tolerance develops (Mebane 1987). The LD_{50} (defined as a lethal dose in 50% of patients) of alcohol is 500 mg/dL. Signs of life-threatening alcohol overdose are unresponsiveness, slow and shallow breathing, and cardiac dysrhythmia.

Management.   Intubation if respiratory failure appears imminent, aggressive hydration, and other cardiovascular support measures may all be required. Hemodialysis is an option in potentially life-threatening alcohol overdoses.

Alcohol-Induced Psychotic Disorder

A diagnosis of alcohol-induced psychotic disorder requires the presence of psychosis following a history of recent heavy alcohol use (unless the disturbance is accounted for by schizophrenia or a psychotic mood disorder). Auditory hallucinations are more prominent than other withdrawal symptoms, last at least 1 week, and occur while the patient has a clear sensorium.

Management.   When patients develop alcohol-induced psychotic disorder during detoxification, an antipsychotic is typically necessary to control agitation and hallucinations. A conventional agent such as haloperidol offers the advantages of lower cost and more experience in medically ill patients. After symptoms cease, antipsychotics should be discontinued.

Alcohol Withdrawal Seizures

Alcohol withdrawal seizures occur in fewer than 5% of unmedicated patients; individuals with a history of prior brain injury, previous withdrawal seizures, or an existing seizure disorder all incur higher risk. Seizures typically occur 8–36 hours after the last alcohol use, with peak frequency during the second day after cessation of alcohol use. One-third of patients who have withdrawal seizures go on to develop alcohol withdrawal delirium, or delirium tremens (DTs).

Management.   BZDs are the treatment of choice for alcohol withdrawal seizures, but intramuscular administration should be avoided because of variable absorption (lorazepam is an exception). Diazepam, 5–10 mg iv, is an effective choice for immediate seizure control. Some clinicians prefer phenobarbital because its very long half-life provides some protection against withdrawal symptoms even if the patient leaves the hospital before withdrawal has been completed. For underlying seizure disorders, a maintenance anticonvulsant agent is necessary. The most effective way to prevent alcohol withdrawal seizures is to detoxify the patient adequately with appropriate dosages of BZDs. Patients who have histories of alcohol withdrawal seizures warrant particularly close monitoring of serum magnesium, with parenteral replacement if they develop marked hypomagnesemia.

Alcohol Withdrawal Delirium

DTs begin 2–7 days after cessation of drinking. The risk for DTs is highest when the patient has a long history (>10 years) of heavy drinking and a major medical illness, especially liver disease, infection, trauma, poor nutrition, or metabolic disorders. Clinical signs and symptoms of DTs are disorientation, agitation, visual or tactile hallucinations, autonomic hyperactivity, tremor, ataxia, fever, and dilated pupils. Alcohol withdrawal delirium is potentially life threatening. If unrecognized and untreated, mortality can approach 40%; however, the mortality rate for hospitalized patients is less than 5% (Yost 1996). When patients die during DTs, the cause of death is usually heart failure, infection, or traumatic injury.

Management. The management of alcohol withdrawal delirium is similar to that for uncomplicated alcohol withdrawal, except much higher dosages of BZDs are often required, and concomitant antipsychotics are often necessary to adequately control confusion, delusions, hallucinations, or agitation. Administration of thiamine, with careful attention to fluid and electrolyte imbalance, is imperative.

Wernicke-Korsakoff Syndrome

Wernicke-Korsakoff syndrome is rare, occurring in less than 1% of alcohol-dependent individuals, but the consequences can be devastating (Thompson and Marshall 2006). Wernicke's encephalopathy begins with an abrupt onset of truncal ataxia, ophthalmoplegia (usually third nerve palsy), and delirium. Ataxia may precede the delirium, which is marked by lethargy, somnolence, and profound apathy. The clinician should not wait for all three signs; the presence of two suggests Wernicke's encephalopathy. The etiology of the disorder is thiamine deficiency; prompt replacement can begin to reverse ocular symptoms within a few hours and thereby offer confirmation of the diagnosis. Long- and short-term memory impairment (Korsakoff syndrome) usually develops if Wernicke's encephalopathy is unrecognized and goes untreated. In Korsakoff syndrome, memory loss can be profound, but other cognitive functions are relatively spared.

Management.   The patient should be given thiamine, 100 mg/hour iv/im or 500 mg iv three times daily, until ophthalmoplegia begins to resolve, at which point the patient is given thiamine, 100 mg/day parenterally, for at least 7 more days to treat alcohol-induced persisting amnestic disorder. Ocular findings improve first, followed by motor improvement; finally, mental status abnormalities improve if the patient has not developed alcoholic dementia. Although the delirium will almost invariably resolve (one-third in the first week, another one-third in the first month, and the last one-third by 2 months), the amnestic symptoms of Korsakoff syndrome resolve completely in only 25% of patients, with another 25% showing no recovery and the remainder improving somewhat. Thiamine deficiency in alcohol-dependent patients may occur as a direct consequence of alcohol consumption or as a part of the refeeding syndrome that can follow the meager nutritional status of many patients who abuse alcohol (Mehanna et al. 2008).

Suicide

Suicide is the means of death for 1 of every 14 alcoholics (Inskip et al. 1998), and multiple retrospective studies provide an average estimate of prior alcohol abuse or dependence at nearly 50% of those who die by suicide (Conner and Duberstein 2004); one-third of suicide completers had detectable alcohol in their bodies at the time of death (Welte et al. 1988).

Predisposing factors.   Predisposing factors (i.e., persisting vulnerabilities) that reinforce the association of alcoholism and suicide include aggression, impulsivity, hopelessness, negative affect, and severity of alcohol dependence (Conner and Duberstein 2004).

Precipitating factors.   Precipitating factors (i.e., time-limited events or situations) that occur within weeks or months of a suicide and appear to herald junctures of high suicide risk among alcoholics include interpersonal traumatic experiences (especially the threatened or actual loss of a partner or relationship) and depressive episodes (Conner and Duberstein 2004).

Screening Tools

Several brief diagnostic screens are available to assist with diagnosis of alcohol abuse and dependence (Soderstrom et al. 1997). Useful questionnaires and laboratory tests are described.

Questionnaires

However well designed, no survey can yield the contextual perspective provided by an astute interview that focuses on chronic anxiety or dysphoria, past injuries, job loss, financial problems, legal problems, and absenteeism. Nevertheless, several screening instruments are commonly used.

Alcohol Use Disorders Identification Test.   The Alcohol Use Disorders Identification Test (AUDIT) consists of 10 multiple-choice questions regarding the quantity and frequency of a patient's alcohol consumption, drinking behavior, and alcohol-related problems (Reinert and Allen 2007). Although the AUDIT is commonly regarded as the gold standard for screening, not all patients who are acutely ill or otherwise poorly disposed to speaking with a psychiatrist will cooperate with the full AUDIT. The following three-item version, the AUDIT-C, has nearly identical sensitivity to the full AUDIT (Bradley et al. 2007):

1. How often do you have a drink containing alcohol? [Score ranges from 0 (never) to 4 (four or more times per week)]
2. How many drinks containing alcohol do you have on a typical day when you are drinking? [Score ranges from 0 (one or two drinks) to 4 (10 or more drinks)]
3. How often do you have six or more drinks on one occasion? [Score ranges from 0 (never) to 4 (daily or almost daily)]

CAGE screen for diagnosis of alcoholism.   The CAGE screen includes four items, easily recalled using the acronym CAGE. Scores of 2 have a sensitivity of 50% for heavy drinkers and 75% for those with alcohol dependence, and a specificity of about 80% (Schuckit 2009). The examiner begins each of the following questions with "Have you ever…"

C   Thought you should CUT BACK on your drinking?
A   Felt ANNOYED by people criticizing your drinking?
G   Felt GUILTY or bad about your drinking?
E   Had a morning EYE-OPENER to relieve hangover or nerves?

Brief Michigan Alcohol Screening Test.   The Michigan Alcohol Screening Test (MAST) consists of 25 questions answered simply yes or no. The Brief

Michigan Alcohol Screening Test (bMAST) is a shorter, valid 10-item version (Connor et al. 2007).

TWEAK.   A score of 3 or higher on the TWEAK screening questionnaire indicates an alcohol problem (Russell et al. 1996). The acronym TWEAK represents the following questions:

1. Tolerance (2 points): How many drinks can you hold? [≥6 indicates tolerance]
2. Worried (2 points): Does your spouse (or [do your] parents) ever worry or complain about your drinking?
3. Eye openers (1 point): Have you ever had a drink first thing in the morning to steady your nerves or get rid of a hangover?
4. Amnesia (1 point): Have you ever awakened in the morning after some drinking the night before and found that you could not remember a part of the evening before?
5. [K] Cut down (1 point): Have you ever felt you ought to cut down on your drinking?

Single-question screening.   The National Institute on Alcohol Abuse and Alcoholism recommends the following single question to screen for unhealthy alcohol use:

• How many times in the past year have you had X or more drinks in a day? (X = 5 for males and 4 for females)

Any response of 1 or more is regarded as indicative of unhealthy alcohol use (Smith et al. 2009). The single question is about 80% sensitive and specific for detection of unhealthy alcohol use.

Laboratory Tests

Although results from several laboratory tests are highly suggestive of alcohol abuse, no test is diagnostic. The following findings are potentially useful:

• Serum γ-glutamyltransferase is increased in more than half of problem drinkers and in 80% of alcoholic patients with liver dysfunction (Schwan et al. 2004; Trell et al. 1984).

- Carbohydrate-deficient transferrin is likely to increase with sustained heavy drinking (Schuckit et al. 2009).
- Aspartate transaminase (AST) and alanine transaminase (ALT) levels are also increased in heavy drinkers; an AST:ALT ratio of >2 suggests alcoholic hepatitis (Schuckit et al. 2009).
- A very high blood alcohol level (>200 mg/dL) found in a nonintoxicated patient, especially in an emergency department setting, is almost pathognomonic of alcohol dependence (Parker et al. 2008).
- Other laboratory indicators of alcohol abuse include increased uric acid, increased red blood cell mean corpuscular volume, decreased white blood cell and platelet counts, and increased triglycerides.

Sedatives, Hypnotics, and Anxiolytics

All BZDs and sedative-hypnotics induce tolerance to some degree. BZD and barbiturate abuse and dependence may develop secondary to medical use or street abuse. Barbiturates are less frequently abused because their role in anxiolysis has been supplanted by the BZDs, and neurologists now have many other antiepileptic alternatives. Nonetheless, the clinician may encounter butalbital (e.g., in the combination drug Fiorinal) and carisoprodol (e.g., Soma), either of which can precipitate serious difficulties, especially in overdose. Unfortunately, as with alcohol, although the barbiturate dose necessary for intoxication increases with chronic abuse, the lethal dose does not. Whereas the opiate-dependent patient may double the dose and still not experience respiratory depression, barbiturate-addicted patients can develop potentially fatal respiratory depression with a dose only 20%–25% higher than the usual daily dose. BZDs, in contrast, have a much higher LD_{50} than barbiturates. A simple diagnostic aid for abuse or dependence is a positive "shopping bag sign." The psychiatrist asks the patient's family to bring in all the patient's medications. More than one BZD prescription obtained from different physicians and filled at unassociated pharmacies betrays a problem. For managing sedative-hypnotic dependence in medical patients, simplification of medication regimens, agreement that one physician will manage sedative-hypnotic prescriptions, and gradual tapering may suffice. However, not all chronic BZD users are abusing these medications, and these individuals should not be regarded as certain future abusers. Legitimate reasons exist for chronic use of BZDs, and any taper must be accompanied by conscientious assessment for an underlying justifiable clinical indication.

Intoxication

Recognition

Symptoms and signs of intoxication include the following:

- Disinhibition
- Mood lability
- Dysarthria
- Ataxia
- Hyporeflexia
- Nystagmus
- Impaired attention

The symptoms and signs are similar to those of alcohol intoxication. Accidental, iatrogenic, or suicidal overdose may cause respiratory depression. Cross-reactivity occurs between alcohol, BZDs, and sedative-hypnotics.

Management

1. Patient should be monitored closely for respiratory depression.
2. Patient should be moved to intensive care unit if he or she becomes stuporous, hypoxic, or unresponsive.
3. Agitation may be managed with haloperidol administered intravenously or intramuscularly.
4. Flumazenil, a BZD antagonist, can reverse coma in a BZD overdose but requires careful titration in a BZD-dependent patient to avoid inducing seizures.

Withdrawal

Recognition

Symptoms and signs of withdrawal include the following:

- Nausea
- Tremor
- Hyperreflexia
- Hyperphagia

- Tachycardia
- Dilated pupils
- Diaphoresis
- Irritability
- Insomnia
- Restlessness
- Anxiety

Fever, autonomic hyperactivity, seizures, and delirium can occur in severe cases. The features of sedative, hypnotic, or anxiolytic withdrawal are similar to those of alcohol withdrawal and can be life threatening. The time of onset and the duration of sedative-hypnotic withdrawal vary with the half-life of the drugs; withdrawal is sometimes missed in hospitalized patients because of a low index of suspicion or because symptoms can occur 7–10 days after admission with a drug that has a long half-life.

Management

1. Baseline dosage should be established. (The dosage may be higher than patient has acknowledged.)
2. If agent has a short half-life (e.g., alprazolam), patient should be switched to a long-half-life alternative (e.g., clonazepam or diazepam).
3. Average daily dosage should be administered for 2 days; then taper should begin.
4. The rate of taper varies with collateral factors but should not exceed 10% per day (Franklin et al. 2002).

Potential Complications

Long- and short-term memory impairment may occur after prolonged, heavy use of a sedative-hypnotic agent. This disorder, termed *sedative-, hypnotic-, or anxiolytic-induced persisting amnestic disorder,* usually reverses gradually if abstinence is achieved.

Opiates

Narcotics are used to relieve pain, cough, diarrhea, agitation, and severe anxiety for patients in the intensive care unit. Unfortunately, tolerance begins within days, compromising potential effectiveness in long-term treatment. Nonetheless, 20% of patients with chronic pain also use opiates regularly (Chabal et al. 1997). Psychiatrists are often consulted to examine patients in pain who do not appear to respond to an "adequate" narcotic regimen, or to evaluate a patient's perceived overuse of narcotics. In the course of such consultations, underuse rather than abuse of narcotic analgesics is often found. Additionally, more than 90% of opiate-addicted patients have at least one other psychiatric disorder, most commonly depression, alcoholism, or antisocial personality disorder (Khantzian and Treece 1985).

Intoxication

Recognition

Symptoms and signs of opiate intoxication include the following:

- Apathy
- Dysphoria or euphoria
- Psychomotor retardation
- Drowsiness
- Dysarthria
- Pinpoint pupils (except with meperidine)

In severe cases, respiratory depression, stupor, or coma can occur; nystagmus is rare. Clinicians should suspect an opiate overdose in any patient who presents in a coma, especially when accompanied by respiratory depression and pupillary constriction.

Management

1. Patient should be monitored for respiratory depression, pulmonary edema, and seizures.
2. Patient should be given naloxone 0.4 mg iv every 3–5 minutes until symptoms clear. Naloxone has a short duration of action relative to almost every opiate.
3. After stabilization and acute detoxification, patient should be referred for treatment.

4. Methadone programs achieve higher success and retention rates than programs that require abstinence.

Withdrawal

Recognition

Narcotic or opioid withdrawal is uncomfortable but rarely life threatening. Classic features include pupillary dilation, yawning, piloerection, rhinorrhea, nausea, fever, hypertension, tachycardia, cramps, drug craving, insomnia, restlessness, irritability, and seizures. The presentation and course of symptoms in opioid withdrawal vary with the half-life of the agent and the patient's hepatic status; untreated symptoms can last 2–4 weeks in patients dependent on methadone.

Management

1. Baseline dosage needs to be established. Because dosage may be higher or lower than patient has acknowledged, withdrawal needs to be gauged through assessment of objective markers such as heart rate, respiratory rate, and pupillary size.
2. If agent of abuse has a short half-life, patient needs to be switched to a long-half-life alternative.
3. Average daily equivalent dosage should be administered for 2 days; then taper should begin.
4. Rate of taper varies with collateral factors but should not exceed 10% per day.
5. Established methadone-maintenance patients should be maintained on usual daily oral dosage, as confirmed by outpatient program staff.
6. Buprenorphine may be dispensed only by qualified physicians who have completed advanced mandatory training and is available only in selected settings.

Amphetamines

Amphetamines block the reuptake of dopamine, serotonin, and norepinephrine and profoundly affect dopamine storage release. Amphetamines are especially abused by night workers, students, dieters, persons who work long hours, and persons who are chronically dysphoric. Legitimate medical uses of amphetamines include treatment of depression, attention-deficit/hyperactivity disorder, fatigue in multiple sclerosis, and narcolepsy; typical dosages range from 5 to ≥50 mg/day. On the street, daily doses often reach 100 mg or more. Higher doses can cause psychosis or delirium. Repeated use leads to postintoxication depression, which can perpetuate further abuse. The clinician should obtain a toxicology screen because polydrug abuse is common. Poor nutrition may lead to anemia.

Intoxication

Recognition

The following are symptoms and signs of mild amphetamine intoxication:

- Euphoria
- Heightened self-esteem
- Grandiosity
- Anxiety
- Suspiciousness
- Miosis
- Tachycardia
- Nausea
- Perspiration
- Hypertension
- Restlessness

More severe intoxication leads to paranoia, hypervigilance, hallucinations, agitation, delirium, arrhythmias, and convulsions.

Management

1. Staff should try to defuse the tension by talking to the patient.
2. Urine should be acidified with vitamin C to speed elimination.
3. Patient should be observed for dysrhythmias, hypertension, fever, and seizures.
4. Staff should remain alert for violent or suicidal ideation and behavior.

5. Patient should be given lorazepam 2–4 mg iv/im every 2 hours for severe anxiety or agitation.
6. A toxicology screen should be done to assess for other drug use.
7. Disruptive paranoia or delusions warrant antipsychotic use.

Withdrawal

Recognition

When amphetamines are abruptly discontinued, various treatable postintoxication findings can occur:

- Depression (especially if the patient has prior existing risk for depression)
- Irritability
- Anxiety
- Fatigue
- Insomnia or hypersomnia
- Drug craving
- Psychomotor agitation
- Hyperphagia

Management

1. Acute management strategies for amphetamine withdrawal are the same as for intoxication.
2. Patient should be watched for potential emergence of acute rebound depression.
3. Patient should be watched for suicidal and drug-seeking behavior.
4. The consultant should not reinitiate amphetamine to ameliorate withdrawal symptoms.

Potential Complications

Amphetamine Intoxication Delirium

Amphetamine intoxication delirium, or an agitated confusional state, may develop within 24 hours of amphetamine use. Hallucinations, delusions, and signs of autonomic hyperactivity are frequently present.

Management.   Management of amphetamine intoxication delirium mirrors the approach to amphetamine intoxication, with one important exception: instead of verbal efforts to calm the patient, an antipsychotic should be administered.

Amphetamine-Induced Psychotic Disorder

Amphetamine-induced psychotic disorder can last several days in a patient with a clear sensorium. Amphetamine psychosis resembles acute paranoid schizophrenia.

Management.   Management of amphetamine-induced psychotic disorder is the same as for amphetamine intoxication delirium.

Street Names for Amphetamines

Street names for amphetamines include black beauties, crank, crystals, cat, ice, meth, pep pills, smart drug, speed, and uppers. Street names for 3,4-methylenedioxymethamphetamine (MDMA, commonly called ecstasy) include Adam, E, lollies, love drug, smarties, vitamin E, and XTC (Erickson et al. 2007).

Cocaine

Cocaine blocks the reuptake of neuronal dopamine, serotonin, and norepinephrine. Cocaine has a fairly specific activating effect on mesocortical and mesolimbic dopaminergic pathways. Dopamine is an important neurotransmitter in limbic pleasure centers, including those related to food and sexual activity. A patient's inability to control cocaine intake is probably related to the highly rewarding properties of the drug. With repeated cocaine use, tolerance develops secondary to decreased reuptake inhibition and altered receptor sensitivity. Cocaine also causes cortical kindling (Halikas et al. 1991), the process by which brief bursts of central nervous system stimulation at regular intervals result in lasting changes in brain excitability. Limbic areas of the brain are uniquely sensitive to kindling. The chronic cocaine user may have severe financial problems because of the large amounts of the drug needed to "chase another high" or stave off the cocaine "crash." When a patient who abuses cocaine is admitted to the hospital, the staff should watch for drug-seeking behavior, depression, suicidal behavior, and insomnia. A toxicology screen can help make the diagnosis (but may be negative if the patient last used cocaine 36 hours before) and rule out potential contributions by other drugs of abuse. After the patient is medically stabilized, he or she should be referred for treatment. Inpatient drug rehabilitation is indicated if outpatient treatment has failed, the patient is unmotivated, concurrent psychiatric illness is present, or a complicating psychosocial situation exists.

Intoxication

Recognition

Features of cocaine intoxication vary but may include the following:

- Euphoria
- Grandiosity
- Hypervigilance
- Increased libido
- Psychomotor agitation
- Tachycardia
- Miosis
- Hypertension
- Perspiration
- Nausea
- Delirium
- Hallucinations

Sudden death has been reported with acute cocaine intoxication; death usually is the result of cardiac arrest or ventricular fibrillation. Cocaine binges can last a few hours to several days. Tolerance to the euphoric effects develops rapidly during the course of a binge.

Management

1. Presence of family or friends may suffice for the acute phase.
2. Lorazepam 2–4 mg iv/im should be administered every 2 hours for severe anxiety or agitation.
3. Patient should be observed for dysrhythmias, psychosis, and precipitous suicidality.

4. Cardiac monitoring and prompt access to airway support are necessary only for 4–6 hours because cocaine is rapidly metabolized and acute, life-threatening levels decline rapidly; use of beta-blockers is controversial due to the risk of consequent unopposed alpha activity by cocaine.
5. Prolonged cocaine use is often followed by severe dysphoria.
6. If dysphoria persists, safety may require inpatient psychiatric care.

Withdrawal

Recognition

Although abrupt discontinuation of cocaine is medically safe, postintoxication sequelae can occur after prolonged use. For most patients, the worst dysphoria and craving occur in the first day of abstinence. However, profound dysphoria may last 2 weeks or longer, typically accompanied by strong drug craving and insomnia. After several weeks of improvement, the patient may experience a second period of craving and depression, which resolves slowly over weeks to months (Gawin and Kleber 1986). Episodic craving, often triggered in response to environmental stimuli, can continue indefinitely.

Management

When a patient accustomed to chronic cocaine abuse is obliged to withdraw because he or she is hospitalized for other medical or surgical reasons, the psychiatric consultant should advise the primary team of the phases of abstinence and watch for suicidal and drug-seeking behavior. If persistent dysphoria and associated symptoms meet criteria for major depression, antidepressant therapy is indicated.

Potential Complications

Cocaine Intoxication Delirium

Cocaine intoxication delirium, an agitated confusional state, may appear within 24 hours of cocaine use.

Management.   Management of cocaine intoxication delirium requires obtaining a toxicology screen, monitoring for seizures and dysrhythmias, and proactively treating escalating anxiety and agitation with parenteral lorazepam. Because violence is common, prompt access to antipsychotics, ample security support, and physical restraints may be necessary.

Cocaine-Induced Psychotic Disorder

Paranoid delusions can appear shortly after cocaine use. Unlike the confusional state, psychosis is often prolonged, lasting weeks or months in an occasional patient.

Management. Psychiatric hospitalization is often required at the outset, and ongoing scheduled antipsychotic medication is commonly necessary until the psychotic symptoms dissipate entirely.

Street Names for Cocaine

Street names for cocaine include all-American drug, coke, crack, girl, mother of pearl, nose candy, Peruvian powder, snow, toot, and white lady (Erickson et al. 2007).

References

American Psychiatric Association: Diagnostic and Statistical Manual of Mental Disorders, 4th Edition, Text Revision. Washington, DC, American Psychiatric Association, 2000

Blondell RD: Ambulatory detoxification of patients with alcohol dependence. Am Fam Physician 71:495–502, 2005

Bradley KA, DeBenedetti AF, Volk RJ, et al: AUDIT-C as a brief screen for alcohol misuse in primary care. Alcohol Clin Exp Res 31:1208–1217, 2007

Chabal C, Erjavec MK, Jacobson L, et al: Prescription opiate abuse in chronic pain patients: clinical criteria, incidence and predictors. Clin J Pain 13:150–155, 1997

Conner KR, Duberstein PR: Predisposing and precipitating factors for suicide among alcoholics: empirical review and conceptual integration. Alcohol Clin Exp Res 28:6S–17S, 2004

Connor JP, Grier M, Feeney GF, et al: The validity of the Brief Michigan Alcohol Screening Test (bMAST) as a problem drinking severity measure. J Stud Alcohol Drugs 68:771–779, 2007

Curtis JR, Geller G, Stokes EG, et al: Characteristics, diagnosis, and treatment of alcoholism in elderly patients. J Am Geriatr Soc 37:310–316, 1989

Erickson TB, Thompson TM, Lu JJ: The approach to the patient with an unknown overdose. Emerg Med Clin North Am 25:249–281, 2007

Franklin JE Jr, Leamon MH, Frances RJ: Substance-related disorders, in The American Psychiatric Publishing Textbook of Consultation-Liaison Psychiatry: Psychiatry in the Medically Ill, 2nd Edition. Edited by Wise MG, Rundell JR. Washington, DC, American Psychiatric Publishing, 2002, pp 417–453

Gawin FH, Kleber HD: Abstinence symptomatology and psychiatric diagnosis in cocaine abusers. Arch Gen Psychiatry 43:107–113, 1986

Gerke P, Hapke U, Rumpf HJ, et al: Alcohol-related diseases in general hospital patients. Alcohol Alcohol 32:179–184, 1997

Halikas JA, Crosby RD, Carlson GA, et al: Cocaine reduction in unmotivated crack users using carbamazepine versus placebo in a short term, double-blind crossover design. Clin Pharmacol Ther 50:81–95, 1991

Hasin DS, Stinson FS, Ogburn E, et al: Prevalence, correlates, disability, and comorbidity of DSM-IV alcohol abuse and dependence in the United States. Arch Gen Psychiatry 64:830–842, 2007

Inskip HM, Harris EC, Barraclough B: Lifetime risk of suicide for affective disorder, alcoholism and schizophrenia. Br J Psychiatry 172:35–37, 1998

Jaeger TM, Lohr RH, Pankratz VS: Symptom-triggered therapy for alcohol withdrawal syndrome in medical inpatients. Mayo Clin Proc 76:695–701, 2001

Katz A, Goldberg D, Smith J, et al: Tobacco, alcohol, and drug use among hospital patients: concurrent use and willingness to change. J Hosp Med 3:369–375, 2008

Khantzian IF, Treece C: DSM-III psychiatric diagnoses of narcotic addicts. Arch Gen Psychiatry 42:1067–1071, 1985

McKeon A, Frye MA, Delanty N: The alcohol withdrawal syndrome. J Neurol Neurosurg Psychiatry 79:854–862, 2008

Mebane AH: Drug abuse issues in critically ill patients, in Problems in Critical Care. Edited by Wise MG. Philadelphia, PA, JB Lippincott, 1987, pp 623–685

Mehanna JM, Moledina J, Travis J: Refeeding syndrome: what it is and how to treat it. BMJ 336:1495–1498, 2008

Moos RF, Moos BS: Rates and predictors of relapse after natural and treated remission from alcohol use disorders. Addiction 101:212–222, 2006

Parker AJR, Marshall EJ, Ball DM: Diagnosis and management of alcohol use disorders. BMJ 336:496–501, 2008

Reinert DF, Allen JP: The Alcohol Use Disorders Identification Test: an update of research findings. Alcohol Clin Exp Res 31:185–199, 2007

Rumpf HJ, Bischof G, Hapke U, et al: Stability of remission from alcohol dependence without formal help. Alcohol Alcohol 41:311–314, 2006

Russell M, Martier SS, Sokol RJ, et al: Detecting risk drinking during pregnancy: a comparison of four screening questionnaires. Am J Public Health 86:1435–1439, 1996

Saitz R: Clinical practice: unhealthy alcohol use. N Engl J Med 352:596–607, 2005

Schuckit MA: Drug and Alcohol Abuse: A Clinical Guide to Diagnosis and Treatment, 6th Edition. New York, Springer, 2006

Schuckit MA: Alcohol use disorders. Lancet 373:492–501, 2009

Schwan R, Albuisson E, Malet L, et al: The use of biological laboratory markers in the diagnosis of alcohol misuse: an evidence-based approach. Drug Alcohol Depend 74:273–279, 2004

Self D: Drug dependence and addiction: neural substrates. Am J Psychiatry 161:223, 2004

Seppa K, Makela R: Heavy drinking in hospital patients. Addiction 88:1377–1382, 1993

Smith PC, Schmidt SM, Allensworth-Davies D, et al: Primary care validation of a single-question alcohol screening test. J Gen Intern Med 24:783–788, 2009

Soderstrom CA, Smith GS, Kufera JA, et al: The accuracy of the CAGE, the Brief Michigan Alcoholism Screening Test, and the Alcohol Use Disorder Identification Test in screening trauma center patients for alcoholism. J Trauma 43:962–969, 1997

Sullivan JT, Sykora K, Schneiderman J, et al: Assessment of alcohol withdrawal: the revised Clinical Institute Withdrawal Assessment for Alcohol (CIWA-Ar) scale. Br J Addict 84:1353–1357, 1989

Thompson AD, Marshall EJ: The natural history and pathophysiology of Wernicke's encephalopathy and Korsakoff's psychosis. Alcohol Alcohol 41:151–158, 2006

Trell E, Kristenson H, Fex G: Alcohol-related problems in middle-aged men with elevated serum gamma-glutamyltransferase: a preventive medical investigation. J Stud Alcohol 45:302–309, 1984

Welte JW, Abel EL, Wieczorek W: The role of alcohol in suicides in Erie County, NY 1972–1984. Public Health Rep 103:648–652, 1988

Williams D, Lewis J, McBride A: A comparison of rating scales for the alcohol withdrawal syndrome. Alcohol Alcohol 36:104–108, 2001

Yates WR: Epidemiology of psychiatric disorders in medically ill patients, in The American Psychiatric Publishing Textbook of Consultation-Liaison Psychiatry: Psychiatry in the Medically Ill, 2nd Edition. Edited by Wise MG, Rundell JR. Washington, DC, American Psychiatric Publishing, 2002, pp 237–256

Yost DA: Alcohol withdrawal syndrome. Am Fam Physician 54:657–664, 1996

PART III

Treatments

14

Biological Treatments

A medically ill patient almost always receives medications. The patient's well-being is already threatened by the medical illness, and the patient's health should not be further compromised by medication-related adverse events. Therefore, appropriate use of biological treatments in patients who are medically ill requires careful consideration of the underlying medical illness, potential alterations to pharmacokinetics, and drug-drug interactions.

Adherence to Pharmacological Treatment

Therapeutic Alliance

Developing a therapeutic alliance with the patient during the consultation and follow-up is fundamental to achieving the best possible outcome. The patient has beliefs about psychiatric medications that must be explored and clarified. Many patients are affected by feelings of failure about needing a medication, fear of addiction, magical hopes for cure, and transference toward the physician. A discussion that includes the patient as a partner facilitates formation of the doctor-patient alliance.

Education About the Medication

Patients benefit from education about medication. An integral part of this process includes a realistic discussion of potential adverse effects, proper administration of the medication, expected time to response, and guidelines for missed doses. Discussions such as these have been found to improve patients' attitudes toward medication, increase confidence that the side effects can be managed, and improve adherence (Lin et al. 2003). Table 14–1 includes medication principles to improve patient care and adherence.

Pharmacokinetics in Medically Ill Patients

Absorption

Orally administered drugs absorbed through the gastrointestinal tract may be altered by first-pass hepatic metabolism before entering the systemic circulation. Sublingual or topical administration of drugs decreases the first-pass effect, and rectal administration may reduce first-pass effect by 50%. Parenteral administration generally results in rapid effects, but it is difficult to carry out in adults, especially elderly patients, and the erratic absorption of some medications given intramuscularly makes their clinical benefits less predictable. Absorption may be affected by gastrointestinal diseases that result in changes in gastric pH, rate of gastric emptying, or dysfunction or resection of the small intestine. Liquid formulations may be better or more quickly absorbed than solid drug preparations in patients with gastrointestinal disease. In patients with renal disease, the alkalinizing effects of excess urea may increase absorption of psychotropic medications, but due to other physiological changes in uremia, the effect is unpredictable. Absorption of drugs through the gastrointestinal tract may be decreased in patients with congestive heart failure (Robinson and Owen 2005).

Drug Distribution

With the exception of lithium, psychotropic medications are lipophilic and drawn to fatty tissues. Thus, psychotropic medications generally have large volumes of distribution. As a person ages, the water content of the body decreases and the fat content rises, so the distribution volume of hydrophilic

Table 14–1. Medication principles in the psychosomatic medicine setting

Review all medications the patient is taking, including herbal and over-the-counter medications.

Keep the medication regimen simple. Whenever possible, use only one medication to treat a symptom or disorder.

Educate the patient about the medication. A therapeutic alliance is your best guarantee of adherence.

Monitor target symptoms and side effects closely when starting a medication.

Remember that discontinuing a medication is often a valuable intervention, especially when an elderly patient is taking multiple medications.

Avoid prescribing medications on an as-needed basis, particularly in patients with pain, withdrawal syndromes, and delirium.

When as-needed medication dosing is required, monitor frequency of use to determine a standing dosage.

Change one medication at a time, and use the minimum dose necessary to obtain the desired response.

Treat prophylactically if a clear rationale exists (e.g., can give benztropine to avoid a dystonic reaction from antipsychotics in an anxious young man with first-break psychosis).

Use a medication that was previously effective for the patient or a family member who had the same disorder.

If treatment fails, reexamine your diagnosis. Always reconsider the possibility of occult substance abuse.

Note that serum drug levels are not a certification of efficacy or toxicity.

Be aware that generic drugs are cost-effective, but bioavailability can vary.

Recognize that social and characterological issues strongly influence treatment acceptance and adherence.

Remember that each patient is unique.

Source. Reprinted from Fait ML, Wise MG, Jachna JS, et al.: "Psychopharmacology," in *The American Psychiatric Publishing Textbook of Consultation-Liaison Psychiatry: Psychiatry in the Medically Ill,* 2nd Edition. Edited by Wise MG, Rundell JR. Washington, DC, American Psychiatric Publishing, 2002, pp 939–987. Used with permission.

compounds is reduced in elderly patients, whereas that of lipophilic drugs is increased. In addition, most psychiatric medications are bound to plasma proteins, such as albumin and glycoproteins. When medication is bound to proteins, it is not available for biological activity, such as occupying receptors in the brain (Fait et al. 2002). Protein binding also complicates removal of toxic levels of medications (e.g., by dialysis). The frequency of drug administration is estimated by the length of its half-life. A steady-state drug level is generally achieved after four to five half-lives of a drug.

Drug Metabolism

Hepatic Metabolism

When absorbed drugs first pass through the liver before entering the systemic circulation, liver enzymes act on them; the metabolites produced may be psychopharmacologically active or inert. Once in the liver, a medication, whether on a first or a subsequent pass, is exposed to two main groups of metabolizing enzymes.

- *Phase I metabolism* includes oxidation, reduction, and hydrolysis reactions, although the oxidative process, which occurs via the monooxygenase or cytochrome P450 (CYP) enzyme system, is most relevant to psychiatric medications.
- *Phase II metabolism* consists of many conjugation pathways, the most common being glucuronidation; the medication or its metabolites are coupled with polar groups to form more easily excreted (i.e., more hydrophilic) compounds.

Most psychotropic drugs are metabolized primarily in the liver, so hepatic insufficiency reduces their clearance. Hepatic clearance of the drug may be influenced by either the rate of delivery of the drug to the hepatic metabolizing enzymes or by the intrinsic capacity of the enzymes to metabolize the substrate.

Cytochrome P450 System

Four CYP isoenzymes—CYP1A2, CYP2C (2C9/2C19), CYP2D6, and CYP3A3/4—are especially important in the oxidative metabolism of medications. Many genetic polymorphisms exist in the CYP isoenzymes and are seen in a significant portion of the population. These genetic alterations may contribute to either diminished metabolism, lack of metabolism, or excessive metabolism of a compound. This genetic variability may explain some individual sensitivity to specific drugs or failure to respond to others. Table 14–2 lists some of the more common interactions among these enzymes and medications. Medications are often metabolized by a particular enzyme, can compete for metabolism with other substrates, or can inhibit an enzyme without being metabolized by it. Hepatic enzyme inhibition slows metabolism (i.e., increases the half-life) and increases the concentration and potential toxicity of psychotropic and other drugs affected.

Drug Elimination

Nearly all psychotropic drugs are metabolized by the liver and eliminated in bile, which is then excreted in feces. Some medications are metabolized to active compounds that are excreted in the urine. (Specific drugs and their use in patients with renal and liver failure are described later in this chapter under "Psychotropic Use in Renal Disease" and "Psychotropic Use in Liver Disease," respectively.) Drug excretion via the kidneys declines with age; therefore, elderly patients may need dose adjustments (Turnheim 2003). Creatinine clearance is a more reliable indicator of renal function than serum creatinine.

Drug Interactions

Recognizing drug interactions is a crucial part of consultation work (see Table 14–2). The effect of one drug on another can be *pharmacokinetic* (i.e., affecting the absorption, distribution, biotransformation, and excretion of the other drug) or *pharmacodynamic* (i.e., changing the effect of the drug at its point of action) (Fait et al. 2002). The clinician should obtain a complete medication list, including medications recently discontinued, over-the-counter medications used, and herbal or other alternative drug preparations used. The clinician should also ask a family member to bring in all medications from the patient's house.

Table 14–2. Cytochrome P450 (CYP)–drug interactions

	Substrates	Inhibitors	Inducers
CYP1A2			
Psychotropic	Caffeine Clozapine Duloxetine Haloperidol Olanzapine Propranolol Tertiary-amine TCAs (amitriptyline, imipramine)	Fluoxetine Fluvoxamine	Caffeine Carbamazepine Tobacco Modafinil
Nonpsychotropic	Cyclobenzaprine Propranolol Tamoxifen Theophylline Verapamil Warfarin	Cimetidine Ciprofloxacin Erythromycin Ketoconazole Grapefruit juice Isoniazid	Charbroiled foods Cruciferous vegetables Lansoprazole Omeprazole Phenobarbital Phenytoin Rifampin
CYP2C (2C9/2C19)			
Psychotropic	Barbiturates Cannabinoids Diazepam Propranolol Tertiary-amine TCAs	Fluoxetine Fluvoxamine Modafinil Tranylcypromine	Carbamazepine St. John's wort Valproate

Table 14–2. Cytochrome P450 (CYP)–drug interactions *(continued)*

	Substrates	Inhibitors	Inducers
CYP2C (2C9/2C19) *(continued)*			
Nonpsychotropic	Lansoprazole	Cimetidine	Phenobarbital
	NSAIDs	Fluconazole	Phenytoin
	Omeprazole	Miconazole	Rifampin
	Oral hypoglycemics	Omeprazole	
	Losartan	Phenylbutazone	
	Phenytoin	Simvastatin	
	Propranolol	Sulfonamides	
	Tamoxifen	Ticlopidine	
	Tolbutamide		
	Valsartan		
	Warfarin		
CYP2D6			
Psychotropic	Clozapine	Atomoxetine	Not induced
	Duloxetine	Bupropion	
	Haloperidol[a]	Duloxetine	
	Olanzapine	Fluoxetine	
	Paroxetine	Fluphenazine	
	Phenothiazines[b]	Fluvoxamine	
	Risperidone	Haloperidol	
	TCAs	Methylphenidate[c]	
	Trazodone	Norfluoxetine	
	Venlafaxine	Paroxetine	
		Phenothiazines[b]	
		Sertraline	
		TCAs	

Table 14–2.   Cytochrome P450 (CYP)–drug interactions
(continued)

	Substrates	Inhibitors	Inducers
CYP2D6 *(continued)*			

Nonpsychotropic	Beta-blockers
	Cyclobenzaprine
	Codeine
	Hydrocodone
	Oxycodone
	Type 1C
	  antiarrhythmics
	  (flecainide,
	  propafenone)
		Amiodarone
		Cimetidine
		Quinidine[d]	

CYP3A3/4			
Psychotropic	Alprazolam Aripiprazole Bupropion Buspirone Caffeine Cannabinoids Clonazepam Fluoxetine Carbamazepine Clozapine Midazolam Modafinil Quetiapine Sertraline Tertiary-amine TCAs Triazolam Venlafaxine Ziprasidone	Cannabinoids Fluoxetine Fluvoxamine Norfluoxetine Sertraline	Carbamazepine Modafinil St. John's wort

Table 14–2. Cytochrome P450 (CYP)–drug interactions *(continued)*

	Substrates	Inhibitors	Inducers
CYP3A3/4 *(continued)*			
Nonpsychotropic	Anticancer drugs	Amiodarone	Dexamethasone
	Antiretroviral agents	Cimetidine	Isoniazid
	Astemizole	Ciprofloxacin	Phenobarbital
	Calcium channel	Cyclosporine	Phenytoin
	blockers	Diltiazem	Primidone
	Cisapride	Erythromycin[d]	Rifabutin
	Cyclosporine	Fluconazole	Rifampin
	Cyclobenzaprine	Grapefruit juice	
	Erythromycin	Itraconazole[d]	
	HMG-CoA reductase	Ketoconazole[d]	
	inhibitors	Miconazole	
	Itraconazole	Protease inhibitors	
	Ketoconazole		
	Lidocaine		
	Omeprazole		
	Tamoxifen		
	Quinidine		
	Steroids		
	Warfarin		

Note. Table includes both in vivo and in vitro data. Tricyclic antidepressants (TCAs) are metabolized by CYP2D6, CYP3A, CYP2C, and CYP1A2. HMG-CoA=3-hydroxy-3-methylglutaryl-coenzyme A; NSAIDs=nonsteroidal anti-inflammatory drugs.
[a]Complex interaction.
[b]Phenothiazines include chlorpromazine, prochlorperazine, perphenazine, trifluoperazine, fluphenazine, thioridazine, and mesoridazine.
[c]Methylphenidate likely has CYP effects, but particular isoenzymes have not been identified.
[d]Extraordinarily powerful inhibitors of CYP enzymes, sometimes referred to as "killers."
Source. Reprinted from Robinson MJ, Owen JA: "Psychopharmacology," in *The American Psychiatric Publishing Textbook of Psychosomatic Medicine.* Edited by Levenson JL. Washington, DC, American Psychiatric Publishing, 2005, pp. 871–922.

Serotonin Syndrome

Non-Idiopathic Drug Reaction

In contrast to neuroleptic malignant syndrome (NMS), serotonin syndrome is not an idiosyncratic drug reaction and is generally dose related. Therefore, the risk factors for serotonin syndrome are pharmacologically related, although constitutional factors may alter the threshold. Table 14–3 lists the most common drugs associated with serotonin syndrome.

Table 14–3.   Drugs associated with serotonin syndrome

Selective serotonin reuptake inhibitors: citalopram, escitalopram, fluoxetine, fluvoxamine, paroxetine, sertraline

Tricyclic antidepressants: amitriptyline, desipramine, doxepin, imipramine, maprotiline, nortriptyline, protriptyline, trimipramine

Monoamine oxidase inhibitors: phenelzine, tranylcypromine, isocarboxazid

Serotonin-norepinephrine reuptake inhibitors: venlafaxine, desvenlafaxine, duloxetine, milnacipran

Other antidepressants: bupropion, mirtazapine, trazodone

Anxiolytic: buspirone

Mood stabilizer: lithium

Herbal products: St. John's wort (*Hypericum perforatum*), tryptophan, ginseng

Amphetamines and amphetamine derivatives

L-Dopa

Drugs of abuse: cocaine, methylenedioxymethamphetamine (MDMA), lysergic acid diethylamide (LSD), Syrian rue

Analgesics: fentanyl, tramadol, meperidine

Antimigraine drugs: triptans

Antiemetic agents: ondansetron, metoclopramide, granisetron

Over-the-counter cold remedies: dextromethorphan

Antibiotics: linezolid (monoamine oxidase inhibitor)

Bariatric medications: sibutramine

Spectrum of Findings

Clinical manifestations of serotonin syndrome range from barely perceptible to fatal (Figure 14–1).

Clinical Triad

Manifestations of serotonin syndrome are described in a clinical triad: mental status changes, autonomic hyperactivity, and neuromuscular abnormalities. Findings, however, are not consistent across patients.

Mental Status Changes

Changes in mental status range from mild restlessness to elevated mood and agitated delirium. Progression to coma may occur in severe cases.

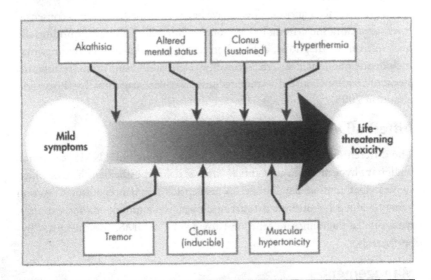

Figure 14–1.   Serotonin syndrome: spectrum of clinical findings.

Manifestations of serotonin syndrome range from mild to life-threatening. The vertical arrows suggest the approximate point at which clinical findings initially appear in the spectrum of the disease, but all findings may not be consistently present in a single patient with serotonin syndrome. Severe signs may mask other clinical findings. For example, muscular hypertonicity can overwhelm tremor and hyperreflexia.

Source.   Reprinted from Boyer EW, Shannon M: "The Serotonin Syndrome." *New England Journal of Medicine* 352:1113, 2005. Used with permission.

Autonomic Hyperactivity

Vital sign abnormalities include tachycardia in mild to moderate cases, and hypertension or hypotension and hyperthermia in severe cases. Physical examination reveals diaphoresis, mydriasis, hyperactive bowel sounds, and shivering. Symptoms of diarrhea and nausea are also common.

Neuromuscular Abnormalities

Neuromuscular abnormalities include tremor, hyperreflexia, clonus (inducible, spontaneous, and ocular), and muscular rigidity, which are often more pronounced in the lower extremities than in the upper extremities.

Diagnosis

Although several diagnostic criteria have been developed, no formal consensus exists regarding the criteria for serotonin syndrome. Laboratory findings do not confirm the diagnosis, although in severe cases, laboratory findings may include metabolic acidosis, rhabdomyolysis, elevated serum aminotransferase, elevated creatinine, and disseminated intravascular coagulopathy (Boyer and Shannon 2005).

Differential Diagnosis

The differential diagnosis for serotonin syndrome includes NMS, catatonia, malignant hyperthermia, and anticholinergic delirium (the first three of which are described in more detail in the "Neuroleptic Malignant Syndrome" section below). Table 14–4 outlines the varying clinical presentations among serotonin syndrome, anticholinergic delirium ("toxidrome"), NMS, and malignant hyperthermia.

Management

Serotonin syndrome is usually self-limited and resolves after discontinuation of the offending agents. The consulting psychiatrist should do the following:

1. Provide necessary supportive care.
2. Discontinue serotonergic agents.
3. Consider administration of antiserotonergic agents. Cyproheptadine has been recommended, but its efficacy has not been established.

4. Control agitation with benzodiazepines and avoid physical restraints to minimize muscle contractions that are associated with lactic acidosis and hyperthermia.
5. Evaluate the need for psychopharmacological therapy before restarting drug therapy. Limited data have been reported on drug rechallenge in patients who have developed serotonin syndrome (Boyer and Shannon 2005).

Neuroleptic Malignant Syndrome

Idiopathic Drug Reaction

In contrast to serotonin syndrome, NMS is an idiopathic drug reaction possibly caused by a decrease in central nervous system (CNS) dopamine activity, but this theory has not been proven. Incidence rates as high as 3% have been reported, but more recent data suggest an incidence of 0.01%–0.02% (Stubner et al. 2004). The decreased frequency likely reflects better awareness of the disorder and perhaps also a shift from use of typical to use of atypical antipsychotics (Strawn et al. 2007). Although antipsychotics that are potent dopamine blockers have generally been implicated, atypical antipsychotics are also known to cause NMS. Nonpsychotropic medications such as metoclopramide, droperidol, and promethazine may also cause NMS. An identical syndrome has been reported after abrupt discontinuation of dopamine agonists in patients with Parkinson's disease.

Risk Factors

Clinical, systemic, and metabolic factors have been associated with an increased risk of NMS. Dehydration and conditions that promote dehydration, such as poor oral intake, agitation, and fever, heighten risk (Levenson 1985). Underlying brain abnormalities, concomitant use of lithium, and parenteral administration or rapid dose escalation of antipsychotic medication also correlate with NMS (Berardi et al. 1998; Pelonero et al. 1998; Smith et al. 2008).

Time Course

NMS most often develops over several days, and the majority of cases present within 1 week from the initiation of an antipsychotic. NMS is less likely to de-

Table 14–4. Characteristics of serotonin syndrome and related clinical conditions

	Serotonin syndrome	Anticholinergic "toxidrome"	Neuroleptic malignant syndrome	Malignant hyperthermia
Medication history	Proserotonergic drug	Anticholinergic agent	Dopamine antagonist	Inhalational anesthesia
Time needed for condition to develop	<12 hours	<12 hours	1–3 days	30 minutes to 24 hours after administration of inhalational anesthesia or succinylcholine
Vital signs	Hypertension, tachycardia, tachypnea, hyperthermia (>41.1°C)	Hypertension (mild), tachycardia, tachypnea, hyperthermia (typically 38.8°C or less)	Hypertension, tachycardia, tachypnea, hyperthermia (>41.1°C)	Hypertension, tachycardia, tachypnea, hyperthermia (can be as high as 46.0°C)
Pupils	Mydriasis	Mydriasis	Normal	Normal
Mucosa	Sialorrhea	Dry	Sialorrhea	Normal
Skin	Diaphoresis	Erythema, hot and dry to touch	Pallor, diaphoresis	Mottled appearance, diaphoresis
Bowel sounds	Hyperactive	Decreased or absent	Normal or decreased	Decreased
Neuromuscular tone	Increased, predominantly in lower extremities	Normal	"Lead-pipe" rigidity present in all muscle groups	Rigor mortis–like rigidity

Table 14–4. Characteristics of serotonin syndrome and related clinical conditions *(continued)*

	Serotonin syndrome	Anticholinergic "toxidrome"	Neuroleptic malignant syndrome	Malignant hyperthermia
Reflexes	Hyperreflexia, clonus (unless masked by increased muscle tone)	Normal	Bradyreflexia	Hyporeflexia
Mental status	Agitation, coma	Agitated delirium	Stupor, alert mutism, coma	Agitation

Source. Reprinted from Boyer EW, Shannon M: "The Serotonin Syndrome." *New England Journal of Medicine* 352:1118, 2005. Used with permission.

velop 1 month or more after treatment initiation unless the dosage was increased or an additional dopamine-blocking drug was added (Strawn et al. 2007). The mean recovery time is 7–10 days after discontinuation of the offending agent (significantly longer if the antipsychotic was given as a depot injection), although Caroff et al. (2000) reported that residual catatonia and parkinsonism can persist for weeks after other symptoms have resolved.

Clinical Manifestations

- *Hyperthermia* is a cardinal feature of NMS, with a temperature typically >38°C, and commonly >40°C.
- *Muscular rigidity.* Increased tone is an essential feature of NMS; superimposed tremor may result in a cogwheel phenomenon.
- *Autonomic instability* primarily includes tachycardia, hypertension or labile blood pressure, and tachypnea. Autonomic volatility is a poor prognostic sign.
- *Altered mental status.* Retrospective analyses indicate that mental status changes or other neurological signs precede the systemic signs in 80% of patients (Velamoor et al. 1994). Decreased levels of consciousness, including stupor or progression to coma, commonly occur.

Laboratory Findings

No laboratory findings are specific for NMS, but elevated serum creatinine kinase is associated with the syndrome. Other laboratory findings may include increased white blood cell count, low serum iron, metabolic acidosis, and mild elevations of lactate dehydrogenase and liver transaminases. Myoglobinuric renal failure can develop from rhabdomyolysis (Strawn et al. 2007).

Differential Diagnosis

NMS is one disorder in a group of related conditions that share common features of rigidity, hyperthermia, and autonomic dysregulation (see Table 14–4). Other medical and neurological disorders, which have symptom overlap with NMS but are unrelated to NMS, need to be considered in the differential diagnosis.

- *Serotonin syndrome* and NMS have similar presentations, although patients with serotonin syndrome are more likely to have myoclonus, hyperreflexia, shivering, nausea, and diarrhea.
- *Malignant catatonia* can appear indistinguishable from NMS (Mann et al. 1986), and some researchers have suggested that NMS is a drug-induced form of malignant catatonia with the same underlying pathophysiology (Fink 1996; Mann et al. 1986). The clinical history may include a psychiatric prodrome of psychosis, agitation, or catatonic excitement. The motor findings in malignant catatonia are more likely to include dystonic posturing, waxy flexibility, and stereotyped repetitive behaviors. Regardless of the diagnosis, any dopamine receptor antagonists should be discontinued.
- A rare genetic disorder, *malignant hyperthermia,* is primarily differentiated from NMS by the history of administration of a potent halogenated inhalational anesthetic agent or succinylcholine.
- *Anticholinergic toxicity* is not associated with rigidity or diaphoresis, and elevated body temperatures are less severe than in NMS. Mydriasis, flushing, and bladder distention are more frequent than in NMS.
- *Medical or neurological disorders with extrapyramidal symptoms* from concomitant antipsychotic use are especially challenging to differentiate from NMS. Diagnoses to consider include CNS infections, anatomic lesions that affect the midbrain and brain stem structures, prodromal viral illnesses, seizures, heatstroke, thyrotoxicosis, drug intoxication, and withdrawal from dopamine agonists, baclofen, sedative-hypnotics, and alcohol (Strawn et al. 2007).

Treatment

In many cases, discontinuation of the offending agent and supportive care are sufficient for the resolution of NMS. Limited evidence suggests that specific pharmacotherapy can facilitate recovery and decrease mortality. Especially because NMS has been conceptualized as a severe form of catatonia, the use of benzodiazepines has been tried, with conflicting results (Caroff et al. 1998). Given the relative risks and benefits, a trial of lorazepam administered parenterally is a reasonable intervention, particularly for patients with less severe or primarily catatonic symptoms (Strawn et al. 2007). Dopaminergic agents, including bromocriptine and amantadine, and the muscle relaxant dantrolene have been reported to hasten recovery and decrease mortality (Rosenberg and Green 1989; Sakkas et al. 1991). If supportive management and pharmacotherapy are not adequate or malignant catatonia cannot be ruled out, electroconvulsive therapy (ECT) is an effective treatment, even late in the course of NMS (Addonizio and Susman 1987; Trollor and Sachdev 1999).

Antipsychotic Use Following NMS

Although estimates of up to 30% have been reported for the likelihood of developing NMS with antipsychotic use following an NMS episode, long-term follow-up data have shown that the majority of patients can be safely restarted on antipsychotic treatment (Levenson and Fisher 1988; Pope et al. 1991). At least 2 weeks should elapse after recovery from NMS before rechallenge, and low dosages of a low-potency typical antipsychotic or atypical antipsychotic are preferred (Strawn et al. 2007).

Psychotropic Use and Cardiac Complications

Arrhythmias, QTc Prolongation, and Risk of Sudden Cardiac Death

Antidepressants

Tricyclic antidepressants. Tricyclic antidepressants (TCAs) have quinidine-like effects that may result in cardiac conduction delay, increased heart rate, and prolongation of the QT, QRS, and PR intervals. Among patients without cardiovascular disease, these effects are often insignificant, although they may lead to ventricular arrhythmias in patients with preexisting conduction abnormalities or those taking type Ia antiarrhythmic drugs (Robinson and Levenson 2000). One study found that the risk of sudden cardiac death was not increased with dosages less than 100 mg amitriptyline equivalents (Ray et al. 2004) (see also Chapter 10, "Mood Disorders").

Selective serotonin reuptake inhibitors. In addition to the long-established capacity of all of the TCAs to prolong the QTc interval, the U.S. Food and Drug Administration (FDA) recently advised clinicians that the selective serotonin reuptake inhibitor (SSRI) citalopram should no longer be used at dosages greater than 40 mg/day. This recommendation was based on an as-yet-unpublished prospective trial demonstrating that citalopram causes dose-dependent QT interval prolongation (FDA Drug Safety Communication 2011).

Antipsychotics

The use of antipsychotics can result in QTc prolongation and risk of sudden cardiac death (see also Chapter 7, "Delirium").

Typical antipsychotics. All antipsychotics have the potential to produce electrocardiographic changes, but not all drugs that prolong the QTc interval result in torsade de pointes and sudden death. QTc prolongation is a warning of the possibility of torsade de pointes and sudden death, but it is not the risk itself. The evidence for torsade de pointes and sudden death is most robust with thioridazine, pimozide, droperidol, and haloperidol. The risk is higher if haloperidol is administered intravenously, given at high dosages, or used in patients with cardiomyopathy (Di Salvo and O'Gara 1995; Hunt and Stern 1995; Reilly et al. 2000; Robinson and Levenson 2000).

Atypical antipsychotics. Although fewer data are available regarding atypical antipsychotics, emerging evidence suggests that atypical antipsychotics are associated with elevated risk for sudden cardiac death (Jolly et al. 2009; Ray et al. 2009). Among the atypical antipsychotics, ziprasidone appears to be the most likely to cause QTc prolongation, and olanzapine and aripiprazole are the least likely. A large retrospective cohort study showed that typical and atypical antipsychotics have similar elevated risks of sudden cardiac death; the risks were dose related for all agents (Ray et al. 2009). The incidence rate ratios among users of high-dose antipsychotics compared with nonusers varied from

1.72 for haloperidol to 5.05 for thioridazine (Ray et al. 2009). The ratios correlate with an incidence rate of 3.3 events per 1,000 patient years among patients receiving higher dosages (Schneeweiss and Avorn 2009).

Factors Associated With QTc Prolongation

In addition to antiarrhythmics, antidepressants, and antipsychotics, certain antihistamines and antimicrobial drugs are known to increase the QTc interval. A careful review of medications is crucial to determine whether coadministration of drugs inhibits the metabolism of arrhythmogenic medications. Factors that increase the likelihood of arrhythmia include congenital long QT syndrome, age, preexisting cardiac disease, female gender, hypomagnesemia, and hypokalemia (Elming et al. 2003).

Orthostatic Hypotension

TCAs, trazodone, and monoamine oxidase inhibitors commonly cause orthostasis. Low-potency antipsychotics are more likely to cause orthostatic hypotension than are high-potency antipsychotics, and among the atypical antipsychotics, clozapine carries the greatest risk. Patients with congestive heart failure or dehydration are particularly vulnerable to changes in blood pressure (Smith et al. 2008).

Myocarditis and Cardiomyopathy

Myocarditis and cardiomyopathy are rare complications of clozapine, often occurring early after treatment initiation, with one study showing a median onset of 17 days (Haas et al. 2007; Mackin 2008).

Psychotropic Use and Endocrine-Related Complications

Metabolic Syndrome

Metabolic syndrome is based on the co-occurrence of metabolic risk factors for both type 2 diabetes mellitus and coronary vascular disease. These risk factors include abdominal obesity, hyperglycemia, dyslipidemia, and hypertension. Questions have been raised about the concept of metabolic syndrome and whether the components of the syndrome warrant classification as an actual syndrome.

This uncertainty is partly due to the absence of a unifying pathogenesis for the syndrome and lack of consensus regarding the definition (Kahn et al. 2005). Olanzapine and clozapine, and to a lesser extent, quetiapine and risperidone, are associated with weight gain, dyslipidemia, and new-onset diabetes mellitus (De Hert et al. 2006; Henderson 2002; Henderson et al. 2000). Prior to initiation of these atypical antipsychotics, minimum baseline screening should include fasting blood glucose and lipid profile. Thereafter, the patient's weight, blood pressure, serum glucose, and lipids must be monitored, with testing frequency determined by the patient's medical history and risk factors. If a patient develops impaired fasting glucose or dyslipidemia, consideration should be given to switching to an atypical antipsychotic with lower risk of metabolic side effects (e.g., ziprasidone or aripiprazole) or a typical antipsychotic (De Hert et al. 2006).

Thyroid Dysfunction

Among the psychotropics, lithium is the most commonly associated with thyroid dysfunction, including goiter, hypothyroidism, chronic autoimmune thyroiditis, and possibly hyperthyroidism. Subclinical hypothyroidism has been reported in up to 25% of patients, and prevalence estimates for overt hypothyroidism range from 10% to 20%. Hypothyroidism can be treated and should not be considered a contraindication to continued lithium therapy (Robinson and Owen 2005).

Psychotropic Use in Renal Disease

Antidepressants

Studies are limited regarding treatment with antidepressants of patients with end-stage renal disease (ESRD). The SSRIs have a more favorable side-effect profile than the TCAs, especially because the hydroxylated metabolites of the TCAs can be elevated in dialysis patients, potentially causing toxicity even at therapeutic levels (Robinson and Levenson 2000). Dosage adjustments of fluoxetine, sertraline, or citalopram are generally not required for patients with ESRD. Plasma levels of paroxetine are increased in patients with renal impairment, and the recommended dosage is one-half of that for adults with normal renal function. Clearances of venlafaxine and mirtazapine are reduced by about 50% in patients with renal failure; therefore, a dosage reduction is recommended (L. M. Cohen et al. 2004; S. D. Cohen et al. 2007).

Mood Stabilizers

Lithium is dialyzable and is therefore given to patients undergoing renal dialysis *after* their dialysis treatments; the usual dose is 300–600 mg/day. Dialysis patients do not eliminate lithium naturally, so they do not require daily lithium supplementation aside from their postdialysis dose. Serum levels of lithium are tested several hours after dialysis because plasma levels may actually rise in the postdialysis period when equilibration between blood and tissue stores occurs. Long-term lithium use rarely leads to renal insufficiency and ESRD, although renal function can improve if the drug is discontinued. Valproate may be used in patients with ESRD, although free valproic acid levels need to be monitored because ESRD can result in increased free serum levels (L. M. Cohen et al. 2004).

Antipsychotics

All antipsychotics may be used in patients with renal disease, and most do not require a dosage adjustment, although clearance of risperidone and its metabolites, including paliperidone, is reduced by 60% (L. M. Cohen et al. 2004).

Benzodiazepines

Because benzodiazepines are metabolized by the liver, a dosage reduction is generally not required, although the half-life of benzodiazepines is higher in patients with ESRD (Wagner and O'Hara 1997).

Psychotropic Use in Liver Disease

Antidepressants

Most antidepressants undergo phase I hepatic oxidative metabolism and require dosage adjustment in patients with liver disease. Citalopram, fluoxetine, paroxetine, and sertraline have been studied in patients with hepatitis C, usually in the setting of interferon-α treatment, and have been found safe (Robinson and Owen 2005). Dosage modification depends on the severity of the liver disease; as a general rule, patients with hepatic insufficiency should receive one-third to one-half the usual dosage for healthy patients (Robinson and Levenson 2000).

Benzodiazepines

The metabolism of oxazepam, lorazepam, and temazepam are phase II dependent; their clearance is less affected by liver disease, and they should therefore be considered first if a benzodiazepine is required (Wilkinson 1978). The clearance of other benzodiazepines is substantially reduced in patients with liver disease because of metabolism by phase I reactions. In patients with hepatic encephalopathy, benzodiazepines can exacerbate mental status changes, including subclinical or latent encephalopathy (Branch 1987).

Antipsychotics

The data are sparse regarding the use of antipsychotics in patients with liver disease, although haloperidol and the atypical antipsychotics are commonly used (Schlatter et al. 2009). Atypical antipsychotics have been associated with pancreatitis, most commonly with clozapine, but pancreatitis has also been reported with olanzapine and risperidone (Koller et al. 2003).

Mood Stabilizers

Valproic acid and carbamazepine are relatively contraindicated in patients with liver disease because of the risk of hepatotoxicity. Valproic acid is associated with elevated liver enzymes in acute and chronic use, and acute liver failure most often occurs within the first 6 months of treatment (Smith et al. 2008). Hyperammonemic encephalopathy has been reported even in the context of normal liver enzymes, with improvement in mental status after discontinuation of the drug (Wadzinski et al. 2007). Valproic acid can also cause pancreatitis.

Nonpharmacological Treatments

Electroconvulsive Therapy

ECT is a first-line treatment for depressed patients who are severely malnourished or dehydrated, who have either catatonia or psychotic depression, or who have a previously documented good response to ECT. ECT has no absolute contraindications; however, some medical conditions increase the morbidity associated with ECT and require thoughtful review of the risks and benefits. These medical conditions include 1) those that cause increased intracranial pressure; 2) those that increase the risk of serious hemorrhage; and 3) pathophysiological states that cause hemodynamic compromise, such as an acute myocardial infarction or malignant arrhythmias. Cardiac complications are the most common etiology of significant morbidity and mortality during ECT. The addition of beta-blockers and antiarrhythmics before ECT reduces some of these risks (Rasmussen et al. 2002a, 2002b).

Other Neuropsychiatric Treatments

For many years, ECT was the only nonpharmacological psychiatric procedure available to treat severe or medication-refractory depression and other psychiatric conditions. Data are emerging regarding other forms of therapeutic brain stimulation, such as transcranial magnetic stimulation (TMS), vagal nerve stimulation (VNS), and deep brain stimulation (DBS). It is not in the scope of this book to review these treatments in detail, but the consulting psychiatrist needs to be aware of the potential psychiatric implications of VNS and DBS, particularly in neurological patients.

Vagal Nerve Stimulation

VNS is delivered from a small pacemaker-like generator implanted in the chest that sends preprogrammed, intermittent, mild electrical pulses through the vagus nerve to the brain. VNS was approved by the U.S. Food and Drug Administration in 1997 for adjunctive treatment for patients whose partial-onset seizures are refractory to antiepileptic drugs. In 2005, VNS was approved for patients with treatment-resistant depression. Studies regarding its effect on depressive symptoms have had mixed results, but generally have shown that the treatment response is delayed and gradual in onset (Elger et al. 2000; Milby et al. 2008; Rush and Siefert 2009). Optimal dosing strategies have not been determined, and clinically useful predictors of who will respond to treatment have not been identified (Rush and Siefert 2009).

Deep Brain Stimulation

The effective use of high-frequency DBS for treatment of various neurological diseases, particularly Parkinson's disease, is well established. Therapeutic trials have been conducted to examine the effectiveness of DBS in treatment-resistant depression, obsessive-compulsive disorder, and Tourette's disorder. Surgical targets for electrode placement are in the subgenual cingulate cortex for depression, the anterior internal capsule for obsessive-compulsive disorder, and the thalamic nucleus for Tourette's disorder. Although immediate relief of symptoms has been reported, a significant proportion of symptom improvement occurs after months of long-term stimulation (Tye et al. 2009).

References

Addonizio G, Susman VL: ECT as a treatment alternative for patients with symptoms of neuroleptic malignant syndrome. J Clin Psychiatry 48:102–105, 1987

Berardi D, Amore M, Keck PE Jr, et al: Clinical and pharmacologic risk factors for neuroleptic malignant syndrome: a case-control study. Biol Psychiatry 44:748–754, 1998

Boyer EW, Shannon M: The serotonin syndrome. N Engl J Med 352:1112–1120, 2005

Branch RA: Is there increased cerebral sensitivity to benzodiazepines in chronic liver disease? Hepatology 7:773–776, 1987

Caroff SN, Mann SC, Keck PE Jr: Specific treatment of the neuroleptic malignant syndrome. Biol Psychiatry 44:378–381, 1998

Caroff SN, Mann SC, Keck PE Jr, et al: Residual catatonic state following neuroleptic malignant syndrome. J Clin Psychopharmacol 20:257–259, 2000

Cohen LM, Tessier EG, Germain MJ, et al: Update on psychotropic medication use in renal disease. Psychosomatics 45:34–48, 2004

Cohen SD, Norris L, Acquaviva K, et al: Screening, diagnosis, and treatment of depression in patients with end-stage renal disease. Clin J Am Soc Nephrol 2:1332–1342, 2007

De Hert M, van Eyck D, De Nayer A: Metabolic abnormalities associated with second generation antipsychotics: fact or fiction? Development of guidelines for screening and monitoring. Int Clin Psychopharmacol 21 (suppl 2):S11–S15, 2006

Di Salvo TG, O'Gara PT: Torsade de pointes caused by high-dose intravenous haloperidol in cardiac patients. Clin Cardiol 18:285–290, 1995

Elger G, Hoppe C, Falkai P, et al: Vagus nerve stimulation is associated with mood improvements in epilepsy patients. Epilepsy Res 42:203–210, 2000

Elming H, Sonne J, Lublin HKF: The importance of the QT interval: a review of the literature. Acta Psychiatr Scand 107:96–101, 2003

Fait ML, Wise MG, Jachna JS, et al: Psychopharmacology, in The American Psychiatric Publishing Textbook of Consultation-Liaison Psychiatry: Psychiatry in the Medically Ill, 2nd Edition. Edited by Wise MG, Rundell JR. Washington, DC, American Psychiatric Publishing, 2002, pp 939–987

FDA Drug Safety Communication: Abnormal heart rhythms associated with high doses of Celexa (citalopram hydrobromide). 8/24/2011. Available at: http://www.fda.gov/Drugs/DrugSafety/ucm269086.htm. Accessed August 26, 2011.

Fink M: Neuroleptic malignant syndrome and catatonia: one entity or two? Biol Psychiatry 39:1–4, 1996

Haas SJ, Hill R, Krum H, et al: Clozapine-associated myocarditis: a review of 116 cases of suspected myocarditis associated with the use of clozapine in Australia during 1993–2003. Drug Saf 30:47–57, 2007

Henderson DC: Diabetes mellitus and other metabolic disturbances induced by atypical antipsychotic agents. Curr Diab Rep 2:135–140, 2002

Henderson DC, Cagliero E, Gray C, et al: Clozapine, diabetes mellitus, weight gain, and lipid abnormalities: a five-year naturalistic study. Am J Psychiatry 157:975–981, 2000

Hunt N, Stern TA: The association between intravenous haloperidol and torsades de pointes: three cases and a literature review. Psychosomatics 36:541–549, 1995

Jolly K, Gammage MD, Cheng KK, et al: Sudden death in patients receiving drugs tending to prolong the QT interval. Br J Clin Pharmacol 68:743–751, 2009

Kahn R, Buse J, Ferrannini E, et al: The metabolic syndrome: time for a critical appraisal: joint statement from the American Diabetes Association and the European Association for the Study of Diabetes. Diabetes Care 28:2289–2304, 2005

Koller EA, Cross JT, Doraiswamy PM, et al: Pancreatitis associated with atypical antipsychotics: from the Food and Drug Administration's MedWatch surveillance system and published reports. Pharmacotherapy 23:1123–1130, 2003

Levenson JL: Neuroleptic malignant syndrome. Am J Psychiatry 142:1137–1145, 1985

Levenson JL, Fisher JG: Long-term outcome after neuroleptic malignant syndrome. J Clin Psychiatry 49:154–156, 1988

Lin EHB, Von Korff M, Ludman EJ, et al: Enhancing adherence to prevent depression relapse in primary care. Gen Hosp Psychiatry 25:303–310, 2003

Mackin P: Cardiac side effects of psychiatric drugs. Hum Psychopharmacol 23 (suppl 1): 3–14, 2008

Mann SC, Caroff SN, Bleier HR, et al: Lethal catatonia. Am J Psychiatry 143:1374–1381, 1986

Milby AH, Halpern CH, Baltuch GH: Vagus nerve stimulation for epilepsy and depression. Neurotherapeutics 5:75–85, 2008

Pelonero AL, Levenson JL, Pandurangi AK: Neuroleptic malignant syndrome: a review. Psychiatr Serv 49:1163–1172, 1998

Pope HG Jr, Aizley HG, Keck PE Jr, et al: Neuroleptic malignant syndrome: long-term follow-up of 20 cases. J Clin Psychiatry 52:208–212, 1991

Rasmussen KG, Rummans TA, Richardson JW: Electroconvulsive therapy in the medically ill. Psychiatr Clin North Am 25:177–193, 2002a

Rasmussen KG, Sampson SM, Rummans TA: Electroconvulsive therapy and newer modalities for the treatment of medication-refractory mental illness. Mayo Clin Proc 77:552–556, 2002b

Ray WA, Meredith S, Thapa PB, et al: Cyclic antidepressants and the risk of sudden cardiac death. Clin Pharmacol Ther 75:234–241, 2004

Ray WA, Chung CP, Murray KT, et al: Atypical antipsychotic drugs and the risk of sudden cardiac death. (Erratum in N Engl J Med 361:1814, 2009.) N Engl J Med 360:225–235, 2009

Reilly JG, Ayis SA, Ferrier IN, et al: QTc-interval abnormalities and psychotropic drug therapy in psychiatric patients. Lancet 355:1048–1052, 2000

Robinson MJ, Levenson JL: The use of psychotropics in the medically ill. Curr Psychiatry Rep 2:247–255, 2000

Robinson MJ, Owen JA: Psychopharmacology, in The American Psychiatric Publishing Textbook of Psychosomatic Medicine. Edited by Levenson JL. Washington, DC, American Psychiatric Publishing, 2005, pp 871–922

Rosenberg MR, Green M: Neuroleptic malignant syndrome: review of response to therapy. Arch Intern Med 149:1927–1931, 1989

Rush AJ, Siefert SE: Clinical issues in considering vagus nerve stimulation for treatment-resistant depression. Exp Neurol 219:36–43, 2009

Sakkas P, Davis JM, Janicak PG, et al: Drug treatment of the neuroleptic malignant syndrome. Psychopharmacol Bull 27:381–384, 1991

Schlatter C, Egger SS, Tchambaz L, et al: Pharmacokinetic changes of psychotropic drugs in patients with liver disease: implications for dose adaptation. Drug Saf 32:561–578, 2009

Schneeweiss S, Avorn J: Antipsychotic agents and sudden cardiac death—how should we manage the risk? N Engl J Med 360:294–296, 2009

Smith FA, Wittmann CW, Stern TA: Medical complications of psychiatric treatment. Crit Care Clin 24:635–656, 2008

Strawn JR, Keck PE Jr, Caroff SN: Neuroleptic malignant syndrome. Am J Psychiatry 164:870–876, 2007

Stubner S, Rustenbeck E, Grohmann R, et al: Severe and uncommon involuntary movement disorders due to psychotropic drugs. Pharmacopsychiatry 37 (suppl 1):S54–S64, 2004

Trollor JN, Sachdev PS: Electroconvulsive treatment of neuroleptic malignant syndrome: a review and report of cases. Aust NZ J Psychiatry 33:650–659, 1999

Turnheim K: When drug therapy gets old: pharmacokinetics and pharmacodynamics in the elderly. Exp Gerontol 38:843–853, 2003

Tye SJ, Frye MA, Lee KH: Disrupting disordered neurocircuitry: treating refractory psychiatric illness with neuromodulation. Mayo Clin Proc 84:522–532, 2009

Velamoor VR, Norman RM, Caroff SN, et al: Progression of symptoms in neuroleptic malignant syndrome. J Nerv Ment Dis 182:168–173, 1994

Wadzinski J, Franks R, Roane D, et al: Valproate-associated hyperammonemic encephalopathy. J Am Board Fam Med 20:499–502, 2007

Wagner BK, O'Hara DA: Pharmacokinetics and pharmacodynamics of sedatives and analgesics in the treatment of agitated critically ill patients. Clin Pharmacokinet 33:426–453, 1997

Wilkinson GR: The effects of liver disease and aging on the disposition of diazepam, chlordiazepoxide, oxazepam and lorazepam in man. Acta Psychiatr Scand Suppl (274):56–74, 1978

15

Psychosocial Management

Beyond the symptoms, signs, personality style, and medical or surgical co-morbidities that each patient brings to a psychiatric consultation are psychosocial elements that shape a patient's experience of illness. These factors may present challenges, interfere with care, or provide additional means of support, but they may not be ignored by the psychiatrist who hopes to understand the patient's dilemma and thereby advise or assist constructively.

Culture, Ethnicity, and Language

Trainees in psychosomatic medicine may feel uncertain or ill at ease during moments when their émigré-tourist status in medical-surgical territory is exposed. Their expectations, disposition, vocabulary, or goals may feel out of place. Similarly, patients may feel that the hospital or a psychiatrist's office is foreign territory, particularly when their identity is shaped by distinctive cultural, ethnic, and language characteristics.

Culture

Culture involves the history, traditions, expressions (whether in art, literature, music, clothing, architecture, etc.), values, social structures, behaviors, and achievements of a particular group of people. Cultural elements may be expansive and transcend national or continental boundaries (e.g., aspects of Islamic or Western European culture), but patients may also present with idiosyncrasies that reflect a select subculture shaped by vocation, age, geography, conviction, or singular practices (Ahmed et al. 2007; Betancourt 2006; Hobbs 2008; Juckett and Rudolf-Watson 2010). DSM-IV-TR (American Psychiatric Association 2000) recommends that a clinician consider the following facets (Lewis-Fernandez and Diaz 2002).

- *Cultural identity*—the patient's perception of cultural background, day-to-day practices that reflect the patient's association with a cultural group, languages spoken, language(s) preferred now (and in which settings), sense of identifying with "mainstream" American culture (and in what practical ways), circumstances of immigration (whether personal or ancestral), and vocational consequences of culture, if any
- *Cultural explanations*—the patient's choice of words to communicate his or her symptoms, the meaning of those symptoms within the patient's cultural group or the family's explanation of the symptoms, the patient's past experience and current expectation of consultation with a psychiatrist, and whether the patient has sought help from alternative sources
- *Psychosocial environment and function*—how current stressors and symptoms have interfered with daily function, and what sources of social support are available within the culture
- *Consequent relationship between patient and clinician*—the difficulties that the cultural and other differences (e.g., socioeconomic, educational, ethnic, gender) between the patient and clinician may cause in diagnosis and treatment (e.g., limited communication because of language, understanding of symptoms, discerning whether a given behavior is pathological)

Ethnicity

Ethnicity is associated with challenges in both diagnosis and treatment.

Differential Diagnosis

Differential diagnosis can be altered by ethnic propensities and prejudice. Ethnicity may influence the timing of a patient's presentation for medical care (prompting a perception of more severe disease), affect a patient's emphasis on psychotic symptoms but denial of mood symptoms (complicating accurate distinction between schizophrenia and bipolar disorder, for example), or shape a physician's bias as expressed in the choice of questions asked of the patient or family (Huang et al. 2006; McGilloway et al. 2010).

Psychopharmacology
Psychopharmacological riddles may arise from ethnic factors.

Genomics.   Genetic variations in hepatic cytochrome P450 isoenzymes may affect efficacy of treatment, side effects, therapeutic dosage requirements, and potential drug-drug interactions. This science is in its infancy, with differing perspectives on the evidence base for widespread clinical application (de Leon et al. 2009; Zhou 2009a, 2009b). Nonetheless, sufficient studies have been reported to warrant the need for the consultation psychiatrist to remain alert to the possibility that unexpected clinical sensitivity (i.e., brisk development of side effects at low doses), apparent absence of effect (i.e., absence of both efficacy and side effects despite unusually high dosages), and other apparent pharmacokinetic aberrations (e.g., unusual reactivity to warfarin) may result from pharmacogenomic variations that affect the metabolism of psychotropic agents.

Herbal and alternative preparations.   Individuals of some ethnic, cultural, or religious groups may perceive herbal and alternative preparations as less toxic (not to mention less expensive and unencumbered by the necessity of a prescription) than medicines associated with Western medicine. Also, these individuals may not disclose the use of these agents to conventional physicians, further obscuring the diagnostic task (Feng et al. 2010; Li et al. 2004).

Language

Language Barriers
Effective communication is a skill that rewards refinement throughout a clinician's career, even when patient and physician are native to the same language. The dismay, frustration, or even resignation that a patient or physician might experience when confronted with a language barrier can be a substantial obstacle to accurate assessment and effective care.

Interpreters

Interpreters are essential and invaluable when providing consultations with individuals who speak other languages (Bauer and Alegria 2010; Diamond and Jacobs 2010; Karliner et al. 2004). The following recommendations will strengthen the patient-physician relationship and improve the interview yield when an interpreter is used to bridge a language gap:

1. Avoid use of family members. Despite the convenience, patients may not be forthcoming with family members, and family members may filter or even falsify sensitive or embarrassing information.
2. Avoid use of nonprofessional staff. Although secretarial or other nonmedical employees may be helpful in providing cultural insight, their absence of medical training may result in inaccurate translation and a diminished awareness of the necessity of strict confidentiality.
3. Welcome "cultural consultation" from the interpreter if time allows before the interview. The interpreter may be able to help the psychiatrist avoid an unnecessary cultural faux pas.
4. Speak to the patient and focus on nonverbal behavior. Although turning to and addressing the interpreter feels natural, the psychiatrist can preserve the advantage of his or her experience in assessing nonverbal communication by remaining assiduously attentive to the patient.
5. Use short sentences and frequent pauses. This style decreases the risk of distraction and helps the interpreter to avoid paraphrasing to summarize a lengthy question.
6. Beware of colloquialisms or informal slang. The interpreter may feel obligated to provide a literal translation or may be unfamiliar with a particular expression. Similarly, the psychiatrist needs to allow the interpreter to rephrase formal terms, such as *depression*, which may not have a precise counterpart in the patient's language.
7. Avoid jargon or technical terms. Even if translated accurately, a patient who does not understand may not feel free to say so.
8. If treatment has been discussed, ask the patient to repeat what he or she understands. The response serves as a comprehension check and may also give a clue regarding the patient's intention to follow through with the recommendations.

9. Ask the interpreter for his or her observations and thoughts after the session. The interpreter may have translated for the patient with several other teams or during previous hospitalizations and may have valuable collateral history to provide.

10. Whenever possible, use the same interpreter in subsequent visits with the patient. This consistency can increase accuracy and trust.

Spiritual, Existential, and Religious Factors

Multiple surveys confirm that most people indicate they have a spiritual life (Mueller et al. 2001) and that the majority of hospitalized patients express appreciation for the religious and supportive attention of chaplains (Piderman et al. 2008). Spirituality commonly involves a pursuit of transcendent meaning or purpose, values, and an experience of connectedness. Medical illness often accentuates these interests and moves them to the fore of a patient's thoughts. Although psychiatrists are less likely than either their patients or other U.S. physicians to describe themselves as religious (Curlin et al. 2007), the consultation psychiatrist misses an important opportunity to better understand the full context of a patient's life and better mobilize appropriate internal and external resources if he or she overlooks a patient's perspective on spiritual matters (Galanter 2010). The goal is not to intrude on the patient's questions with either conviction or skepticism, but rather to elicit the patient's feelings and thoughts in a manner that reinforces the patient's experience of having been heard and, thereby, encourages the patient to seek further appropriate resources. The following questions may inform a patient that a psychiatrist respects and hopes to better understand this dimension of the patient's life (Breitbart 2002; Grossman et al. 2005; Puchalski and Romer 2000):

1. Do you see yourself as a spiritual or religious person?

2a. (If no) Has that always been so, or have your beliefs and/or practice changed over time?

2b. (If yes) For you, is this a personal, private exercise? Are you part of a spiritual or religious community?

3. If you identify with a particular religious community, how does this community support you?

4. Has spirituality or religion helped you? How? Or hurt you in any way? How?

5. How important are your religious or spiritual beliefs to you now?
6. How might those beliefs influence your choices or behavior during this illness?
7. Are you at peace? (Steinhauser et al. 2006)
8. How would you like me to help address these issues in your care?
9. Would you appreciate the opportunity to visit with a hospital chaplain?

Patient's Practical Concerns

Practical concerns may weigh on a patient's mind, influence his or her willingness to consider diagnostic and treatment options, moderate adherence to recommendations, and possibly determine long-term outcome. In the hospital, these issues may be addressed by the primary team or a social worker; however, in outpatient consultation or in situations where a patient perceives that the hospital team's focus is solely on medical or surgical issues, these concerns may not receive optimal attention unless the psychiatrist opens the subject.

Financial Worries

Financial worries may be elicited by questions such as the following:

1. Do you spend time thinking about your financial affairs or stressors most days?
2. Have you looked for or taken on additional work to ease your financial situation?
3. Are there other people (e.g., aging parents, unemployed child or relative) who depend on you for financial support?
4. Have you chosen to postpone medical care or decided to stop a medication in the past because of cost?

Safety

Safety may be compromised for multiple reasons, with or without the patient's awareness. The patient's initial hospital presentation may have resulted from an injury or illness that alerts medical staff to a particular safety risk; at other times, the underlying problem remains obscure unless deliberately pursued.

Domestic Abuse or Violence

The psychiatrist should interview the patient without family members present and broach the subject of domestic abuse or violence in a respectful, gentle tone that avoids arousing shame and subsequent silence.

Incapacity

Insidious but progressive cognitive decline (or the burden of caring for a partner with debilitating dementia), decreasing mobility and independence by virtue of age and dwindling vigor, or a confluence of psychosocial stressors may render an individual increasingly isolated and incapable of making effective decisions in his or her own best interest. The psychiatrist may need to activate necessary medical, family, community, or legal resources to clarify the patient's situation and explore alternative living arrangements.

Postconsultation Care

Physicians are on familiar ground in the hospital, but most patients are not. They may not understand the role of different teams or different members of the same team; they may be confused and feel less secure about their care when a particular physician appears to vanish without a word; the lexicon of medicine may be foreign and important questions occur only after the consulting team has left the room. The psychiatrist can improve the patient's confidence and lower anxiety by addressing the following:

- The role of the consultation team and its various members
- Communication between successive team members if a rotation will introduce a change for the patient
- Subsequent follow-up:
    - *Guidance regarding psychotropic adjustments or termination.* To avoid either an inadequate trial or the risk of ongoing use of a psychotropic that may require only time-limited use, consider printing a patient education information sheet about the relevant medication(s) and briefly annotating it with the same recommendations given to the primary medical-surgical team caring for the patient.

- *Psychiatric follow-up.* Clarify for the patient if his or her diagnosis and treatment plan warrant psychiatric follow-up or if follow-up from a primary care physician will be appropriate and sufficient.
- *Community resources.* When community resources are available, specify the particular resources and tell the patient how to access the help; be realistic about possible obstacles, waiting lists, and other issues.

Promoting Resilience Rather Than Vulnerability

Demoralization is common among patients in the general hospital and is often mistaken for depression, with which demoralization may share features. The hallmark of demoralization consists of a subjective appraisal of one's own impotence; typically, the multiple or prolonged uncertainties of medical illness so deplete an individual that he or she loses confidence in his or her capacity to endure. Feelings of worthlessness and hopelessness may follow, but when the tide of adversity is turned, patients who feel demoralized can recapture hope, confidence, and purpose much more rapidly than can patients with severe depression.

Griffith and colleagues (Griffith and Gaby 2005; Griffith and Griffith 2002) have proposed a helpful and practical schema of eight existential postures (Table 15–1). A healthy person may enjoy a position of resilience in all or most of these domains, whereas a patient oppressed by illness may slip toward the opposing pole of vulnerability. The psychiatrist has an opportunity to identify what themes of vulnerability dominate a patient's perception of his or her illness, and to structure the interview to help the patient move instead toward postures of greater resilience. The eight existential postures and suggested questions listed in the table are intended as instruments of respectful inquiry, not exhortation (Griffith and Gaby 2005; Griffith and Griffith 2002). The reader is strongly encouraged to consult the source material, in which each question is further explained and illustrated with clinical examples.

Additional Supportive Tools

Additional supportive tools, including education, psychotherapy, hypnosis, and relaxation, can be used to help a patient manage the trials and tensions that emerge when medical and surgical problems disrupt life.

Education

Education need not be formal, comprehensive, or physician delivered to play an important part in easing a patient's experience of alienation and fear in the medical arena.

Hospital Bedside

At the hospital bedside, the psychiatrist may observe that a patient's distress is aggravated by ignorance, inaccurate assumptions, distorted communication, or a limited coping reservoir. Remaining aware that information alone may increase anxiety and stress for some patients, the therapist may use the bedside consultation for the following functions:

- Informing the patient who is unaware of the procedure involved in a forthcoming diagnostic test, or translating a medical acronym the patient heard as the team discussed his or her situation in rounds
- Correcting misunderstandings or perhaps public prejudice regarding particular medical or psychiatric conditions
- Affirming permission for the patient to pose particular questions to his or her primary physician, or offering practical tips to improve communication and reinforce a sense of participation with the primary team
- Illustrating a coping technique, such as reframing or distraction, that the patient might use to help endure a noxious procedure or a setback in clinical prognosis

Outpatient Setting

In the outpatient setting, educational intervention and support more commonly occur in group settings and are often organized according to disease (e.g., pulmonary disease, diabetes mellitus) or treatment (e.g., organ transplantation, radiation therapy). Elements of effective group psychoeducation include the following:

- Accurate medical knowledge and associated management tips
- Recognition of the emotional challenges common to most patients who are adjusting to the disease and encouragement of mutual expression to reduce individual isolation

Table 15–1.   Existential postures: themes of resilience versus vulnerability

Coherence Versus Confusion

- How do you make sense of what you are going through?
- When you are uncertain, how do you deal with moments of feeling confused?
- To whom do you turn for help when you feel confused?
- To whom do you turn for help when you feel confused?

Communion Versus Isolation

- Who really understands your situation?
- When you have difficult days, with whom do you talk?
- In whose presence do you feel a bodily sense of peace?

Hope Versus Despair

- From what sources do you draw hope?
- On difficult days, what keeps you from giving up?
- Who have you known in your life who would not be surprised to see you hopeful despite adversity?
- What did this person understand about you that we do not know?

Purpose Versus Meaninglessness

- What keeps you going on difficult days?
- For whom, or for what, does it matter that you continue to live?
- What is your best sense as to what your life is about and how this illness fits in it?
- What do you hope to contribute with your life in whatever time you have remaining? (for the terminally ill patient)

Agency Versus Helplessness

- What is your prioritized list of concerns? What concerns you most?
- What most helps you to stand strong against the challenges of this illness?
- What should I know about you as a person that lies beyond your illness?
- How have you kept this illness from taking charge of your entire life?

Table 15–1. Existential postures: themes of resilience versus vulnerability *(continued)*

Courage Versus Cowardice

- Have there been moments when you felt tempted to give up but didn't? How did you make a decision to persevere?
- If you saw someone else taking such a step even though feeling afraid, would you consider that an act of courage?
- Can you imagine viewing yourself as courageous? Is that a description of yourself you would desire?
- Can you imagine that others who see how you are coping with this illness might describe you as courageous?

Gratitude Versus Resentment

- For what are you most grateful?
- Are there moments when you can still feel joy despite the sorrow you have been through?
- What sustains your capacity to experience joy in the midst of pain?
- If you could look back on this illness from some future time, what would you say that you took from the experience that added to your life?

Trust Versus Fear

- Who has given you a shoulder to lean on?
- Who relies on you? How did he or she first decide to trust you?

Source. Adapted with permission from Griffith JL, Gaby L: "Brief Psychotherapy at the Bedside: Countering Demoralization From Medical Illness." *Psychosomatics* 46:109–116, 2005.

- Collaborative support and strategies to reinforce adherence to treatment regimens that may be demanding or have unpleasant side effects
- The experience of giving to one another, which provides a tonic infusion of refreshed purpose and meaning for individuals whose illness has left them feeling impotent and dependent

Psychotherapy

Psychotherapy involves a relationship and the psychiatrist's effort to see the world through the patient's eyes. Even brief inpatient encounters can either serve and advance these goals or erode connection and hope. More formal, structured psychotherapy with medically ill patients is most often conducted in an outpatient setting.

Group Psychotherapy

Group psychotherapy, like psychoeducational groups, is most frequently organized according to type of illness, age group, or treatment modality. Regardless of the common ground shared by the patients, group processes give patients important opportunities for the following:

- *Emotional expression*—Shared expression in a group can reduce isolation and moderate the intensity of emotion shared with a spouse or family members.
- *Social support*—Patients have often experienced social losses as a consequence of illness; group psychotherapy can form the nidus for a new social network.
- *Shared coping strategies and resources*—Patients can learn a great deal from one another and may award peers with singular credibility and understanding.

Individual Therapy

Individual therapy, whether brief and focused or open-ended with evolving goals, may be largely supportive, interpersonal, or psychodynamic, depending on the unique circumstances of each patient. The patient's and clinician's choice of therapy includes consideration of the following:

- *Disease characteristics*—acute versus chronic, indolent versus life threatening, consequent disruptions in function (e.g., mobility, vocational, sexual), potential lifestyle modifications necessary
- *Psychiatric history*—previous anxiety or depression, illness-related experiences, family history
- *Goals*—for example, management of acute symptoms only versus resolving conflict at home or work brought to the fore by illness versus adjustment to major reorganization of life and priorities

Cognitive-Behavioral Therapy

Cognitive-behavioral therapy, provided in either group psychoeducational formats or in individual sessions that allow greater focus on each patient's situation and symptoms, has earned a broad evidence base for efficacy in reducing anxiety and depression (Hollon and Ponniah 2010; Zinbarg et al. 2010).

Family Therapy

Family therapy, although not often used, is a useful adjunct when a patient's diagnosis may force significant role changes, introduce new financial stressors, exhaust family caregivers, unmask prior dysfunction, or pose an imminent loss (Hartmann et al. 2010).

Hypnosis and Relaxation

Hypnosis is limited by the relative paucity of experienced and certified practitioners, the time commitment necessary, and the fact that a minority of patients (perhaps 25%) are able to fully engage in the process. However, a broader range of patients can be taught relaxation strategies and may, with diligent repetition, enable themselves to achieve deep relaxation that can provide adjunctive relief or assistance in situations in which hypnosis has also been successfully applied (Patterson and Jensen 2003; Surman and Baer 2008). Hypnosis and/or relaxation may be beneficial for patients experiencing the following:

- *Nausea and vomiting*—By recruiting an intensified focus away from the sensations and thoughts associated with nausea (i.e., displacing nausea from the patient's center stage of awareness), hypnosis and/or relaxation helps to diminish the symptom and interrupt a behavioral cycle (Miller and Whorwell 2009).
- *Pain*—Similarly, through hypnosis and/or relaxation, pain is relegated to the periphery of a patient's awareness, enabling the patient to deliberately replace the sensation with a more relaxing image or focus of attention. Although pain is not ablated, a patient may tolerate procedures more easily with less analgesic requirement (Lang et al. 2000; Stoelb et al. 2009).
- *Anxiety*—The benefit of hypnosis and/or relaxation is further enhanced when nausea or pain has exacerbated anxiety.
- *Problems with compliance and control*—To the extent that procedural pain or anxiety has impeded patient adherence to recommended diagnostic or therapeutic measures, hypnosis and/or relaxation can facilitate a successful outcome; this tool has the further advantage of providing the patient some sense of control over his or her circumstances.

References

Ahmed K, Mohan RA, Bhugra D: Self-harm in South Asian women: a literature review informed approach to assessment and formulation. Am J Psychother 61:71–81, 2007

American Psychiatric Association: Diagnostic and Statistical Manual of Mental Disorders, 4th Edition, Text Revision. Washington, DC, American Psychiatric Association, 2000

Bauer AM, Alegria M: Impact of patient language proficiency and interpreter service use on the quality of psychiatric care: a systematic review. Psychiatr Serv 61:765–773, 2010

Betancourt JR: Cultural competency: providing quality care to diverse populations. Consult Pharm 21:988–995, 2006

Breitbart W: Spirituality and meaning in supportive care: spirituality- and meaning-centered group psychotherapy interventions in advanced cancer. Support Care Cancer 10:272–280, 2002

Curlin FA, Odell SV, Lawrence RE, et al: The relationship between psychiatry and religion among U.S. physicians. Psychiatr Serv 58:1193–1198, 2007

de Leon J, Susce MT, Johnson M, et al: DNA microarray technology in the clinical environment: the AmpliChip CYP450 test for CYP2D6 and CYP2C19 genotyping. CNS Spectr 14:19–34, 2009

Diamond LC, Jacobs EA: Let's not contribute to disparities: the best methods for teaching clinicians how to overcome language barriers to health care. J Gen Intern Med 25 (suppl 2):S189–S193, 2010

Feng L, Chiam PC, Kua EH, et al: Use of complementary and alternative medicines and mental disorders in community-living Asian older adults. Arch Gerontol Geriatr 50:243–249, 2010

Galanter M: Spirituality in psychiatry: a biopsychosocial perspective. Psychiatry 73:145–157, 2010

Griffith JL, Gaby L: Brief psychotherapy at the bedside: countering demoralization from medical illness. Psychosomatics 46:109–116, 2005

Griffith JL, Griffith ME: Living beyond medical and psychiatric illness, in Encountering the Sacred in Psychotherapy. New York, Guilford Press, 2002, pp 258–300

Grossman S, Wyszynski AA, Barkin L, et al: When patients ask about the spiritual, in Manual of Psychiatric Care for the Medically Ill. Edited by Wyszynski AA, Wyszynski B. Washington, DC, American Psychiatric Publishing, 2005, pp 237–244

Hartmann M, Bazner E, Wild B, et al: Effects of interventions involving the family in the treatment of adult patients with chronic physical diseases: a meta-analysis. Psychother Psychosom 79:136–148, 2010

Hobbs K: Reflections on the culture of veterans. AAOHN J 56:337–341, 2008

Hollon SD, Ponniah K: A review of empirically supported psychological therapies for mood disorder in adults. Depress Anxiety 27:891–932, 2010

Huang B, Grant BF, Dawson DA, et al: Race-ethnicity and the prevalence and co-occurrence of Diagnostic and Statistical Manual of Mental Disorders, 4th Edition, alcohol and drug use disorders and Axis I and II disorders: United States, 2001 to 2002. Compr Psychiatry 47:252–257, 2006

Juckett G, Rudolf-Watson L: Recognizing mental illness in culture-bound syndromes. Am Fam Physician 81:206–210, 2010

Karliner LS, Perez-Stable EJ, Gildengorin G: The language divide: the importance of training in the use of interpreters for outpatient practice. J Gen Intern Med 19:175–183, 2004

Lewis-Fernandez R, Diaz N: The cultural formulation: a method for assessing cultural factors affecting the clinical encounter. Psychiatr Q 73:271–295, 2002

Li JZ, Quinn JV, McCulloch CE, et al: Patterns of complementary and alternative medicine use in ED patients and its association with health care utilization. Am J Emerg Med 22:187–191, 2004

Lang EV, Benotsch EG, Fick LJ, et al: Adjunctive non-pharmacological analgesia for invasive medical procedures: a randomized trial. Lancet 355:1486–1490, 2000

McGilloway A, Hall RE, Lee T, et al: A systematic review of personality disorder, race and ethnicity: prevalence, aetiology and treatment. BMC Psychiatry 10:33–47, 2010

Miller V, Whorwell PJ: Hypnotherapy for functional gastrointestinal disorders: a review. Int J Clin Exp Hypn 57:279–292, 2009

Mueller PS, Plevak DJ, Rummans TA: Religious involvement, spirituality, and medicine: implications for clinical practice. Mayo Clin Proc 76:1225–1235, 2001

Patterson DR, Jensen MP: Hypnosis and clinical pain. Psychol Bull 129:495–521, 2003

Piderman KM, Marek DV, Jenkins SM, et al: Patients' expectations of hospital chaplains. Mayo Clin Proc 83:58–65, 2008

Puchalski C, Romer AL: Taking a spiritual history allows clinicians to understand patients more fully. J Palliat Med 3:129–137, 2000

Steinhauser KE, Voils CI, Clipp EC, et al: "Are you at peace?" One item to probe spiritual concerns at the end of life. Arch Intern Med 166:101–105, 2006

Stoelb BL, Molton IR, Jensen MP, et al: The efficacy of hypnotic analgesia in adults: a review of the literature. Contemp Hypn 26:24–39, 2009

Surman OS, Baer L: Hypnosis, in Massachusetts General Hospital Comprehensive Clinical Psychiatry. Edited by Stern TA, Rosenbaum JF, Fava M, et al. Philadelphia, PA, Mosby, 2008, pp 183–188

Zhou SF: Polymorphism of human cytochrome P450 2D6 and its clinical significance: part I. Clin Pharmacokinet 48:689–723, 2009a

Zhou SF: Polymorphism of human cytochrome P450 2D6 and its clinical significance: part II. Clin Pharmacokinet 48:761–804, 2009b

Zinbarg RE, Mashal NM, Black DA, et al: The future and promise of cognitive behavioral therapy: a commentary. Psychiatr Clin North Am 33:711–727, 2010

PART IV

Unique Issues in Psychosomatic Medicine Settings

16

Bariatric Surgery

The number of bariatric surgical procedures performed in the United States has steadily increased. Several factors have contributed to this increase (Collazo-Clavell et al. 2006):

- The prevalence of extreme obesity continues to increase.
- Medical therapies for obesity have limited effectiveness.
- Weight loss after bariatric surgery has demonstrated positive effects on obesity-related medical complications. Benefits of surgery usually outweigh risks when there are at least partially remediable obesity-related medical complications in a reasonably suitable surgical candidate. Many measures of psychological and physical functioning convincingly improve after bariatric surgery (Powers and Santana 2011).

Types of Bariatric Surgery

Restrictive Procedure

A small pouch is created at the top of the stomach. Restrictive procedures include vertical-banded gastroplasty and adjustable gastric banding. Both procedures produce less dramatic weight loss over time than combination procedures.

319

Combined Restrictive and Malabsorptive Procedure

The most commonly performed combination procedures include biliopan-creatic diversion and the Roux-en-Y gastric bypass. Roux-en-Y gastric bypass is the most frequently performed bariatric surgery in the United States (Miller and Smith 2006), accounting for 80% of bariatric procedures (Adams et al. 2007). By bypassing the lower stomach and a majority of the small intestine, pH changes and malabsorption occur. Patients are at risk for nutrient deficiencies and require supplementation postoperatively. The surgery also has significant effects on drug absorption.

Criteria for Bariatric Surgery

No criteria have been published that completely address all of the complicated factors that must be collectively weighed before a patient gives informed consent for bariatric surgery. Bariatric surgery is never either risk-free or unquestioningly effective. Generally accepted guidelines (Collazo-Clavell et al. 2006; National Institutes of Health 1991) include the following:

- High body mass index (i.e., BMI≥40, or >35 if two or more serious remediable complications are present)
- Presence of obesity-related medical complications (e.g., diabetes, arthropathy, obstructive sleep apnea, stroke, cardiovascular disease)
- Documented or high probability of failure of nonsurgical weight loss interventions
- Demonstrated motivation and adherence
- High level of education about risks and benefits and ability to give informed consent

Medical Assessment of the Potential Bariatric Surgery Patient

1. Obtain comprehensive weight and nutrition history. Domains include current dietary habits, current physical activity, exercise habits, previous

weight loss efforts, medical treatments, duration of weight loss maintenance, and obstacles to successful weight loss maintenance.
2. Identify obesity-related medical comorbidities
3. Identify medical comorbidities that might affect surgical risk. Bariatric
surgery has few absolute medical contraindications. Certainly, patients
who cannot give informed consent because of disabling cognitive impairment and patients who have advanced liver disease with portal hypertension would not qualify as surgical candidates (Collazo-Clavell et al.
2006). Unstable coronary artery disease and uncontrolled severe obstructive sleep apnea cause great concern as well, particularly if accompanied
by other medical risks.
4. Identify medical causes of obesity (e.g., thyroid disorder, Cushing's syndrome).
5. Identify medications that may promote weight gain (especially antipsychotics, mood stabilizers, and antidepressants).
6. Review family history of obesity.
7. Identify harmful lifestyle habits (e.g., smoking, alcohol use, illicit drug
use).

Psychiatric Assessment of the Potential Bariatric Surgery Patient

Lack of Evidence-Based Evaluative Models or Consensus Guidelines

No evidence-based evaluative models or consensus guidelines currently exist
to guide psychiatric evaluation of bariatric surgery candidacy. Different centers have different methodologies and thresholds (Fabricatore et al. 2006;
Marcus et al. 2009). In practice, most centers would list only a few absolute
psychiatric contraindications for bariatric surgery. Most centers would include the following (Bauchowitz et al. 2005):

- Active alcohol abuse
- Inability to maintain adherence to medical treatments and medications
- Active anorexia or bulimia nervosa

- Significant current suicidality or self-harm impulses requiring psychiatric hospitalization
- Severe personality disorder
- Active psychosis
- Current manic episode
- Inability to provide informed consent

Negative Effects of Presurgical Psychiatric Disorders on Postsurgical Weight Loss

The presence of presurgical psychiatric disorders negatively impacts postsurgical weight loss. Recent psychiatric hospitalization and the presence of a psychiatric disorder have each been associated with suboptimal weight loss after surgery (Herpetz et al. 2004; Kinzl et al. 2006). Bariatric surgery candidates who have two or more psychiatric diagnoses have significantly less postsurgical weight loss than patients with one or no psychiatric disorder (weight loss of 10.8, 14.0, and 16.0 BMI units, respectively, $P=0.047$; Kinzl et al. 2006). Often, the recommendation is to delay surgery until a psychiatric disorder or behavioral disturbance is more stable or better managed.

High Rates of Psychiatric Disorders Among Bariatric Surgery Candidates

High rates of psychiatric disorders exist among bariatric surgery candidates. Up to 70% of patients referred for weight loss surgery have a lifetime history of a psychiatric disorder, and up to 50% have a current psychiatric disorder (Black et al. 1992; Herpetz et al. 2004; Kalarchian et al. 2007; Mauri et al. 2008; Rosenberger et al. 2006; Rosik 2005; Sarwer et al. 2005). Half are taking psychotropic medications at the time of presurgical evaluation (Pawlow et al. 2005). The following are the most common psychiatric diagnoses:

- Major depressive disorder
- Generalized anxiety disorder
- Posttraumatic stress disorder
- Obsessive-compulsive disorder
- Social anxiety disorder
- Substance use disorder

- Binge-eating disorder
- Night eating syndrome
- Somatoform disorders

Psychological Issues That May Be Associated With Poor Outcomes

Some specific psychological issues may be associated with poor outcomes. Although no level 1 evidence is available yet, case series, case reports, and expert consensus all strongly suggest that the following psychosocial factors predict suboptimal postsurgical weight loss and psychological adjustment (Black et al. 1992; Herpetz et al. 2004; Rosik 2005; Sarwer et al. 2005):

- Binge eating pattern.
- Night eating pattern.
- History of past or current physical, sexual, or emotional abuse that is associated with a positive aspect of obesity (i.e., avoidance of intimacy). History of childhood maltreatment is associated with elevated risk for psychiatric hospitalization after gastric bypass. Patients who derive positive psychological benefit from obesity related to abuse history need to be identified and treated with psychotherapy (Clark et al. 2007).
- Nonadherence to medical, medication, and nutritional advice. Demonstrating that behavioral changes can be made prior to surgery, even if weight is not actually lost preoperatively, improves patient confidence that the changes can be maintained after surgery.

Elements of Psychiatric Evaluation of a Bariatric Surgery Candidate

At least 20% of patients being evaluated for weight loss surgery have active psychiatric illness that should be addressed prior to proceeding with bariatric surgery (Wildes et al. 2008; Zimmerman et al. 2007). The following clinical domains are derived from reported reasons for recommending surgery deferral for psychiatric reasons:

- Current and past psychiatric diagnoses and treatments, especially of mood, eating, anxiety, substance use, and personality disorders.

- Psychiatric predisposition (i.e., family history, past history).
- Medical history, including potential toxic or metabolic contributors to psychiatric symptoms and signs.
- Nutritional and weight loss history, including self-described barriers to maintenance of weight loss in the past.
- Eating patterns, focusing on history of binge eating, night eating, and image of food as comforting. Questions about a patient's capacity to self-soothe, relax, and manage stress should be included.
- Current and past physical, emotional, or sexual abuse history, along with documentation about whether the patient derives positive psychological benefit to being overweight. Questions about intimacy and desire for intimacy are important and appropriate. Up to 66% of bariatric surgery candidates report childhood history of emotional, sexual, or physical abuse (Wildes et al. 2008). History of childhood maltreatment is associated with risk for psychiatric hospitalization after gastric bypass (Clark et al. 2007).
- Evidence for adherence and nonadherence to medical, medication, and nutritional advice.
- Assessment of locus of control. A patient with an external locus of control may minimize his or her view that he or she can exert significant influence on outcome of weight loss attempts, including surgery. For example, the patient may minimize the roles of physical exercise, nutrition-related behavioral changes, and social support.
- Documentation of available supports, including both perioperative physical assistance and postoperative sources of emotional support.
- Lifestyle considerations, including physical activity, eating habits of others in the house, smoking, and alcohol and drug use patterns.
- Current medications. After surgery, a patient may experience changes in absorption and distribution of medications, including, and perhaps especially, psychotropic medications.
- Careful mental status examination. The psychiatrist must establish that the patient's self-harm risk is low and that the patient has sufficient cognitive capacity to provide informed consent.

Presurgical Psychiatric Management

1. *Optimally manage psychiatric disorders.* In the Mayo Clinic integrated bariatric surgery practice (Collazo-Clavell et al. 2006), patients must not have had psychiatric hospitalization for 12 months prior to surgery. Also, for patients with a diagnosed substance use disorder, 12 months of abstinence must be documented before surgery proceeds.

2. *Document completion of indicated psychotherapy interventions.* In the Mayo Clinic bariatric surgery practice, patients are required to have documentation of successful completion of psychotherapy by a licensed mental health professional for identified psychosocial barriers to postsurgical confidence in ability to maintain weight loss (Collazo-Clavell et al. 2006). The content of most psychotherapy focuses on trauma survivorship issues, adherence issues, extreme internal locus of control, and difficulties with impulse control that lead to stress eating and night eating.

3. *Prescribe behavioral and lifestyle interventions that build patient confidence that postsurgical weight loss can be maintained.* To assess motivation, predict adherence to postsurgical recommendations, and build confidence in providers and patients, some programs mandate that patients achieve behavioral milestones (and sometimes actual weight loss) prior to surgery. Although no published randomized controlled trial has examined the benefits of receiving behavioral therapy before bariatric surgery with regard to postsurgical weight loss, some programs require completion of presurgical behavioral structured interventions that focus on improved nutrition, eating patterns, social support, exercise, and stress management. Patients are told that making necessary lifestyle and eating pattern changes before surgery should give them increased confidence they can maintain those necessary changes postoperatively.

4. *Consider presurgery psychotropic medication drug levels.* Drug solubility and surface area for absorption are affected by gastric bypass:

   • *Potential for reduced drug absorption.* Reductions in the amount of functioning gastrointestinal tract lead to reduced drug bioavailability because of decreased surface area for drug absorption and reduced transit time (Miller and Smith 2006).

- *Reduced solubility of drugs.* The solubility of drugs is affected by pH. Drugs that are more soluble in an acidic pH are absorbed in the stomach, and those soluble in alkaline environments are absorbed in the small intestine. The solubility of both types of drugs is affected by gastric bypass.

Perioperative Psychiatric Management

During the perioperative period, consulting psychiatrists should watch for evidence of changes in the effects of psychotropic medications, due to absorptive and metabolic changes that occur as a result of bypass procedures. Ensuring ongoing availability of sources of social support and providing supportive psychotherapy may be important for helping some patients. Other reasons for psychiatric consultation during the perioperative period include delirium management and pain control.

Postoperative Psychiatric Management

1. *Make postoperative support groups and individual psychotherapy available.* Psychological issues may not have been completely resolved during preoperative psychotherapy, or may reemerge with body image changes precipitated by postsurgical weight loss.
2. *Follow patients as indicated.* Even with optimal preoperative psychiatric management, this patient population has an elevated baseline level of psychiatric illness and will frequently have psychiatric disorders recur postoperatively.
3. *Consider postoperative psychotropic medication drug levels.* In the postoperative periods, absorptive area losses and pH changes may affect bioavailability and absorption of medications, including psychotropic medications. With metabolic changes and adipose tissue loss come the possibilities for changes in volume of distribution and in amounts of drugs, particularly lipophilic drugs, stored in body fat. At the Mayo Clinic, psychotropic medication levels are routinely measured 1 week before surgery

and again 1 and 12 months after surgery, even if blood has to be sent out to specialty laboratories. Medication dosage changes are sometimes required postoperatively.

4. *Change extended-release preparations to regular-release formulations.* Many psychotropic medications are available in extended-release preparations and therefore have long absorptive phases. Because of the large loss of surface area for absorption and reduced transit time, extended-release medications have even greater likelihood of being affected by bypass procedures than do regular-release preparations (Miller and Smith 2006). Liquid or orally disintegrating tablet versions of drugs, if available, are likely to be better absorbed.

References

Adams TD, Gress RE, Smith SC, et al: Long-term mortality after gastric bypass surgery. N Engl J Med 357:753–761, 2007

Bauchowitz AU, Gonder-Frederick LA, Olbrisch ME, et al: Psychosocial evaluation of bariatric surgery candidates: a survey of present practices. Psychosom Med 67:825–832, 2005

Black DW, Goldstein RB, Mason EE: Prevalence of mental disorder in 88 morbidly obese bariatric clinic patients. Am J Psychiatry 149:227–234, 1992

Clark MM, Hanna BK, Mai JL, et al: Sexual abuse survivors and psychiatric hospitalization after bariatric surgery. Obes Surg 19:465–469, 2007

Collazo-Clavell ML, Clark MM, McAlpine DE, et al: Assessment and preparation of patients for bariatric surgery. Mayo Clin Proc 81 (suppl):S11–S17, 2006

Fabricatore AN, Crerand CE, Wadden T, et al: How do mental health professionals evaluate candidates for bariatric surgery? Obes Surg 16:567–573, 2006

Herpetz S, Kielmann R, Wolf AM, et al: Do psychosocial variables predict weight loss or mental health after obesity surgery: a systematic review. Obes Res 12:1554–1569, 2004

Kalarchian MA, Marcus MD, Levine MD, et al: Psychiatric disorders among bariatric surgery candidates: relationship to obesity and functional health status. Am J Psychiatry 164:328–334, 2007

Kinzl JF, Schrattenencker M, Traweger C, et al: Psychosocial predictors of weight loss after bariatric surgery. Obes Surg 16:1609–1614, 2006

Marcus MD, Kalarchian MA, Courcoulas AP: Psychiatric evaluation and follow-up of bariatric surgery patients. Am J Psychiatry 166:285–291, 2009

Mauri M, Rucci P, Calderone A, Santini F, et al: Axis I and II disorders and quality of life in bariatric surgery candidates. J Clin Psychiatry 69:295–301, 2008

Miller AD, Smith KM: Medication and nutrient administration considerations after bariatric surgery. Am J Health Syst Pharm 63:1852–1857, 2006

National Institutes of Health Consensus Development Conference Panel: NIH Conference: gastrointestinal surgery for severe obesity. Ann Intern Med 115:956–961, 1991

Pawlow LA, O'Neill PM, White MA, et al: Findings and outcomes of psychological evaluations of gastric bypass applicants. Surg Obes Relat Dis 1:523–527, 2005

Powers PS, Santana CA: Surgery, in The American Psychiatric Publishing Textbook of Psychosomatic Medicine, 2nd Edition. Edited by Levenson JL. Washington, DC, American Psychiatric Publishing, 2011, pp 691–724

Rosenberger PH, Henderson KE, Grilo CM: Psychiatric disorder comorbidity and association with eating disorders in bariatric surgery patients: a cross-sectional study using structured interview-based diagnosis. J Clin Psychiatry 67:1080–1085, 2006

Rosik CH: Psychiatric symptoms among prospective bariatric surgery patients: rates of prevalence and their relation to social desirability, pursuit of surgery, and follow-up attendance. Obes Surg 15:677–683, 2005

Sarwer DB, Wadden TA, Fabricatore AN: Psychosocial and behavioral aspects of bariatric surgery. Obes Res 13:639–648, 2005

Wildes JE, Kalarchian MA, Marcus MD, et al: Childhood maltreatment and psychiatric morbidity in bariatric surgery candidates. Obes Surg 18:306–313, 2008

Zimmerman M, Rancione-Witt C, Chelminski I, et al: Presurgical psychiatric evaluations of candidates for bariatric surgery, part I: reliability and reasons for and frequency of exclusion. J Clin Psychiatry 68:1557–1562, 2007

17

Cardiology

Cardiovascular disease (CVD) is highly prevalent in the general population. The lifetime risk at age 40 is one in two for men and one in three for women (Lloyd-Jones et al. 1999). The relationship between CVD and psychiatric illness is complex: psychosocial factors have effects on the cardiovascular system, and cardiac disease influences psychiatric symptoms. Depression is associated with the development of CVD and predicts cardiac hospital admissions and death, as well as increased health care costs and utilization of services; however, mental health treatment has not been shown to change cardiac outcomes. Given the prevalence of CVD, the psychosomatic medicine psychiatrist must be aware of the interrelationship of psychiatric illness and CVD and recognize the potential impact of psychiatric interventions on the cardiovascular system (Shapiro 2011).

Relationship Between Depression and Cardiovascular Disease

Prevalence of Comorbidity

The prevalence rates of depression in patients with CVD range from 17% to 27% (Evans et al. 2005).

Depression and Increased Risk for Onset of Cardiovascular Disease

Substantial evidence demonstrates that depression is associated with an elevated risk for the development of CVD in initially healthy individuals. The effect sizes range from 1.5 to 2.7 depending on the definition of CVD and the measure of depression, with major depression a stronger predictor than depressive mood (Lett et al. 2004; Rugulies 2002; Wulsin and Singal 2003). Depression is often described as a "cardiac risk factor," but caution is advised in using this terminology because it can imply a causal relationship. Although the evidence is robust that depression is correlated with the incidence of CVD, whether depression may reflect preclinical cardiac disease is unknown (Frasure-Smith and Lespérance 2010).

Depression Independently Associated With Poor Prognosis

Depression predicts morbidity and death in patients with existing CVD, and this relationship remains significant after statistical adjustment for covariates reflecting cardiac disease severity. For patients with stable CVD, both anxiety and depression have been shown to predict greater major cardiac events at 2-year follow-up (Frasure-Smith and Lespérance 2008).

Myocardial Infarction

A number of studies have examined the relationship of depression and outcome in patients after myocardial infarction (MI); the majority of the studies have demonstrated increased mortality (Carney et al. 2003; Frasure-Smith et al. 1993; Lett et al. 2004). Among hospitalized patients following MI, major depression predicts mortality at 6 months and its impact is at least equivalent to that of left ventricular dysfunction and a history of previous MI (Frasure-Smith et al. 1993). The risk of death is four times greater for depressed patients than for nondepressed control patients (Frasure-Smith et al. 1993), and patients 5 years after acute MI who were depressed during the time of admission have a greater than 3.5-fold increased risk of cardiac death (Lespérance et al. 2002).

Congestive Heart Failure

Depression is associated with an increased incidence of congestive heart failure in patients with coronary artery disease, regardless of antidepressant treatment (May et al. 2009), and depression predicts long-term mortality in patients with comorbid congestive heart failure and atrial fibrillation (Frasure-Smith et al. 2010).

Cardiac Surgery

Compared with cardiac coronary bypass graft surgery patients without depression, patients who have moderate to severe depression at baseline or persistent depression 6 months after the surgery have more than a twofold increase in mortality independent of the number of grafts, diabetes, smoking, left ventricular ejection fraction, and previous MI (Blumenthal et al. 2003). Depression also predicts mortality in patients who undergo cardiac valve surgery (Ho et al. 2005).

Comorbidity Mechanisms

A number of mechanisms linking depression to CVD have been proposed, although none of the factors individually provides an explanation for the association. If CVD and depression are causally related, it is likely to be multifactorial (Frasure-Smith and Lespérance 2010).

Nonadherence

Depressed patients are less likely to adhere to treatment recommendations, and nonadherence to treatment and recommended lifestyle changes are associated with worse cardiac outcomes (Horwitz et al. 1990; McDermott et al. 1997).

Shared Risk Factors

A number of factors have been identified with an increased risk of CVD; these include smoking, hypertension, obesity, and high levels of alcohol consumption. Depressed individuals are more likely than nondepressed individuals to have one or more of these risk factors, and therefore the link between CVD and depression could be due to shared risk factors (Blumenthal et al. 2003; Joynt et al. 2003; Lett et al. 2004).

Platelet Activity

Platelets play an important role in the development of atherosclerosis and acute coronary syndromes, and depression has been linked to increased platelet activation and hypercoagulability (Kop et al. 2002; Musselman et al. 1996).

Hypothalamic-Pituitary-Adrenal and Sympathoadrenal Activation

Hypothalamic-pituitary-adrenal (HPA) axis dysregulation is associated with depression, and HPA axis hyperactivity augments sympathoadrenal hyperactivity, manifested by elevated plasma norepinephrine. HPA and sympathoadrenal hyperactivity may promote the development of CVD and worsen prognosis (Joynt et al. 2003).

Autonomic Nervous System Dysfunction

The association between impaired autonomic function and depression among CVD patients has been demonstrated, and decreased heart rate variability is a risk factor for sudden death and ventricular arrhythmias in patients with CVD (Kleiger et al. 1987). Evidence suggests an association between depression and decreased heart rate variability (Carney et al. 2001); the decreased heart rate variability partially mediates the effect of depression on increased mortality after MI (Carney et al. 2005), although not all studies support a correlation (Gehi et al. 2005).

Inflammation

Depressed patients with or without CVD have elevated plasma levels of inflammatory markers. An accelerated inflammatory response may contribute to CVD, or CVD may induce physiological changes that result in depression (Joynt et al. 2003; Kop et al. 2002).

Anxiety

Prevalence

Anxiety has not been studied as extensively as depression, but anxiety symptoms appear to be elevated in patients with acute coronary disease, and anxiety occurs in 5%–10% of patients with chronic CVD (Frasure-Smith and Lespérance 2008; Sullivan et al. 2010). Although anxiety is often underdiagnosed in hospitalized patients, some evidence suggests that anxiety is better recognized than depression by the medical staff in patients after MI (Huffman et al. 2006).

Association With Reduced Adherence

Anxiety is associated with reduced adherence to many risk-reducing recommendations after MI, particularly smoking cessation (Kuhl et al. 2009).

Predictive Value of Cardiac Mortality

Some data suggest that anxiety is a predictor of cardiac morbidity and mortality, but, overall, the evidence is much stronger linking depression and increased cardiac mortality than anxiety (Eaker et al. 2005; Frasure-Smith and Lespérance 2008; Meyer et al. 2010; Phillips et al. 2009).

Atypical Chest Pain and Palpitations

Atypical chest pain and palpitations commonly occur in patients who have psychiatric illness, including panic disorder, somatoform disorders, or depression. Characteristics predictive of a diagnosis of panic disorder in patients with chest pain include absence of coronary artery disease, atypical chest pain quality, female sex, younger age, and high self-reported anxiety (Huffman and Pollack 2003).

Special Issues

Implantable Cardioverter-Defibrillator

Studies examining psychopathology and quality of life after implantable cardioverter-defibrillator placement have increased in recent years, although the results have been contradictory (Bostwick and Sola 2007). Avoidance and nonspecific somatic worry can develop, and new-onset panic disorder and posttraumatic stress disorder have been reported. Preimplantation psychological variables, such as history of depression, trait anxiety, and dispositional optimism, may account for as much of the variance in quality of life outcomes as do ejection fraction and age (Sears et al. 2005). Data are conflicting regarding whether increased frequency of shocks is associated with the development of psychiatric disorders, but patient concern about being shocked, regardless of whether the shock occurs, appears to be correlated with psychological morbidity (Pedersen et al. 2005). The literature regarding treatment is limited, but findings are encouraging for the effectiveness of psychosocial interventions, including preimplantation education programs and cognitive-behavioral therapy (CBT), in reducing anxiety and improving quality of life (Lewin et al. 2009; Salmoirago-Blotcher and Ockene 2009; Sears et al. 2007).

Left Ventricular Assist Device

Left ventricular assist devices (LVADs) are used as an alternative therapy for patients with end-stage heart failure who do not qualify for cardiac transplantation or as a bridge for patients awaiting transplantation. LVADs as destination therapy were approved by the U.S. Food and Drug Administration in 2003. As the use of LVADs continues to rise, understanding the psychiatric and quality of life issues involved for patients and transplant selection teams has become increasingly important. The specific self-care behaviors required for LVAD patients are different from those for transplant patients, but both groups have many similarities, including the need to take multiple medications for a lifetime and to adhere to prescribed health behaviors, cardiac rehabilitation, frequent lab tests, and ongoing physician visits. The LVAD patient also needs to perform technical tasks related to the device, which require the cognitive ability to follow complex instructions. Patients receiving destination therapy may initially feel hope and relief, but if they functionally decline, their feelings may change to anger or disappointment that transplant is not an option (Eshelman et al. 2009).

Treatment Issues

Treatment of Depression and Reduction of Cardiovascular Risk

Despite the link between CVD and depression, studies have not been able to demonstrate a reduction in cardiovascular risk by treating depression (Thombs et al. 2008).

- The Sertraline Antidepressant Heart Attack Randomized Trial (SADHART) was the first trial to examine the safety and efficacy of sertraline treatment for depressed patients hospitalized with acute MI or unstable angina. The study's major contribution was to demonstrate the safety of treatment with sertraline. Mortality was not significantly different between the treated and untreated groups, and the efficacy data were mixed, with improvement primarily found in the patients with severe or recurrent depression (Glassman et al. 2002).

- The Enhancing Recovery in Coronary Heart Disease (ENRICHD) study found that CBT improved depression and social isolation in patients after MI, but the effect size was small and CBT had no impact on cardiovascular morbidity or mortality (Berkman et al. 2003).

- The Canadian Cardiac Randomized Evaluation of Antidepressant and Psychotherapy Efficacy (CREATE) trial demonstrated efficacy of citalopram plus weekly clinical management for major depression among patients with CVD, and found no benefit of interpersonal therapy over clinical management (Lespérance et al. 2007).

- The Myocardial INfarction and Depression-Intervention Trial (MIND-IT), an effectiveness trial to determine whether an active treatment strategy resulted in better outcomes than usual care, demonstrated that antidepressant treatment did not improve depression or cardiac prognosis (van Melle et al. 2006, 2007), although mirtazapine appeared to be safe in patients after MI (Honig et al. 2007).

Pharmacological Considerations

The selective serotonin reuptake inhibitors (SSRIs) are generally considered first-line treatments for patients with depression and CVD, in contrast to the tricyclic antidepressants, which may delay cardiac conduction, increase heart rate, and prolong the QT and PR intervals. Limited data suggest that SSRIs may be cardioprotective, but further studies are needed (Evans et al. 2005; Glassman et al. 2002). (See also Chapter 14, "Biological Treatments.")

References

Berkman LF, Blumenthal J, Burg M, et al: Effects of treating depression and low perceived social support on clinical events after myocardial infarction: the Enhancing Recovery in Coronary Heart Disease Patients (ENRICHD) randomized trial. JAMA 289:3106–3116, 2003

Blumenthal JA, Lett HS, Babyak MA, et al: Depression as a risk factor for mortality after coronary artery bypass surgery. Lancet 362:604–609, 2003

Bostwick JM, Sola CL: An updated review of implantable cardioverter/defibrillators, induced anxiety, and quality of life. Psychiatr Clin North Am 30:677–688, 2007

Carney RM, Blumenthal JA, Stein PK, et al: Depression, heart rate variability, and acute myocardial infarction. Circulation 104:2024–2028, 2001

Carney RM, Blumenthal JA, Catellier D, et al: Depression as a risk factor for mortality after acute myocardial infarction. Am J Cardiol 92:1277–1281, 2003

Carney RM, Blumenthal JA, Freedland KE, et al: Low heart rate variability and the effect of depression on post-myocardial infarction mortality. Arch Intern Med 165:1486–1491, 2005

Eaker ED, Sullivan LM, Kelly Hayes M, et al: Tension and anxiety and the prediction of the 10-year incidence of coronary heart disease, atrial fibrillation, and total mortality: the Framingham Offspring Study. Psychosom Med 67:692–696, 2005

Eshelman AK, Mason S, Nemeh H, et al: LVAD destination therapy: applying what we know about psychiatric evaluation and management from cardiac failure and transplant. Heart Fail Rev 14:21–28, 2009

Evans DL, Charney DS, Lewis L, et al: Mood disorders in the medically ill: scientific review and recommendations. Biol Psychiatry 58:175–189, 2005

Frasure-Smith N, Lespérance F: Depression and anxiety as predictors of 2-year cardiac events in patients with stable coronary artery disease. Arch Gen Psychiatry 65:62–71, 2008

Frasure-Smith N, Lespérance F: Depression and cardiac risk: present status and future directions. Heart 96:173–176, 2010

Frasure-Smith N, Lespérance F, Talajic M: Depression following myocardial infarction: impact on 6-month survival. (Erratum in JAMA 271:1082, 1994.) JAMA 270:1819–1825, 1993

Frasure-Smith N, Lespérance F, Habra M, et al: Elevated depression symptoms predict long-term cardiovascular mortality in patients with atrial fibrillation and heart failure. Circulation 120:134–140, 2010

Gehi A, Mangano D, Pipkin S, et al: Depression and heart rate variability in patients with stable coronary heart disease: findings from the Heart and Soul Study. Arch Gen Psychiatry 62:661–666, 2005

Glassman AH, O'Connor CM, Califf RM, et al: Sertraline treatment of major depression in patients with acute MI or unstable angina. (Erratum in JAMA 288:1720, 2002.) JAMA 288:701–709, 2002

Ho PM, Masoudi FA, Spertus JA, et al: Depression predicts mortality following cardiac valve surgery. Ann Thorac Surg 79:1255–1259, 2005

Honig A, Kuyper AMG, Schene AH, et al: Treatment of post-myocardial infarction depressive disorder: a randomized, placebo-controlled trial with mirtazapine. Psychosom Med 69:606–613, 2007

Horwitz RI, Viscoli CM, Berkman L, et al: Treatment adherence and risk of death after a myocardial infarction. Lancet 336:542–545, 1990

Huffman JC, Pollack MH: Predicting panic disorder among patients with chest pain: an analysis of the literature. Psychosomatics 44:222–236, 2003

Huffman JC, Smith FA, Blais MA, et al: Recognition and treatment of depression and anxiety in patients with acute myocardial infarction. Am J Cardiol 98:319–324, 2006

Joynt KE, Whellan DJ, O'Connor CM: Depression and cardiovascular disease: mechanisms of interaction. Biol Psychiatry 54:248–261, 2003

Kleiger RE, Miller JP, Bigger JT Jr, et al: Decreased heart rate variability and its association with increased mortality after acute myocardial infarction. Am J Cardiol 59:256–262, 1987

Kop WJ, Gottdiener JS, Tangen CM, et al: Inflammation and coagulation factors in persons >65 years of age with symptoms of depression but without evidence of myocardial ischemia. Am J Cardiol 89:419–424, 2002

Kuhl EA, Fauerbach JA, Bush DE, et al: Relation of anxiety and adherence to risk-reducing recommendations following myocardial infarction. Am J Cardiol 103:1629–1634, 2009

Lespérance F, Frasure-Smith N, Talajic M, et al: Five-year risk of cardiac mortality in relation to initial severity and one-year changes in depression symptoms after myocardial infarction. Circulation 105:1049–1053, 2002

Lespérance F, Frasure-Smith N, Koszycki D, et al: Effects of citalopram and interpersonal psychotherapy on depression in patients with coronary artery disease: the Canadian Cardiac Randomized Evaluation of Antidepressant and Psychotherapy Efficacy (CREATE) trial. (Erratum in JAMA 298:40, 2007.) JAMA 297:367–379, 2007

Lett HS, Blumenthal JA, Babyak MA, et al: Depression as a risk factor for coronary artery disease: evidence, mechanisms, and treatment. Psychosom Med 66:305–315, 2004

Lewin RJ, Coulton S, Frizelle DJ, et al: A brief cognitive behavioural preimplantation and rehabilitation programme for patients receiving an implantable cardioverter-defibrillator improves physical health and reduces psychological morbidity and unplanned readmissions. Heart 95:63–69, 2009

Lloyd-Jones DM, Larson MG, Beiser A, et al: Lifetime risk of developing coronary heart disease. Lancet 353:89–92, 1999

May HT, Horne BD, Carlquist JF, et al: Depression after coronary artery disease is associated with heart failure. J Am Coll Cardiol 53:1440–1447, 2009

McDermott MM, Schmitt B, Wallner E: Impact of medication nonadherence on coronary heart disease outcomes: a critical review. Arch Intern Med 157:1921–1929, 1997

Meyer T, Buss U, Herrmann-Lingen C: Role of cardiac disease severity in the predictive value of anxiety for all-cause mortality. Psychosom Med 72:9–15, 2010

Musselman DL, Tomer A, Manatunga AK, et al: Exaggerated platelet reactivity in major depression. Am J Psychiatry 153:1313–1317, 1996

Pedersen SS, van Domburg RT, Theuns DA, et al: Concerns about the implantable cardioverter defibrillator: a determinant of anxiety and depressive symptoms independent of experienced shocks. Am Heart J 149:664–669, 2005

Phillips AC, Batty GD, Gale CR, et al: Generalized anxiety disorder, major depressive disorder, and their comorbidity as predictors of all-cause and cardiovascular mortality: the Vietnam experience study. Psychosom Med 71:395–403, 2009

Rugulies R: Depression as a predictor for coronary heart disease: a review and meta-analysis. Am J Prev Med 23:51–61, 2002

Salmoirago-Blotcher E, Ockene IS: Methodological limitations of psychosocial interventions in patients with an implantable cardioverter-defibrillator (ICD): a systematic review. BMC Cardiovasc Disord 9:56, 2009

Sears SF, Lewis TS, Kuhl EA, et al: Predictors of quality of life in patients with implantable cardioverter defibrillators. Psychosomatics 46:451–457, 2005

Sears SF, Sowell LD, Kuhl EA, et al: The ICD shock and stress management program: a randomized trial of psychosocial treatment to optimize quality of life in ICD patients. Pacing Clin Electrophysiol 30:858–864, 2007

Shapiro PA: Heart disease, in The American Psychiatric Publishing Textbook of Psychosomatic Medicine, 2nd Edition. Edited by Levenson JL. Washington, DC, American Psychiatric Publishing, 2011, pp 407–440

Sullivan MD, LaCroix AZ, Spertus JA, et al: Five-year prospective study of the effects of anxiety and depression in patients with coronary artery disease. Am J Cardiol 86:1135–1138, 2010

Thombs BD, de Jonge P, Coyne JC, et al: Depression screening and patient outcomes in cardiovascular care: a systematic review. JAMA 300:2161–2171, 2008

van Melle JP, de Jonge P, Kuyper AM, et al: Prediction of depressive disorder following myocardial infarction data from the Myocardial INfarction and Depression–Intervention Trial (MIND-IT). Int J Cardiol 109:88–94, 2006

van Melle JP, de Jonge P, Honig A, et al: Effects of antidepressant treatment following myocardial infarction. Br J Psychiatry 190:460–466, 2007

Wulsin LR, Singal BM: Do depressive symptoms increase the risk for the onset of coronary disease? A systematic quantitative review. Psychosom Med 65:201–210, 2003

18

Dermatology

Psychiatric disorders are frequent among dermatology patients. The prevalence of DSM-IV-TR (American Psychiatric Association 2000) conditions in these patients may be as high as 40% (Picardi et al. 2006). Several groups of psychocutaneous conditions cut across DSM-IV-TR categories. Psychocutaneous conditions may be delusional (e.g., delusional parasitosis), somatoform (e.g., body dysmorphic disorder), functional (e.g., unexplained pruritus), factitious (e.g., dermatitis artefacta), or psychophysiological (e.g., atopic dermatitis), or related to another psychiatric disorder (e.g., trichotillomania).

Delusional Psychocutaneous Conditions

Delusional psychocutaneous conditions share the characteristic that a fixed false belief that defies reality testing is central to the clinical presentation. Psychocutaneous disorders of delusional severity are among the most treatment-resistant conditions encountered by psychosomatic medicine psychiatrists. Evidence from randomized controlled treatment trials is lacking because many people who believe or fear that they have a dermatological condition doubt or reject the possibility that psychological factors may be relevant; therefore, they are unlikely to participate in psychiatric treatment research. Limited knowledge about effective management, coupled with the density of patients' beliefs about their skin symptoms, creates challenges in clinical management (Lepping et al. 2007). Some psychosomatic medicine outpatient consultants report anecdotal success in gaining access to patients by seeing them in the dermatology clinic instead of in a psychosomatic medicine or general psychiatry clinic (Rundell 2008; Woodruff et al. 1997).

Delusional Parasitosis

Clinical Presentation

Delusional parasitosis typically has a monosymptomatic presentation. Patients with delusional parasitosis seek dermatological care because they believe, despite compelling evidence to the contrary, that they have been invaded by parasites. They vigorously assert their beliefs about what the organisms are doing to their skin. Patients usually have a specific theory about how they came to be infected; they see or sense skin lesions that others, including medical professionals, cannot appreciate. Medical evaluations are normal.

Delusional parasitosis patients may generate high health care costs. Patients typically make multiple attempts at evaluation and treatment, often moving from physician to physician and center to center in repeated attempts to gain definitive evaluation and treatment. Each physician and clinic repeats a comprehensive evaluation, often under substantial pressure from patients and sometimes their families or friends.

Clinical Management

Pharmacological approaches.   Advice regarding clinical management of delusional parasitosis is based on small case series, case reports, and one very small double-blind, placebo-controlled crossover study in 1982 (Hamann and Avnstorp 1982; Lepping et al. 2007). In the controlled study, 10 of 11 patients who received pimozide improved; this study was limited by small sample size and lack of randomization. Antipsychotic medications said to be effective in case reports or series include haloperidol, risperidone, quetiapine, trifluoperazine, fluphenazine, aripiprazole, olanzapine, and chlorpromazine (Lepping et al. 2007; Sambhi and Lepping 2010). These case reports must be interpreted cautiously, however, because unsuccessful treatments are not likely to be reported or accepted for publication. Use of antipsychotic medication requires attention to the possibility of QTc prolongation and motor and metabolic adverse effects.

Nonpharmacological approaches. Psychotherapy has minimal efficacy in treatment of delusional parasitosis. Advice to dermatologists and general internists should include emphases on empathically listening to patients, conducting appropriate and regular examinations so patients will not feel compelled to "doctor shop," and focusing on each patient's ability to function. The physicians should make an effort not to reinforce the delusional beliefs; however, they should also avoid taking a completely neutral stance that will make a patient guarded (Sandoz et al. 2008). Asking how the condition has affected the patient's life may lead to recommendations to the patient and family about improving social or occupational functioning.

Other Delusional Disorders With Skin Manifestations

When anxiety or fear about a perceived skin-related condition becomes a fixed false belief, the psychiatrist diagnoses delusional disorder, somatic type.

Clinical Presentations

Delusions apart from parasitosis can take the form of beliefs that ingested or inhaled motile substances or shards may be forcing their way out through the skin or beliefs about defects in appearance (akin to body dysmorphic disorder) or skin odor (olfactory reference syndrome).

Clinical Management

Principles of treating delusions of motile substances or shards are the same as principles of managing delusional parasitosis. Authors report anecdotal success with managing delusional beliefs about defects in skin appearance with selective serotonin reuptake inhibitors (SSRIs) (Phillips 1996; Phillips et al. 2002). If symptoms do not respond to SSRI medications, an antipsychotic may be helpful.

Somatoform Psychocutaneous Conditions

Body Dysmorphic Disorder

Clinical Presentation

Body dysmorphic disorder is a preoccupation with an imagined defect in appearance. Although the disorder may not be delusional in quality or severity, it may be quite disabling and is surprisingly common in dermatology (Arnold

2005) and otorhinolaryngology clinics. (Body dysmorphic disorder is discussed in more detail in Chapter 12, "Somatoform and Related Disorders.")

Clinical Management

Dermatological treatments and reassurance do not commonly result in improvements in body dysmorphic disorder. SSRI medications and cognitive-behavioral therapy (CBT) can be helpful (Phillips et al. 2002).

Idiopathic (Unexplained) Pruritus

Clinical Presentation

Pruritus (itching) can occur with many medical conditions, allergies, and medication adverse effects. When exhaustive investigation has not revealed a plausible etiology (particularly if a patient has a history of psychological trauma, a high stress level, or both), a shift toward psychiatric treatment can help prevent a secondary dermatological problem from excessive scratching or self-administered topical agents.

Clinical Management

Case reports and case series suggest that tricyclic antidepressants, habit reversal training, and CBT are often effective, at least in preventing complications of scratching and in improving function (Rosenbaum and Ayllon 1981; Welkowitz et al. 1989).

Factitious Psychocutaneous Conditions

Patients with psychocutaneous factitious disorder intentionally produce skin lesions to assume an ongoing patient role. Arnold (2005) describes two main categories of factitious disorders relevant to dermatology: factitious dermatitis and psychogenic purpura. (See also Chapter 12, "Somatoform and Related Disorders.")

Factitious Dermatitis

In factitious dermatitis, also called dermatitis artefacta, patients assume the sick role by intentionally producing skin lesions. Patients typically deny that the lesions are self-inflicted (Arnold 2005; Sambhi and Lepping 2010).

Clinical Presentation

Several methods of self-inflicted injury have been reported, including scratching, biting, picking, cutting, puncturing, or rubbing; applying heat, suction cups, or caustic substances to the skin; and injecting foreign material such as blood or feces (Gupta et al.1987; Koblenzer 1987). Lesions depend on methods used and may include excoriations, blisters, ulcers, erythema, edema, or nodules (Koblenzer 1987).

Clinical Management

Anecdotal evidence suggests that patients may respond positively to efforts to protect the doctor-patient relationship. By maintaining a supportive relationship with the patient over time, a primary care physician or dermatologist may increase the chance that a patient will accept a psychotherapy referral (Koblenzer 1987).

Psychogenic Purpura

Spontaneous and unexplained appearance of recurrent purpura (bruising) is considered most often to be a manifestation of factitious behavior (Arnold 2005). However, competing theories suggest that many cases may be the result of conversion (no intentional behavior causing the bruising) or of autoerythrocyte sensitization after trauma, such as an injury or surgery. Skin trauma may result in future easy bruising because of sensitization to the stroma of extravasated erythrocytes (Koblenzer 1987). When a patient presents with unexplained bruising, consideration of nonfactitious explanations is important.

Psychiatric Disorders With Dermatological Consequences

Trichotillomania

Chronic trichotillomania (pulling out of one's hair) is classified in DSM-IV-TR as an impulse-control disorder, but it frequently occurs in the context of obsessive-compulsive disorder (OCD) (Stein et al. 1995a, 1995b). The importance of compulsivity-related trichotillomania may be particularly relevant in dermatology because the frequency of OCD in patients who consult dermatologists may be four to five times higher than in the general population (Ebrahimi et al. 2007).

Clinical Presentation

Patients with trichotillomania may impulsively or compulsively pull hair from the scalp, eyelashes, eyebrows, pubic areas, and armpits. When the behaviors are impulsive, the patient may feel dissociation or a detached state of mind during the pulling behaviors (Gupta 2006). When the behaviors are compulsive or occur in the context of OCD, the patient may experience anxiety relief. Patients with trichotillomania may have, in addition to OCD, concurrent mood disorders, anxiety disorders, or personality disorders.

Clinical Management

Pharmacological approaches.   Several controlled trials of antidepressant medications have been conducted in patients with trichotillomania. Results are mixed, but the most impressive results appear to have been achieved with clomipramine, in terms of both outcome and study design (double-blind crossover) (Swedo et al. 1989). Most SSRIs have been used to treat trichotillomania; in case reports and case series, favorable results have been reported. Interpreting the large number of positive cases reported is limited by publication bias, and controlled trials of SSRIs are mixed in terms of outcome. In a few case reports, improved outcomes in treatment-resistant cases were reported when low doses of antipsychotics such as olanzapine or risperidone were added to SSRI medication (Arnold 2005). Higher than usual dosages of antidepressant medications may also be helpful.

Nonpharmacological approaches.   Controlled trials have demonstrated that habit reversal training and CBT are efficacious for trichotillomania (Ninan et al. 2000; van Minnen et al. 2003). Behavioral treatment may have better results than medication for many patients (van Minnen et al. 2003). A reasonable assumption is that the combination of pharmacotherapy and behavioral management may have better outcomes than medication alone for trichotillomania, as has been demonstrated for other conditions.

Onychophagia

Onychophagia (nail biting) is common in childhood and adolescence. Like trichotillomania, onychophagia may have both impulsive and compulsive drivers (Arnold 2005). Evidence-based treatments include antidepressant medication and habit reversal training (Twohig et al. 2003). Symptoms may respond better to clomipramine than to other antidepressant medications.

Dermatological Conditions Exacerbated by Psychological Factors

Classified in DSM-IV-TR as examples of psychological factors affecting medical conditions, a number of dermatological conditions can be sensitive to psychological factors, as well as exacerbated by them.

Psoriasis

Clinical Presentation

Stress has been reported to trigger and exacerbate psoriasis (Arnold 2005). Mechanisms of stress-induced exacerbations likely involve interactions between the nervous, immune, and endocrine systems. Up to 40% of psoriasis patients may have mood or anxiety disorders, or clinically significant mood or anxiety symptoms (Sharma et al. 2003). Some psychopharmacological medications, especially lithium, may cause or exacerbate psoriasis (Levenson 2008).

Clinical Management

Controlled studies have demonstrated that a number of behavioral interventions—CBT, meditation, hypnosis, relaxation training, and stress management training—result in reduced psoriasis activity (Fortune et al. 2002). No controlled psychopharmacological trials for psoriasis treatment have been reported, but the diagnosis and treatment of comorbid mood and anxiety disorders are important.

Acne

Stress may aggravate acne, possibly through the increased release of adrenal steroids, which affect sebaceous glands (Strauss and Thiboutot 1999). Acne, in turn, causes increased anxiety and stress. Behavioral interventions, such as biofeedback and relaxation training, may reduce acne severity, especially when anxiety levels are high (Hughes et al. 1983).

Atopic Dermatitis

Atopic dermatitis is characterized by inflammation and itching that may spontaneously appear and spontaneously resolve, and may recur in many episodes over a lifetime. Atopic dermatitis often has its onset in childhood.

Clinical Presentation

Allergies, contact irritants, airborne irritants, sweating, hormones, and stress have all been linked to triggering or exacerbating episodes of dermatitis (Morren et al. 1994). Flare-ups may be influenced by proinflammatory cytokines, which in turn are modulated by psychosocial stressors (Davis 2007). Controlled studies have found that as a group, patients with adult atopic dermatitis are more anxious and depressed than are disease-free controls and comparison groups with other medical conditions (Ehlers et al. 1995; Schmitt et al. 2009).

Clinical Management

Addressing distress, anxiety, and depression may improve health-related quality of life for patients with atopic dermatitis (Kiebert et al. 2002). Pharmacological strategies center on treating comorbid mood or anxiety disorders and attempting to treat dermatological, anxiety, and distress symptoms with antidepressants that have histamine receptor antagonism (e.g., doxepin, trimipramine) (Savin et al. 1979). Controlled trials have demonstrated effectiveness of habit reversal training, relaxation training, CBT, and stress management training as adjuncts to standard medical care for atopic dermatitis when a patient has associated depression and anxiety (Ehlers et al. 1995).

References

American Psychiatric Association: Diagnostic and Statistical Manual of Mental Disorders, 4th Edition, Text Revision. Washington, DC, American Psychiatric Association, 2000

Arnold LM: Dermatology, in The American Psychiatric Publishing Textbook of Psychosomatic Medicine. Edited by Levenson JL. Washington, DC, American Psychiatric Publishing, 2005, pp 629–646

Davis LS: Psychodermatology: the psychological impact of skin disorders (book review). JAMA 297:97–98, 2007

Ebrahimi AA, Salehi M, Tafti AK: Obsessive compulsive disorder in dermatology outpatients. Int J Psychiatry Clin Pract 11:218–221, 2007

Ehlers A, Stangier U, Gieler U: Treatment of atopic dermatitis: a comparison of psychological and dermatological approaches to relapse prevention. J Consult Clin Psychol 63:624–635, 1995

Fortune DG, Richards HL, Kirby B, et al: A cognitive-behavioral symptom management programme as an adjunct in psoriasis therapy. Br J Dermatol 146:458–465, 2002

Gupta MA: Somatization disorders in dermatology. Int Rev Psychiatry18:41–47, 2006

Gupta MA, Gupta AK, Haberman HF: The self-inflicted dermatoses: a critical review. Gen Hosp Psychiatry 9:45–52, 1987

Hamann K, Avnstorp C: Delusions of infestation treated by pimozide: a double-blind crossover clinical study. Acta Derm Venereol 62:55–58, 1982

Hughes H, Brown BW, Lawlis GF, et al: Treatment of acne vulgaris by biofeedback relaxation and cognitive imagery. J Psychosom Res 27:185–191, 1983

Kiebert G, Sorensen SV, Revicki D, et al: Atopic dermatitis is associated with a decrement in health-related quality of life. Int J Dermatol 41:151–158, 2002

Koblenzer CS: Psychocutaneous Disease. Orlando, FL, Grune & Stratton, 1987

Lepping P, Russell I, Freudenmann RW: Antipsychotic treatment of primary delusional parasitosis. Br J Psychiatry 191:198–205, 2007

Levenson JL: Psychiatric issues in dermatology, part 1: atopic dermatitis and psoriasis. Prim Psychiatry 15:35–38, 2008

Morren MA, Przybilla B, Bamelis M, et al: Atopic dermatitis: triggering factors. J Am Acad Dermatol 31:467–473, 1994

Ninan PT, Rothbaum BO, Marsteller FA, et al: A placebo-controlled trial of cognitive-behavioral therapy and clomipramine in trichotillomania. J Clin Psychiatry 61:47–50, 2000

Phillips KA: Body dysmorphic disorder: diagnosis and treatment of imagined ugliness. J Clin Psychiatry 57:61–65, 1996

Phillips KA, Albertinie RS, Rasumessen SA: A randomized placebo-controlled trial of fluoxetine in body dysmorphic disorder. Arch Gen Psychiatry 59:381–388, 2002

Picardi A, Porcelli P, Pasquini P, et al: Integration of multiple criteria for psychosomatic assessment of dermatological patients. Psychosomatics 47:122–128, 2006

Rosenbaum MS, Ayllon T: The behavioral treatment of neurodermatitis through habit-reversal. Behav Res Ther 19:313–318, 1981

Rundell JR: Toward defining the scope of psychosomatic medicine practice: psychosomatic medicine in the tertiary care practice setting. Psychosomatics 49:487–493, 2008

Sambhi R, Lepping P: Psychiatric treatments in dermatology: an update. Clin Exp Dermatol 35:120–125, 2010

Sandoz A, LoPiccolo M, Kusnir D, et al: A clinical paradigm of delusions of parasitosis. J Am Acad Dermatol 59:698–704, 2008

Savin JA, Patterson WE, Adam K, et al: Effects of trimeprazine and trimipramine on nocturnal scratching in patients with atopic eczema. Arch Dermatol 115:313–315, 1979

Schmitt J, Romanos M, Pfennig A, et al: Psychiatric comorbidity in adult eczema. Br J Dermatol 161:878–883, 2009

Sharma N, Koranne RV, Singh RK: A comparative study of psychiatric morbidity in dermatological patients. Indian J Dermatol 48:137–141, 2003

Stein DJ, Mullen L, Islam MN, et al: Compulsive and impulsive symptomatology in trichotillomania. Psychopathology 28:208–213, 1995a

Stein DJ, Simeon D, Cohen LJ, et al: Trichotillomania and obsessive-compulsive disorder. J Clin Psychiatry 56:28–34, 1995b

Strauss JS, Thiboutot DM: Diseases of the sebaceous glands, in Fitzpatrick's Dermatology in General Medicine, 5th Edition. Edited by Freedberg IM, Eisen AZ, Wolff K, et al. New York, McGraw-Hill, 1999, pp 769–784

Swedo SE, Leonard HL, Rapoport JL, et al: A double-blind comparison of clomipramine and desipramine in the treatment of trichotillomania (hair pulling). N Engl J Med 321:497–501, 1989

Twohig MP, Woods DW, Marcks BA, et al: Evaluating the efficacy of habit reversal: comparison with a placebo control. J Clin Psychiatry 64:40–48, 2003

van Minnen A, Hoogduin KA, Keijsers GP, et al: Treatment of trichotillomania with behavioral therapy or fluoxetine. Arch Gen Psychiatry 60:517–522, 2003

Welkowitz LA, Held JL, Held AL, et al: Management of neurotic scratching with behavioral therapy. J Am Acad Dermatol 21:802–804, 1989

Woodruff PW, Higgins EM, duVivier AW, Wessely S: Psychiatric illness in patients referred to a dermatology-psychiatry clinic. Gen Hosp Psychiatry 19:29–35, 1997

19

Disaster and
Terrorism Casualties

Following a disaster or terrorist attack, individuals with surgical injuries or medical conditions have an increased likelihood of having a psychiatric condition. Many times more patients go to medical facilities because of fear of exposure to toxic agents than because of actual toxic exposure (Rundell 2003, 2005). The following list includes useful information for consultation psychiatrists working with disaster and terrorism casualties.

- *Psychiatric symptoms.* Psychiatric symptoms in victims of disasters should be evaluated within the context of concurrent medical-surgical assessment and treatment (Rundell 2005).
- *Health systems.* Careful differential diagnosis and timely communication to the public lessen the risk of misdiagnosis and mass hysterical reactions, thereby protecting health care systems from being overwhelmed (Rundell and Christopher 2004).
- *Patient categories.* Following a potential mass toxic exposure, three types of patients present themselves for medical evaluation:

1. People with disease due to the toxic agent
2. People who have disease due to the toxic agent in addition to a concurrent psychiatric condition
3. People who have not been exposed but fear they have

Unique Considerations in Clinical Evaluation

Symptom Overlap

- Anxiety provoked by having been potentially exposed to a substance or disease can complicate diagnosis.
- Physiological signs of autonomic nervous system arousal and dysphoria can mimic symptoms and signs of toxic exposure or other medical diseases.
- Signs and symptoms, and effects of treatment, of chemical and biological attacks can be nonspecific and mimic neuropsychiatric syndromes.
- Differential diagnosis by skilled clinicians is crucial to effective triage of large populations.
- Presence or absence of fever may, in many cases, be the only reliable early differentiator between those exposed to a biological agent and those not exposed but fearful they may have been.

Triage Concepts

Advanced Trauma Life Support

The underlying concept of Advanced Trauma Life Support (ATLS) is simple: the greatest threats to life—loss of airway, loss of breathing ability, loss of circulating blood volume, and effects of an expanding intracerebral mass—are treated first (American College of Surgeons 2004). This standardized approach to handling trauma patients involves two surveys:

- The primary survey is a rapid, targeted examination necessary to identify life-threatening injuries to the airway and blood circulation. The purpose is to assess whether the patient is alert, responsive to verbal stimuli, responsive to painful stimuli, or unresponsive.

- The secondary survey is a head-to-toe evaluation of the trauma patient in which each region of the body is systematically examined and all available medical history (allergies, current medications, significant past illnesses, and events related to the injury or exposure) is reviewed.

Early Identification of Psychiatric Casualties

The postdisaster or postterrorism psychiatric screening examination that is used for triage and identification of early psychiatric casualties can be thought of as a tertiary survey that focuses on the most common psychiatric sequelae (Rundell 2003) and those most likely to adversely affect outcomes.

- The screening psychiatric examination of the traumatized victim is easier if findings from the primary and secondary ATLS surveys are unremarkable. Psychiatric symptoms are then likely to represent primary psychiatric disorders.
- When psychiatric signs are present in addition to significant primary and secondary survey findings, differential diagnosis can be complex, and the patient may have multiple disorders.

Key principles of psychiatric screening of disaster victims following primary and secondary surveys and medical stabilization are summarized in Table 19–1.

Unique Considerations in Diagnosis and Management

Delirium

Diagnosis

- In the disaster or terrorism victim with major illness or injuries, volume depletion and metabolic derangements can cause delirium: clouded consciousness, agitation or diminished responsiveness, and disorientation.
- Common causes of delirium in disaster settings include hypovolemia, hypoxemia, central nervous system mass effect, infection, and adverse effects of ATLS and Advanced Cardiovascular Life Support (ACLS) medications.

Table 19–1.   Screening psychiatric examination of medical-surgical disaster casualties

Examination parameter	Finding increases likelihood of:
History	
Sustained physical injuries during traumatic event	Secondary psychiatric disorder,[a] ASD, PTSD, dissociation
Past history of psychiatric disorder	That psychiatric disorder
Patient is on routine, ongoing medication	Substance intoxication, substance withdrawal, secondary psychiatric disorder
Received ATLS or ACLS medications	Secondary psychiatric disorder[a]
Physical findings	
Elevated heart rate, blood pressure	Substance withdrawal, generalized anxiety disorder, panic disorder, ASD, PTSD, secondary psychiatric disorder[a]
Easy startle	ASD, PTSD, generalized anxiety disorder
Lateralizing neurological signs	Head or vertebral column injury, secondary psychiatric disorder[a]
Physical complaints out of proportion to objective findings	Conversion disorder, hypochondriasis, factitious disorder, malingering,[b] undiagnosed physical condition
Mental status examination	
Disoriented	Delirium, secondary psychiatric disorder[a]
Clouded consciousness	Delirium, secondary psychiatric disorder,[a] dissociation
Dysarthria	Substance intoxication, head injury
Dysgraphia, dyscalculia	Head injury, delirium
Impaired short-term memory	Head injury, substance intoxication, delirium, generalized anxiety disorder, panic attack

Table 19–1. Screening psychiatric examination of medical-surgical disaster casualties *(continued)*

Examination parameter	Finding increases likelihood of:
Hallucinations or delusions	Substance intoxication, secondary psychiatric disorder,[a] substance withdrawal, primary psychotic disorder

Note. ACLS = Advanced Cardiovascular Life Support; ASD = acute stress disorder; ATLS = Advanced Trauma Life Support; PTSD=posttraumatic stress disorder.
[a]Psychiatric disorders due to general medical conditions or due to toxins/psychoactive substances.
[b]Malingering is not a psychiatric disorder; it is a legal accusation.
Source. Adapted from Rundell JR: "Assessment and Management of Medical-Surgical Disaster Casualties," in *Textbook of Disaster Psychiatry.* Edited by Ursano RJ, Fullerton CS, Weisaeth L, et al. New York, Cambridge University Press, 2005, pp. 164–189. Used with permission.

Management

- Prevention of or resolution of the delirium etiology should be the main goal and requires resolving the metabolic sequelae of the injury.
- Although medication treatment of delirium symptoms can help decrease psychosis and agitation, as well as mitigate a safety problem, this is not the ideal management.
  - Medications used to manage agitation can further complicate both medical assessment and an already difficult clinical course.
  - Symptomatic management of the patient's behavioral problems with sedating medication should be initially reserved to protect the life or safety of the patient and other patients or staff.

Depression

Diagnosis

- Depressed mood or resignation in the aftermath of a disaster or terrorist event may be difficult to distinguish from the malaise and lassitude common among the prodromes of many chemical and bioterrorism exposures.
- Differential diagnosis is based on assessment of the patient's predisposition, timeline of syndrome development, and presence or absence of biological factors that could produce mood symptoms.

Management

Antidepressant medications and cognitive-behavioral psychotherapy are the mainstays of treatment for major depressive disorder following disaster or trauma, and may assist with managing subsyndromal depression.

Acute Stress Disorder and Posttraumatic Stress Disorder

Acute stress disorder (ASD) and posttraumatic stress disorder (PTSD) can be substantial burdens following a major terrorist event. Among 1,008 adults interviewed in New York City between 1 and 2 months after the attacks on the World Trade Center, 7.5% reported symptoms consistent with a diagnosis of current PTSD (Galea et al. 2002).

Diagnosis

- ASD and PTSD are frequently comorbid with major depressive disorder, panic disorder, substance use disorder, and generalized anxiety disorder (Rundell 2005).
- Having a physical injury increases the risk of ASD and PTSD (Rundell 2005).
  - Mild traumatic brain injury is associated with increased frequency of PTSD.
  - Returning Iraq war veterans who reported injuries with loss of consciousness are three times more likely than soldiers who reported no injuries (27% vs. 9%) to report PTSD symptoms (Hoge et al. 2008).

Management

Medication treatment.

- Selective serotonin reuptake inhibitors (SSRIs) are the first-line medication treatment for the PTSD symptoms of reexperiencing, insomnia, and arousal. Five SSRIs have demonstrated efficacy in at least one double-blind, placebo-controlled trial, although up to 50% of patients may be treatment resistant (Lineberry et al. 2006; see Table 19–2).
- Prazosin (mean dosage 9 mg/day at bedtime) was superior to placebo for managing distressing dreams, insomnia, and functional status in a 20-week double blind, placebo-controlled, crossover study of patients with PTSD (Raskind et al. 2003).

Table 19–2. Studies demonstrating efficacy of selective serotonin reuptake inhibitors (SSRIs) in posttraumatic stress disorder

SSRI	Number of studies	Mean dosage
Sertraline	2	133–146 mg/day
Paroxetine	2	20–50 mg/day
Fluoxetine	1	57 mg/day
Fluvoxamine	1	150 mg/day
Citalopram	1	30 mg/day

Source. Lineberry et al. 2006.

- Anecdotal reports suggest that low doses of antipsychotics (e.g., quetiapine 25 mg at bedtime) may help with insomnia and arousal (Lineberry et al. 2006).

Psychotherapy

The two psychotherapies most frequently discussed as helpful for PTSD are cognitive-behavioral therapy and marital therapy (Lineberry et al. 2006).

Health Anxiety and Hypochondriasis

In the generally anxious atmosphere and uncertainty following disasters and terrorist events, patients who are prone to health anxiety or hypochondriasis may have problems managing their anxiety and beliefs.

Diagnosis

- Six months of symptoms are required before making a diagnosis of hypochondriasis.
- The patient with hypochondriasis has bodily preoccupation and vigilance regarding body sensations.

Management

Health anxiety and subsyndromal hypochondriacal fears may be widespread among the general population following a disaster or terrorist event, and should be managed with *reassurance* and a degree of *tolerance* for patients' requests for appointments and examinations by their primary care providers.

Unexplained Physical Symptoms and Conversion Symptoms

Not all unexplained physical symptoms are conversion symptoms, although conversion is well documented anecdotally after terrorist and combat events. Even though little scientific basis exists for future prevention and care of unexplained physical symptoms (Clauw et al. 2003), persons with unexplained symptoms need to be identified in the triage process so that inappropriate and potentially harmful treatments are not conducted and to avoid drawing resources away from victims needing them.

Dissociation and Dissociative Disorder

Dissociation is a disruption in the usually integrated functions of consciousness, memory, identity, or perception of the environment.

- The core feature of dissociative disorder is the presence of significant distress or of significant disruption in social or occupational functioning.
- Dissociation that falls short of diagnostic criteria for dissociative disorder is common in the context of any traumatic or terrorist event.
- Dissociation is generally underrecognized in the immediate aftermath of a traumatic event or terrorist event (Rundell 2005).
- Dissociation may be adaptive in the immediate aftermath of a trauma, because it may prevent the eruption of intolerable affects or the unleashing of potentially dangerous impulses or behaviors (e.g., attempts to flee the scene).
- Identifying otherwise uninjured disaster victims who are simply dissociating frees up scarce evaluation and treatment resources for other emergency patients.
- Dissociation and diminished neurological responsiveness are easily confused. A key role for a consulting psychiatrist in the immediate aftermath of a disaster, while primary and secondary surveys are being done, is to help identify dissociation. The following are helpful in this identification:
  - Gently tap patients on the shoulder and ask if they need anything and whether they know where they are and what day it is.
  - Watch for a muted but appropriate response in a dissociating person; this response indicates that level of consciousness and orientation is grossly intact.

Substance Use Disorders

Following a disaster or terrorism event, people may increase their use of alcohol or drugs as a way to decrease the acute despair or anxiety associated with the event.

- Rescue and health care workers are at risk because of their participation in and exposure to the aftermath of the event.
- Disaster response leaders must educate and model for their workers the avoidance of alcohol and drugs during the disaster management period and its aftermath.
- Patients who have substance-related disorders may present intoxicated or in withdrawal at a triage or patient management area. Health care workers can confuse effects of either intoxication or withdrawal with toxicities associated with chemical agents, biological agents, metabolic derangements, or medications used to treat patients' medical-surgical conditions. Patients may also present seeking prescription medications with the potential for abuse.

Effects of Disaster Medications

An important part of postdisaster psychiatric screening is to find out what medications an injured patient has received, in what amounts, and over what time period. Disaster and resuscitation agents such as intravenous fluids (water), epinephrine, lidocaine, atropine, sedatives, nitroglycerin, and morphine are commonly used and have significant psychiatric or autonomic effects.

- Atropine causes significant anxiety and anticholinergic effects.
- Epinephrine causes blood pressure and heart rate elevations, and causes patients to feel anxious or panicky.
- Morphine causes sedation and impairs orientation and responsiveness.

References

American College of Surgeons: Advanced Trauma Life Support for Doctors—Student Course Manual, 7th Edition. Chicago, American College of Surgeons, 2004

Clauw DJ, Engel CC, Aronowitz R, et al: Unexplained symptoms after terrorism and war: an expert consensus statement. J Occup Environ Med 45:1040–1048, 2003

Galea S, Ahern J, Resnick H, et al: Psychological sequelae of the September 11 terrorist attacks in New York City. N Engl J Med 346:982–987, 2002

Hoge CW, McGurk D, Thomas JL, et al: Mild traumatic brain injury in U.S. soldiers returning from Iraq. N Engl J Med 358:453–463, 2008

Lineberry TW, Ramaswamy S, Bostwick M, et al: Traumatized troops: how to treat combat-related PTSD. Curr Psychiatr 5:53–56, 2006

Raskind MA, Peskind ER, Kanter ED, et al: Reduction of nightmares and other PTSD symptoms in combat veterans by prazosin: a placebo-controlled study. Am J Psychiatry 160:371–373, 2003

Rundell JR: A consultation-liaison psychiatry approach to disaster/terrorism victim assessment and management, in Terrorism and Disaster: Individual and Community Mental Health Interventions. Edited by Ursano RJ, Fullerton CS, Norwood AE. New York, Cambridge University Press, 2003, pp. 107–120

Rundell JR: Assessment and management of medical-surgical disaster casualties, in Textbook of Disaster Psychiatry. Edited by Ursano RJ, Fullerton CS, Weisaeth L, et al. New York, Cambridge University Press, 2005, pp 164–189

Rundell JR, Christopher GW: Differentiating manifestations of infection from psychiatric disorders and fears of having been exposed to bioterrorism, in Bioterrorism. Edited by Ursano RJ and Norwood AE. New York, Cambridge University Press, 2004, pp 88–108

20

Endocrinology

Endocrinopathies arise from and involve a broad array of organs and have far-reaching pathophysiological disruption, both central and peripheral. Initial symptoms may be cryptic and covert or definitive and dramatic. The diverse biochemical sequelae of endocrine disturbances help explain both the frequency and variety of neuropsychiatric consequences, some of which precede discernible somatic disease and may confound even the astute clinician. Only the most prevalent examples are discussed in this chapter.

Diabetes Mellitus

Nearly 10% of adults in the United States have diabetes mellitus, including 20% of those over age 65. The annual incidence of new cases is approaching 1 million; 90%–95% of existing and new cases are type 2. Poorly controlled diabetes mellitus, whether type 1 or type 2, disposes the patient to macrovascular and microvascular sequelae, including retinopathy, cardiovascular disease, nephropathy, nontraumatic limb amputation, and peripheral neuropathy. In the United Kingdom, a large prospective study found that a 1-point shift in hemoglobin A1c (HbA_{1c}) was associated with a 35% shift in development of complications (Goebel-Fabbri et al. 2011). Comorbid depression and diabetes mellitus compound the morbidity and expense associated with each, emphasizing the importance of clinical awareness and intervention.

Depression and Diabetes

The association between diabetes and depression is bidirectional. Depression, independent of multiple confounding factors, is associated with a 60%–65% increased risk for development of type 2 diabetes; however, antidepressant treatment is not associated with an increased risk of diabetes (Campayo et al. 2010; Mezuk et al. 2008; Musselman et al. 2003). A recent review of largely prospective epidemiological studies suggests that anxiety, anger, hostility, sleeping problems, and general emotional distress are also associated with an increased risk for development of type 2 diabetes (Pouwer et al. 2010).

Pathophysiology

Possible pathophysiological mechanisms for the association between diabetes and depression include the following:

- Counterregulatory hormones (catecholamines, glucocorticoids, growth hormone, and glucagon) are released in response to stress and in depression; these hormones oppose the glucoregulatory effect of insulin.
- Alterations in glucose transport and utilization occur.
- Proinflammatory cytokines, which are increased in depression, induce "sickness behavior." One of these cytokines, tumor necrosis factor–alpha, is overproduced in the adipose and muscle tissue of obese individuals, potentially increasing fatigue and leading to decreased physical activity (Golden 2007; Musselman et al. 2003).

Behavioral Consequences

The following behavioral consequences of depression may predispose to diabetes and/or further impede diabetic control (Katon 2008; Katon et al. 2009; Musselman et al. 2003):

- Physical inactivity and obesity
- Nonadherence to dietary guidelines

- Inconsistent blood glucose monitoring
- Poor compliance with medication

Diabetes and Depression

The prevalence of depression in persons with diabetes is two to three times higher than in the general population, although the absolute risk of depression following type 2 diabetes is only 15% (Mezuk et al. 2008). Patients with more extensive complications of diabetes, less education, socioeconomic hardship, and chronic stressors are at higher risk for developing depression (Musselman et al. 2003). The mechanism whereby diabetes may predispose to depression is unclear. Indirect suggestions include the following:

- *Dysglycemia and malaise.* Glycemic control is associated with increased subjective well-being (Lustman and Clouse 2005).
- *Cognitive contribution.* Hyperglycemia is associated with cognitive impairment (Cukierman-Yaffe et al. 2009; Solanki et al. 2009).
- *Treatment effect.* Untreated type 2 diabetes is not associated with an increased risk of depression; the increased association occurs only in patients with treated type 2 diabetes (Golden et al. 2008).

Consequences of Comorbid Depression and Diabetes

The consequences of comorbid depression and diabetes are multiple and substantial:

- The course of depression is intensified, with up to 80% of patients experiencing a depressive relapse within 5 years (Katon 2008).
- Diabetic patients respond less robustly to antidepressants than matched control subjects without diabetes (Bryan et al. 2010).
- Depression is associated with poorer medical outcomes and increased diabetic complications (Lustman et al. 2007).
- Depression is associated with a threefold to fivefold increased risk of mortality in patients with diabetes (Black et al. 2003; Ismail et al. 2007).
- Health care costs are markedly increased. A recent study demonstrated that the annual Medicare patient cost for patients with comorbid diabetes and depression was 4.5 times greater than for nondepressed patients with diabetes (Katon 2008).

Treatment

Treatment is imperative to reduce suffering and conserve resources. Pharmacological treatment, cognitive-behavioral therapy, or both have been studied in patients with comorbid depression and diabetes.

Pharmacological Treatment

- Tricyclic antidepressants are effective for depression and neuropathic pain (Saarto and Wiffen 2010) but are associated with weight gain and cardiac effects.
- Selective serotonin reuptake inhibitors (SSRIs) are tolerated well by diabetic patients, with fewer side effects than among nondiabetic control patients (Bryan et al. 2010). With the possible exception of paroxetine, SSRIs are effective for treatment of depression in patients with diabetes but do not improve medical outcome (Petrak and Herpetz 2009).
- Serotonin-norepinephrine reuptake inhibitors (SNRIs) are more likely to reduce neuropathic pain than SSRIs; duloxetine, milnacipran, and venlafaxine have had favorable results in this population (Abrahamian et al. 2009; Lee and Chen 2010; Sultan et al. 2008).
- Mirtazapine may also reduce neuropathic pain but is generally avoided because it is associated with more weight gain than other newer antidepressants.
- Bupropion is not associated with weight gain and is the least likely to contribute to sexual dysfunction; one study has shown improvement in mood, body mass index, and HbA_{1c} (Toplak and Abrahamian 2009).

Cognitive-Behavioral Therapy

Cognitive-behavioral therapy is effective in the treatment of depression (Petrak and Herpetz 2009) and in one study demonstrated a significant decrease in HbA_{1c} levels at 6-month follow-up (Lustman et al. 1998).

Combined Psychotherapy and Pharmacotherapy

Combined psychotherapy and pharmacotherapy may be prudent for diabetic patients with severe or refractory depression who are unresponsive to trials of either modality alone. Although combined therapy yields greater efficacy, a reflexive recommendation for combined therapy for all depressed patients overlooks individual preferences, probability of adherence, and cost issues. Integrated treatment with interpersonal therapy and citalopram is the only strategy studied to date that has demonstrated a significant decrease in 5-year mortality (Bogner et al. 2007).

Thyroid Disease

Hypothalamic thyrotropin-releasing hormone (TRH) stimulates pituitary production of thyrotropin, which regulates thyroid secretion of thyroxine (T_4), triiodothyronine (T_3), and reverse T_3 (rT_3). Ninety-nine percent of these thyroid hormones are protein bound; only unbound hormones are active. The thyroid gland is the sole source of T_4 and about 20% of T_3, the remainder of which is derived throughout the body by deiodinase enzymes, which strip iodine from T_4. In the brain, the neuron is the principal site of T_3 action. Although thyroid hormone receptors occur throughout the central nervous system (CNS), the amygdala, cortex, and hippocampus are richly supplied, consistent with their integral roles in mood regulation and cognitive function (Bauer et al. 2008; Williams 2008).

Hypothyroidism

Hypothyroidism is associated with neurological and psychiatric disruption (Lass et al. 2008).

Cognitive Dysfunction

Cognitive dysfunction, most commonly in the domains of working memory and executive function, is associated with both hypothyroidism and hyperthyroidism. Individuals with grossly normal thyroid function but elevated free T_4 concentrations demonstrated deterioration in Mini-Mental State Examination scores 2 years later, prompting the proposal that perhaps elevated T_4 leads to oxidative stress and secondary neuronal damage (Hogervorst et al. 2008).

Depression

More often than not, low thyrotropin and low T_3 are associated with depression. However, studies of thyroid function and depression are less uniform than conventional wisdom would suggest. T_4 levels in the high-normal range have also been linked to depression. Thyroid disorders were the only medical comorbidity among rapid cyclers in a sample of 1,090 patients with bipolar I disorder; unfortunately, patient history rather than laboratory confirmation was used to establish thyroid dysfunction (Bunevicius 2009). A tentative conclusion drawn from divergent observations in different studies is that patients with thyroid disorders who develop depression and patients with depression who develop thyroid dysfunction may have different biochemical profiles.

Patients with comorbid depression and thyroid dysfunction may benefit from treatment with antidepressants and/or thyroid augmentation:

- Antidepressants of multiple classes have shown efficacy in patients with comorbid depression and thyroid dysfunction, although different agents appear to promote different thyroid hormone effects (Bunevicius 2009).
- T_4 and/or T_3 augmentation of conventional antidepressants in euthyroid but depressed patients is a time-honored strategy, but studies and attempted meta-analyses have drawn discordant conclusions regarding the degree of efficacy; T_3 is generally regarded as superior to T_4.

Delirium

Hashimoto's encephalopathy is a pleomorphic autoimmune syndrome that may include multiple neuropsychiatric signs and symptoms: aphasia, ataxia, cognitive compromise ranging from confusion to coma, headache, mood disturbance, paranoia, personality change, seizures, sleep disturbances, strokelike episodes, and visual hallucinations. The clinical course may be acute, subacute, chronic, or relapsing-remitting (Mijajlovic et al. 2010; Schiess and Pardo 2008). Thyroid function is almost always normal, biochemically and clinically. The pathogenesis remains unclear, but elevated titers of antithyroid peroxidase antibodies are present in more than 95% of cases, and antithyroglobulin antibodies in more than 70%. The differential diagnosis includes Creutzfeldt-Jakob disease, CNS lupus, paraneoplastic and nonparaneoplastic limbic encephalitis, rapidly progressive dementias, and vasculitis (Mocellin et al. 2007).

Patients with Hashimoto's encephalopathy often benefit from pharmacotherapy.

- High-dose corticosteroids are commonly very effective in treating Hashimoto's encephalopathy, emphasizing the importance of clinician diagnostic vigilance despite the cryptic and often severe presentation of these patients.

- Other immunomodulators, such as cyclophosphamide, immunoglobulin, and methotrexate, as well as plasmapheresis, have been effective when corticosteroids were not (Mocellin et al. 2007).

Hyperthyroidism

Hyperthyroidism is most commonly the result of Graves disease, an autoimmune disorder caused by thyroid-stimulating immunoglobulins that bind to thyroid-stimulating hormone receptors and thereby precipitate production of T_4 and T_3. Uncommonly, a patient may ingest excessive thyroid hormone in hope of boosting energy or enabling weight loss.

Neuropsychiatric consequences of hyperthyroidism include anxiety, apathy, cognitive inefficiency, dysphoria, fatigue, irritability, mood disturbances ranging from depression to mania, memory difficulties, and tremulousness. Elderly patients with hyperthyroidism more commonly experience apathy and depression, whereas younger adult patients are more likely to be kinetically restless and anxiously dysphoric (Goebel-Fabbri et al. 2011).

Restoring normal thyroid function, whether by thyroidectomy, antithyroid medication, or radioactive iodine, is essential to reversing the psychiatric sequelae of thyrotoxicosis.

Parathyroid Disorders

Parathyroid disorders may precipitate a range of psychiatric symptoms, primarily generated by elevated or depleted serum calcium.

Hyperparathyroidism

Hyperparathyroidism is the oversecretion of parathyroid hormone. The consequent hypercalcemia can cause anergia, anxiety, apathy, dysphoria, and impaired concentration and memory; severe hypercalcemia is associated with a full spectrum of psychotic symptoms. Restoration of normal calcium levels brings about resolution of psychiatric and cognitive symptoms for most patients (Roman and Sosa 2007).

Hypoparathyroidism

Hypoparathyroidism, the result of inadequate parathyroid hormone secretion typically caused by prior surgery, presents with hypocalcemia-mediated paresthesias and muscle cramping. Anxiety and irritability often accompany neuromuscular symptoms; if unrecognized and untreated, cognitive difficulties may follow (Goebel-Fabbri et al. 2011).

Adrenal Gland Disorders

Adrenal gland disorders may cause a broad range of psychiatric symptoms.

Cushing's Syndrome

Cushing's syndrome, whether the result of excess corticotropin triggered by a pituitary or adrenal tumor or the result of administered corticosteroids, occurs due to supranormal levels of cortisol. Although depressive symptoms occur in more than 50% of patients with Cushing's syndrome, patients may also be referred to the psychiatric consultation service because of anxiety, cognitive impairment, hypomania, mania, and psychosis (Arnaldi et al. 2003; Brown 2009).

Adrenal Insufficiency

Adrenal insufficiency occurs for many reasons, including Addison's disease (i.e., primary adrenal insufficiency) and chronic glucocorticoid administration. Addisonian crisis may precipitate delirium and psychosis. Patients with gradual development of inadequate adrenal corticosteroid production experience anhedonia, anorexia, apathy, fatigue, and social withdrawal (Goebel-Fabbri et al. 2011).

Osteoporosis

Osteoporosis, as well as the consequent increased risk of fractures, is linked to psychiatric illness and treatments in multiple areas.

Depression

Depression is a significant risk factor for osteoporosis (Bab and Yirmiya 2010; Cizza et al. 2009; Williams et al. 2009).

Selective Serotonin Reuptake Inhibitors

SSRIs are likely an independent risk factor for osteoporosis, although confounding factors make this research challenging (Haney et al. 2010).

Antipsychotic-Induced Hyperprolactinemia

Antipsychotic-induced hyperprolactinemia, which is a greater risk in patients taking first-generation antipsychotics, as well as risperidone and paliperidone, results in decreased bone mineral density (Bostwick et al. 2009; Byerly et al. 2007).

Pheochromocytoma

Pheochromocytomas are very rare tumors, and approximately 10% prove malignant. These tumors secrete excessive catecholamines, resulting in multiple and sometimes paroxysmal hyperadrenergic signs and symptoms. Although pheochromocytoma invariably appears in the textbook differential diagnosis of panic disorder and severe anxiety, laboratory testing for pheochromocytoma is not recommended when the patient presents only with psychiatric symptoms, but should be considered when unresponsive hypertension or persistent headaches are present (Goebel-Fabbri et al. 2011).

Vitamins

Vitamins are essential organic compounds that cannot be produced in sufficient quantities by the body to serve the diverse biochemical tasks necessary, and therefore require dietary or other supply. Vitamins function as antioxidants, coenzymes, immunomodulators, precursors for enzyme cofactors, and hormonelike regulators of metabolism and cell differentiation. Although historically well-known sequelae of many vitamin deficiencies are now rare in the developed world, some deficiencies still affect patients whom the psychosomatic medicine physician will encounter.

Vitamin B_1

Vitamin B_1 (thiamine) may be deficient in patients with alcohol dependence, starvation (e.g., severe anorexia), short gut syndrome, lymphoma (particularly following chemotherapy), and chronic hemodialysis, as well as patients who have had gastric bypass surgery. Administering intravenous glucose to a thiamine-deficient patient may precipitate overt Wernicke's encephalopathy.

Vitamin B_3

Vitamin B_3 (niacin) deficiency results in pellagra, classically characterized by diarrhea, dermatitis, and dementia.

Vitamin B_6

Vitamin B_6 (pyridoxine) deficiency impairs proprioception; supplementation may ameliorate some peripheral neuropathies.

Vitamin B_9

Vitamin B_9 (folic acid) is commonly tested in tandem with vitamin B_{12} because an excess of the former may mask the symptoms of vitamin B_{12} deficiency; however, vitamin B_9 is rarely found to be deficient except in alcohol-dependent patients.

Vitamin B_{12}

Vitamin B_{12} (cyanocobalamin) deficiency causes megaloblastic anemia and a range of neuropsychiatric disorders, including anxiety, delirium, dementia, and mood disturbances.

Vitamin D

Vitamin D (cholecalciferol) has earned renewed interest because recent scrutiny has revealed multiple potential consequences of hypovitaminosis D, ranging from depression to autoimmune and inflammatory conditions, as well as pain and oncological susceptibility (de Abreu et al. 2009).

Vitamin E

Vitamin E (tocopherol) has had fluctuating popularity as a dietary supplement intended to stave off progression of mild cognitive impairment or to reduce the risk of Alzheimer's disease. Although studies continue, at present no compelling evidence has been reported to mandate its use for these purposes.

Other Factors

Careful endocrine assessment is warranted when patients have any of the following (Kornstein et al. 2000):

- Comorbid mood disturbance, unusual behavioral symptoms, and cognitive dysfunction
- Atypical and/or fluctuating psychiatric presentations

- Psychiatric symptoms that are refractory to standard treatment strategies
- Cognitive deterioration and/or dementia
- Affective symptoms following a closed head injury
- Personal or family history of antecedent endocrine or psychiatric dysfunction

References

Abrahamian H, Hofmann P, Prager R, et al: Diabetes mellitus and co-morbid depression: treatment with milnacipran results in significant improvement in both diseases (results from the Austrian MDDM Study Group). Neuropsychiatr Dis Treat 5:261–266, 2009

Arnaldi G, Angeli A, Atkinson AB, et al: Diagnosis and complications of Cushing's syndrome: a consensus statement. J Clin Endocrinol Metab 88:5593–5602, 2003

Bab I, Yirmiya R: Depression, selective serotonin reuptake inhibitors, and osteoporosis. Curr Osteoporos Rep 8:185–191, 2010

Bauer M, Goetz T, Glenn T, et al: The thyroid-brain interaction in thyroid disorders and mood disorders. J Neuroendocrinol 20:1101–1114, 2008

Black SA, Markides KS, Ray LA: Depression predicts increased incidence of adverse health outcomes in older Mexican Americans with type 2 diabetes. Diabetes Care 26:2822–2828, 2003

Bogner HR, Morales KH, Post EP, et al: Diabetes, depression, and death: a randomized controlled trial of a depression treatment program for older adults based in primary care (PROSPECT). Diabetes Care 30:3005–3010, 2007

Bostwick JR, Guthrie SK, Ellingrod VL: Antipsychotic-induced hyperprolactinemia. Pharmacotherapy 29:64–73, 2009

Brown ES: Effects of glucocorticoids on mood, memory, and the hippocampus: treatment and preventive therapy. Ann NY Acad Sci 1179:41–55, 2009

Bryan C, Songer T, Brooks MM, et al: The impact of diabetes on depression treatment outcomes. Gen Hosp Psychiatry 32:33–41, 2010

Bunevicius R: Thyroid disorders in mental patients. Curr Opin Psychiatry 22:391–395, 2009

Byerly M, Suppes T, Tran QV, et al: Clinical implications of antipsychotic-induced hyperprolactinemia in patients with schizophrenia spectrum or bipolar spectrum disorders: recent developments and current perspectives. J Clin Psychopharmacol 27:639–661, 2007

Campayo A, de Jonge P, Roy JF: Depressive disorder and incident diabetes mellitus: the effect of characteristics of depression. Am J Psychiatry 167:580–588, 2010

Cizza G, Primma S, Csako G: Depression as a risk factor for osteoporosis. Trends Endocrinol Metab 20:367–373, 2009

Cukierman-Yaffe T, Gerstein HC, Anderson C, et al: Glucose intolerance and diabetes as risk factors for cognitive impairment in people at high cardiovascular risk: results from the ONTARGET/TRANSCEND research programme. Diabetes Res Clin Pract 83:387–393, 2009

de Abreu DAF, Eyles D, Feron F: Vitamin D, a neuro-immunomodulator: implications for neurodegenerative and autoimmune diseases. Psychoneuroendocrinology 34S:S265–S277, 2009

Goebel-Fabbri A, Musen G, Levenson JL: Endocrine and metabolic disorders, in The American Psychiatric Publishing Textbook of Psychosomatic Medicine, 2nd edition. Edited by Levenson JL. Washington, DC, American Psychiatric Publishing, 2011, pp 503–524

Golden SH: A review of the evidence for a neuroendocrine link between stress, depression and diabetes mellitus. Curr Diabetes Rev 3:252–259, 2007

Golden SH, Lazo M, Carnethon M, et al: Examining a bidirectional association between depressive symptoms and diabetes. JAMA 299:2751–2759, 2008

Haney EM, Warden SJ, Bliziotes MM: Effects of selective serotonin reuptake inhibitors on bone health in adults: time for recommendations about screening, prevention and management? Bone 46:13–17, 2010

Hogervorst E, Huppert F, Matthews FE, et al: Thyroid function and cognitive decline in the MRC Cognitive Function and Ageing Study. Psychoneuroendocrinology 33:1013–1022, 2008

Ismail K, Winkley K, Stahl D, et al: A cohort study of people with diabetes and their first foot ulcer: the role of depression on mortality. Diabetes Care 30:1473–1479, 2007

Katon WJ: The comorbidity of diabetes mellitus and depression. Am J Med 121 (suppl 2): S8–S15, 2008

Katon WJ, Russo J, Lin EH, et al: Diabetes and poor disease control: is comorbid depression associated with mood medication adherence or lack of treatment intensification? Psychosom Med 71:965–972, 2009

Kornstein SG, Sholar EF, Gardner DF: Endocrine disorders, in Psychiatric Care of the Medical Patient, 2nd Edition. Edited by Stoudemire A, Fogel BS, Greenberg DB. New York, Oxford University Press, 2000, pp 801–819

Lass P, Slawek J, Derejko M, et al: Neurological and psychiatric disorders in thyroid dysfunctions. The role of nuclear medicine: SPECT and PET imaging. Minerva Endocrinol 33:75–84, 2008

Lee YC, Chen PP: A review of SSRIs and SNRIs in neuropathic pain. Expert Opin Pharmacother 11:2813–2825, 2010

Lustman PJ, Clouse RE: Depression in diabetic patients. The relationship between mood and glycemic control. J Diabetes Complications 19:113–122, 2005

Lustman PJ, Griffith LS, Freedland KE, et al: Cognitive behavior therapy for depression in type 2 diabetes mellitus: a randomized, controlled trial. Ann Intern Med 129:613–621, 1998

Lustman PJ, Penckofer SM, Clouse RE: Recent advances in understanding depression in adults with diabetes. Curr Diab Rep 7:114–122, 2007

Mezuk B, Eaton WW, Albrecht S, et al: Depression and type 2 diabetes over the lifespan: a meta-analysis. Diabetes Care 31:2383–2390, 2008

Mijajlovic M, Mirkovic M, Dackovic J, et al: Clinical manifestations, diagnostic criteria and therapy of Hashimoto's encephalopathy: report of two cases. J Neurol Sci 288:194–196, 2010

Mocellin R, Walterfang M, Velakoulis D: Hashimoto's encephalopathy: epidemiology, pathogenesis and management. CNS Drugs 21:799–811, 2007

Musselman DL, Betan E, Larsen H, et al: Relationship of depression to diabetes types 1 and 2: epidemiology, biology, and treatment. Biol Psychiatry 54:317–329, 2003

Petrak F, Herpertz S: Treatment of depression in diabetes: an update. Curr Opin Psychiatry 22:211–217, 2009

Pouwer F, Kupper N, Adriaanse MC: Does emotional stress cause type 2 diabetes mellitus? A review from the European Depression in Diabetes (EDID) Research Consortium. Discov Med 9:112–118, 2010

Roman S, Sosa JA: Psychiatric and cognitive aspects of primary hyperparathyroidism. Curr Opin Oncol 19:1–5, 2007

Saarto T, Wiffen P: Antidepressants for neuropathic pain: a Cochrane review. J Neurol Neurosurg Psychiatry 81:1372–1373, 2010

Schiess N, Pardo CA: Hashimoto's encephalopathy. Ann NY Acad Sci 1142:254–265, 2008

Solanki RK, Dubey V, Munshi D: Neurocognitive impairment and comorbid depression in patients of diabetes mellitus. Int J Diabetes Dev Ctries 29:133–138, 2009

Sultan A, Gaskell H, Derry S, et al: Duloxetine for painful diabetic neuropathy and fibromyalgia pain: systematic review of randomized trials. BMC Neurol 8:29, 2008

Toplak H, Abrahamian H: Impact of depression on diabetes mellitus. Obes Facts 2:211–215, 2009

Williams GR: Neurodevelopmental and neurophysiological actions of thyroid hormone. J Neuroendocrinol 20:784–794, 2008

Williams LJ, Pasco JA, Jacka FN, et al: Depression and bone metabolism: a review. Psychother Psychosom 78:16–25, 2009

21

Fatigue and Fibromyalgia

Fatigue

Fatigue is a complex problem with a wide range of conditions and symptoms that may cause or co-occur with it. Assessment requires consideration of both medical and psychological factors. Fatigue is a common medical complaint: one-fourth of patients in primary care settings describe it as a major problem (Kroenke et al. 1988).

Definition

Fatigue is the inability to initiate activity due to the perception of generalized weakness and/or lessened capacity or motivation to maintain activity (Evans and Lambert 2007). It should be distinguished from somnolence or muscle weakness even though these symptoms may occur with fatigue. Fatigue is considered chronic when symptoms persist for at least 6 months.

Epidemiology and Etiology of Fatigue

Prevalence

The prevalence of fatigue in the general population is 7%, and the lifetime rate is 25% (Walker et al. 1993). Fatigue is generally more common in women

373

than men (Kroenke et al. 1988). Medically unexplained fatigue has a lifetime prevalence rate of 15%.

Neurasthenia

The term *neurasthenia* was coined in the 1880s to describe chronic fatigue, and neurasthenia still remains a separate diagnosis in the *International Statistical Classification of Diseases and Related Health Problems,* 10th Revision (ICD-10). It is defined as persistent and distressing complaints of increased fatigue after mental effort, or persistent and distressing complaints of body weakness and exhaustion after minimal effort, with accompanying somatic symptoms in the absence of a depressive or anxiety disorder (World Health Organization 1992). Although significant overlap exists between fatigue and psychiatric disorders, about 7% of adults suffer from fatigue without psychiatric symptoms (Harvey et al. 2009).

Differential Diagnosis

Although only one-half of primary care patients receive a diagnosis that explains their fatigue (Nijrolder et al. 2009), a broad range of medical conditions may result in fatigue. These include congestive heart failure, cancer, chronic obstructive pulmonary disease, renal failure, HIV, sleep disorders, musculoskeletal disorders, and depression (Evans and Lambert 2007). (See Table 21–1 for a longer list.)

Higher Rates of Psychiatric Illness

In the general population, people with fatigue are more likely to have experienced current and lifetime episodes of depression, anxiety, and somatization compared with people without fatigue (Walker et al. 1993). In primary care settings, most patients with chronic fatigue (60%) and chronic fatigue syndrome (75%) have a current psychiatric disorder (Wessely et al. 1996).

Premorbid Predictors of Chronic Fatigue

Higher emotional instability (an individual's tendency to experience psychological distress) and self-reported stress in the premorbid period have been shown to increase the risk for chronic fatigue–like illness, and the effect appears to be modulated by genetic factors (Kato et al. 2006). Excessive childhood energy and adult obesity appear to be risk factors for fatigue without comorbid psychiatric illness (Harvey et al. 2009).

Table 21–1. Differential diagnosis for chronic fatigue

Cardiopulmonary	**Neoplastic-hematological**
Chronic congestive heart failure	Anemia
Chronic obstructive pulmonary	Occult malignancy
disease	**Neurological**
Endocrine-metabolic	Multiple sclerosis
Adrenal insufficiency	Poststroke
Apathetic hyperthyroidism	Spinal stenosis
Chronic renal failure	**Pharmacological**
Diabetes mellitus	Antidepressants
Hepatic failure	Antihypertensives
Hypercalcemia	Benzodiazepines
Hypothyroidism	Chemotherapeutic agents
Idiopathic	Opioids
Chronic fatigue syndrome	Statins
Fibromyalgia	**Psychiatric**
Idiopathic chronic fatigue	Anxiety
Infectious	Depression
Cytomegalovirus	Somatoform disorders
Endocarditis	**Sleep disorders**
Hepatitis C	Obstructive sleep apnea
HIV	**Rheumatological**
Lyme disease	Polymyalgia rheumatica
Mononucleosis	Rheumatoid arthritis
Occult abscess	Systemic lupus

Chronic Fatigue Syndrome

History

Chronic fatigue syndrome (CFS) was named in 1988, but CFS-like cases were described over a century ago. Over the last several decades, controversies have existed about whether CFS is a real condition, and about its pathogenesis and treatment. Debate over whether it is organic or psychogenic has given rise to a dichotomous approach that does not integrate the biological, psychological, and social aspects of the illness, as required for effective treatment. Consensus criteria published in 1994 require that patients have clinically evaluated, unexplained, persistent, or relapsing fatigue plus four or more specifically defined associated symptoms (Fukuda et al. 1994) (see Table 21–2).

Epidemiology

Although chronic fatigue is common in medical patients, CFS is relatively uncommon, accounting for only 1%–9% of chronic fatigue patients, with a prevalence of 0.3% (Bates et al. 1993; Prins et al. 2006). Seventy-five percent of CFS patients are female, and the mean age at onset is between 29 and 35 years; the mean duration of illness is 3–9 years. Patients with psychiatric illness have a poorer prognosis, whereas patients who have less severe fatigue at baseline, demonstrate a sense of control over their symptoms, and do not attribute their illness to a physical cause have a better prognosis (Cairns and Hotopf 2005).

Etiology

Predisposing factors.   Twin studies have shown a familial predisposition to CFS, but no specific genetic abnormalities have been found. Personality characteristics such as neuroticism and introversion may be risk factors (Prins et al. 2006).

Precipitating factors.   Some evidence suggests that infection is associated with the development of CFS. Stressful life events may also precipitate the disorder (Prins et al. 2006).

Perpetuating factors.   Immunological factors, including cytokines, neuroendocrine changes, sleep abnormalities, and chronic infection, may have a role in maintaining the illness. Psychological factors, such as a strong belief in a physical cause of the illness, a focus on bodily sensations, and a sense of loss of control, have been found to perpetuate the symptoms (Prins et al. 2006).

Treatment

Cognitive-behavioral therapy.   Cognitive-behavioral therapy (CBT), which focuses on changing condition-related thoughts and behaviors, and teaches patients how to control their symptoms, is effective in treating CFS (Prins et al. 2006). In a 5-year follow-up study, 70% of patients receiving CBT had sus-

Table 21–2. International Chronic Fatigue Syndrome Study Group consensus criteria for chronic fatigue syndrome

1. Clinically evaluated, unexplained, persistent, or relapsing fatigue that is of new or definite onset; is not the result of ongoing exertion; is not alleviated by rest; and results in substantial reduction in previous levels of occupational, educational, social, or personal activities

and

2. Four or more of the following symptoms that persist or recur during 6 or more consecutive months of illness and that do not predate the fatigue:

   - Self-reported impairment in short-term memory or concentration
   - Sore throat
   - Tender cervical or axillary nodes
   - Muscle pain
   - Multijoint pain without redness or swelling
   - Headaches of a new pattern or severity
   - Unrefreshing sleep
   - Postexertional malaise lasting ≥24 hours

Source. Adapted from Fukuda et al. 1994.

tained improvement, compared with 35% of patients treated with relaxation therapy (Deale et al. 2001).

Graded exercise therapy. Graded exercise therapy is an educational intervention that encourages graded activity, based on a physiological model of deconditioning. A randomized controlled trial (RCT) demonstrated continued benefit for patients with CFS 2 years following treatment (Powell et al. 2004).

Other treatments. Insufficient evidence is available to support the use of pharmacological agents, supplements, or alternative treatments for CFS (Whiting et al. 2001), although treatment of comorbid psychiatric illness is important. Data do not show benefit from treatment of CFS with modafinil (Randall et al. 2005), methylphenidate (Blockmans et al. 2006), or antidepressants (Vercoulen et al. 1996).

Fibromyalgia

Epidemiology

The prevalence of fibromyalgia syndrome (FMS) in the United States is approximately 2%, and FMS is at least six times more common in women than in men (Wolfe et al. 1995). The prevalence increases with age, and patients who present with FMS are, on average, 10 years older than patients who present with CFS. FMS is more prevalent in individuals with less education and lower socioeconomic status (White et al. 1999).

Pathophysiology

Controversy exists about whether FMS is a distinct disorder or the manifestation of an underlying malady ranging from inflammatory arthritic disease to depression (Hauser et al. 2009). A particular pathology has not been found for FMS. One potential explanatory mechanism is that individuals with FMS experience pain differently than do those without FMS. FMS has been considered a rheumatological disease, in part because of prominent muscle and joint pain, although evidence has not supported the presence of musculoskeletal abnormalities. Recent literature has focused on abnormal central pain processing rather than dysfunction in the peripheral tissues (Abeles et al. 2007).

Classification Criteria

The American College of Rheumatology listed the following classification criteria (Wolfe et al. 1990):

1. History of widespread pain involving all four limbs and the trunk
2. Pain in at least 11 of 18 specified tender point sites with digital palpation

Clinical Manifestations

Despite the American College of Rheumatology's criteria (Wolfe et al. 1990), the syndrome is associated with a myriad of other symptoms, the most common of which are fatigue, poor sleep quality, and morning stiffness (Abeles et al. 2007). Frequent neurological symptoms include poor balance or coordination, tingling or weakness in the arms or legs, numbness, and photophobia (Watson et al. 2009). The majority of patients have headaches (Marcus et al.

2005), and many have a variety of other pain symptoms, including abdominal and pelvic pain. Additional symptoms such as night sweats, sexual dysfunction, dyspnea, dysphagia, and urinary urgency may occur.

Increased Rates of Psychiatric Disorders

Depression

Depression is prevalent in patients with FMS and may exceed 50% (Okifuji et al. 2000). Both the rate and familial prevalence of major affective disorder are significantly higher in patients with fibromyalgia than in patients with rheumatoid arthritis (Hudson et al. 1985). Concurrent depressive disorders may be independent of the cardinal features of FMS (i.e., pain severity and hypersensitivity to pressure pain), but depression nonetheless influences the effects of FMS symptoms on patients' daily lives and functional activities (McBeth and Silman 2001; Okifuji et al. 2000).

Anxiety Disorders

Anxiety disorders are twice as prevalent in patients with FMS as in control patients with chronic pain (McBeth and Silman 2001). Patients with FMS have higher rates of posttraumatic stress disorder (PTSD) and are more likely to have experienced childhood trauma or abuse. Patients with FMS who have PTSD-like symptoms have been shown to have significantly greater levels of pain, emotional distress, and disability than FMS patients without those symptoms (Sherman et al. 2000).

Somatization and Onset of Widespread Body Pain

The multiple pain complaints of patients diagnosed with fibromyalgia may represent a somatization process. One prospective study demonstrated that the strongest predictor of the development of chronic widespread pain in patients who had no pain at baseline was high scores on measures of somatization and maladaptive coping mechanisms (McBeth et al. 2001).

Shared Genetic Risk Factors for Fibromyalgia and Major Depressive Disorder

Family aggregation studies suggest that patients with fibromyalgia and major depressive disorder may have genetically or biologically mediated vulnerability to respond to stressful life events with pain-related and affective symptoms (Kato et al. 2009; Raphael et al. 2004).

Pharmacological Treatment

Antidepressants

On the basis of a meta-analysis, researchers concluded that strong evidence exists for the efficacy of antidepressants to reduce pain, sleep disturbance, and depressed mood, as well as to improve health-related quality of life (Hauser et al. 2009). The data on the long-term effects of antidepressants are insufficient to draw conclusions (Uceyler et al. 2008).

Tricyclic antidepressants.   The most robust evidence for medication efficacy in FMS is for the tricyclic antidepressants (TCAs). Amitriptyline, the most widely studied TCA, has demonstrated effects on sleep, fatigue, and pain. Most studies report the use of low dosages of amitriptyline, between 12.5 and 50 mg/day; TCAs have been shown to have an effect on fibromyalgia independent of depressive symptoms. Adverse effects are the primary reason for not increasing the dosage to achieve serum levels in the therapeutic window for depression (Goldenberg et al. 2004; Hauser et al. 2009; Perrot et al. 2008). Cyclobenzaprine is a muscle relaxant with a tricyclic structure, and the evidence is strong for its efficacy at dosages of 10–40 mg/day (Goldenberg et al. 2004).

Serotonin-norepinephrine reuptake inhibitors.   The serotonin-norepinephrine reuptake inhibitors (SNRIs) duloxetine and milnacipran have both been approved by the U.S. Food and Drug Administration (FDA) for the management of FMS. Both are significantly more effective than placebo for pain, dysfunction, dyssomnia, and fatigue. Duloxetine 60–120 mg/day and milnacipran 100–200 mg/day are equally effective for pain (Perrot et al. 2008). The analgesic effect appears to be unrelated to the antidepressant effects and may be due to the modulation of pain pathways in the central nervous system. Venlafaxine has not been studied as extensively as duloxetine and milnacipran for the treatment of FMS.

Selective serotonin reuptake inhibitors.   In the meta-analysis by Hauser et al. (2009), the effect sizes for the selective serotonin reuptake inhibitors were smaller than for the TCAs, but a definitive conclusion could not be made for superior efficacy of one class of antidepressant over another.

Anticonvulsants

Pregabalin and gabapentin are anticonvulsants with analgesic effects thought to be mediated through the $\alpha 2\delta$ protein, a subunit of voltage-dependent calcium channel neurons. These medications modulate the influx of calcium ions and reduce the synaptic release of neurotransmitters believed to have an effect in pain processing. Pregabalin is approved by the FDA for treatment of FMS, and is associated with improvements in pain, sleep, health-related quality of life, and global measures (Crofford et al. 2005). The FDA-indicated dosage of pregabalin is 150–225 mg twice daily. An RCT of gabapentin for FMS used flexible dosing of 1,200–2,400 mg/day (Arnold et al. 2007).

Analgesic Medications

Modest evidence supports the efficacy in patients with FMS of tramadol administered with or without acetaminophen in dosages of 200–300 mg/day. The long-term efficacy and tolerability is unknown, however, and the risk of abuse needs to be considered. Nonsteroidal anti-inflammatory drugs alone are not effective, although they may be useful when combined with TCAs. No RCTs of opioids in the treatment of FMS have been reported (Goldenberg et al. 2004).

Nonpharmacological Treatments

Exercise

Substantial evidence indicates that cardiovascular exercise is effective for increasing aerobic performance, raising tender-point pain pressure thresholds, and decreasing pain in patients with FMS. Exercise combined with education has shown improvement in global well-being, fatigue, sleep, and aerobic performance (Goldenberg et al. 2004).

Cognitive Therapies

In RCTs of CBT, patients with FMS have experienced improved pain, mood, fatigue, and function, and the effects are often sustained beyond 6 months (Goldenberg et al. 2004).

Multidisciplinary Treatment

Treatment that combines education, CBT, relaxation training, and exercise have demonstrated beneficial effects on patient self-efficacy and pain, and reduced physician-rated disease severity. Further studies are needed to evaluate programs that combine medication and nonpharmacological treatment (Goldenberg et al. 2004).

References

Abeles AM, Pillinger MH, Solitar BM, et al: Narrative review: the pathophysiology of fibromyalgia. Ann Intern Med 146:726–734, 2007

Arnold LM, Goldenberg DL, Stanford SB, et al: Gabapentin in the treatment of fibromyalgia: a randomized, double-blind, placebo-controlled, multicenter trial. Arthritis Rheum 56:1336–1344, 2007

Bates DW, Schmitt W, Buchwald D, et al: Prevalence of fatigue and chronic fatigue syndrome in a primary care practice. Arch Intern Med 153:2759–2765, 1993

Blockmans D, Persoons P, Van Houdenhove B, et al: Does methylphenidate reduce the symptoms of chronic fatigue syndrome? Am J Med 119:167.e23–e30, 2006

Cairns R, Hotopf M: A systematic review describing the prognosis of chronic fatigue syndrome. Occup Med (Lond) 55:20–31, 2005

Crofford LJ, Rowbotham MC, Mease PJ, et al: Pregabalin for the treatment of fibromyalgia syndrome: results of a randomized, double-blind, placebo-controlled trial. Arthritis Rheum 52:1264–1273, 2005

Deale A, Husain K, Chalder T, et al: Long-term outcome of cognitive behavior therapy versus relaxation therapy for chronic fatigue syndrome: a 5-year follow-up study. Am J Psychiatry 158:2038–2042, 2001

Evans WJ, Lambert CP: Physiological basis of fatigue. Am J Phys Med Rehabil 86:S29–S46, 2007

Fukuda K, Straus SE, Hickie I, et al: The chronic fatigue syndrome: a comprehensive approach to its definition and study. International Chronic Fatigue Syndrome Study Group. Ann Intern Med 121:953–959, 1994

Goldenberg DL, Burckhardt C, Crofford L: Management of fibromyalgia syndrome. JAMA 292:2388–2395, 2004

Harvey SB, Wessely S, Kuh D, et al: The relationship between fatigue and psychiatric disorders: evidence for the concept of neurasthenia. J Psychosom Res 66:445–454, 2009

Hauser W, Bernardy K, Uceyler N, et al: Treatment of fibromyalgia syndrome with antidepressants: a meta-analysis. JAMA 301:198–209, 2009

Hudson JI, Hudson MS, Pliner LF, et al: Fibromyalgia and major affective disorder: a controlled phenomenology and family history study. Am J Psychiatry 142:441–446, 1985

Kato K, Sullivan PF, Evengård B, et al: Premorbid predictors of chronic fatigue. Arch Gen Psychiatry 63:1267–1272, 2006

Kato K, Sullivan PF, Evengård B, et al: A population-based twin study of functional somatic syndromes. Psychol Med 39:497–505, 2009

Kroenke K, Wood DR, Mangelsdorff AD, et al: Chronic fatigue in primary care: prevalence, patient characteristics, and outcome. JAMA 260:929–934, 1988

Marcus DA, Bernstein C, Rudy TE: Fibromyalgia and headache: an epidemiological study supporting migraine as part of the fibromyalgia syndrome. Clin Rheumatol 24:595–601, 2005

McBeth J, Silman AJ: The role of psychiatric disorders in fibromyalgia. Curr Rheumatol Rep 3:157–164, 2001

McBeth J, Macfarlane GJ, Benjamin S, et al: Features of somatization predict the onset of chronic widespread pain: results of a large population-based study. Arthritis Rheum 44:940–946, 2001

Nijrolder I, van der Windt D, de Vries H, et al: Diagnoses during follow-up of patients presenting with fatigue in primary care. CMAJ 181:683–687, 2009

Okifuji A, Turk DC, Sherman JJ: Evaluation of the relationship between depression and fibromyalgia syndrome: why aren't all patients depressed? J Rheumatol 27:212–219, 2000

Perrot S, Javier RM, Marty M, et al: Is there any evidence to support the use of antidepressants in painful rheumatological conditions? Systematic review of pharmacological and clinical studies. Rheumatology 47:1117–1123, 2008

Powell P, Bentall RP, Nye FJ, et al: Patient education to encourage graded exercise in chronic fatigue syndrome: 2-year follow-up of randomised controlled trial. Br J Psychiatry 184:142–146, 2004

Prins JB, van der Meer JWM, Bleijenberg G: Chronic fatigue syndrome. Lancet 367:346–355, 2006

Randall DC, Cafferty FH, Shneerson JM, et al: Chronic treatment with modafinil may not be beneficial in patients with chronic fatigue syndrome. J Psychopharmacol 19:647–660, 2005

Raphael KG, Janal MN, Nayak S, et al: Familial aggregation of depression in fibromyalgia: a community-based test of alternate hypotheses. Pain 110:449–460, 2004

Sherman JJ, Turk DC, Okifuji A: Prevalence and impact of posttraumatic stress disorder–like symptoms on patients with fibromyalgia syndrome. Clin J Pain 16:127–134, 2000

Uceyler N, Hauser W, Sommer C: A systematic review on the effectiveness of treatment with antidepressants in fibromyalgia syndrome. Arthritis Rheum 59:1279–1298, 2008

Vercoulen JH, Swanink CM, Zitman FG, et al: Randomised, double-blind, placebo-controlled study of fluoxetine in chronic fatigue syndrome. Lancet 347:858–861, 1996

Walker EA, Katon WJ, Jemelka RP: Psychiatric disorders and medical care utilization among people in the general population who report fatigue. J Gen Intern Med 8:436–440, 1993

Watson NF, Buchwald D, Goldberg J, et al: Neurologic signs and symptoms in fibromyalgia. Arthritis Rheum 60:2839–2844, 2009

Wessely S, Chalder T, Hirsch S, et al: Psychological symptoms, somatic symptoms, and psychiatric disorder in chronic fatigue and chronic fatigue syndrome: a prospective study in the primary care setting. Am J Psychiatry 153:1050–1059, 1996

White KP, Speechley M, Harth M, et al: The London Fibromyalgia Epidemiology Study: comparing the demographic and clinical characteristics in 100 random community cases of fibromyalgia versus controls. J Rheumatol 26:1577–1585, 1999

Whiting P, Bagnall AM, Sowden AJ, et al: Interventions for the treatment and management of chronic fatigue syndrome: a systematic review. JAMA 286:1360–1368, 2001

Wolfe F, Smythe HA, Yunus MB, et al: The American College of Rheumatology 1990 Criteria for the Classification of Fibromyalgia: report of the Multicenter Criteria Committee. Arthritis Rheum 33:160–72, 1990

Wolfe F, Ross K, Anderson J, et al: The prevalence and characteristics of fibromyalgia in the general population. Arthritis Rheum 38:19–28, 1995

World Health Organization: International Statistical Classification of Diseases and Related Health Problems, 10th Revision. Geneva, Switzerland, World Health Organization, 1992

22

Gastroenterology

The brain-gut axis challenges the physician, whether psychiatrist or endoscopist. Not long ago, peptic ulcer disease was emblematic of psychosomatic illness, but stress and conflict have been displaced by *Helicobacter pylori* and nonsteroidal anti-inflammatory drugs (NSAIDs) as the causes of peptic ulcers. Nevertheless, a patient's biopsychosocial milieu may leave a morphological trace in the pathologist's description of a small bowel frozen section. Childhood trauma may now find a muted voice in visceral hypersensitivity. In one study, psychotherapy eased somatic symptoms in patients with severe irritable bowel syndrome (IBS), but psychological markers of distress changed little (Creed et al. 2003). The brain-gut axis invites the consultation psychiatrist's study.

Oropharyngeal and Upper Gastrointestinal Disorders

Even when they are not the primary reason for a psychiatric consultation request, oropharyngeal and upper gastrointestinal disorders are common comorbidities with psychiatric disorders.

Dysphagia

Dysphagia affects up to 10% of older adults, precipitated by several neurological conditions (e.g., stroke, multiple sclerosis, Parkinson's disease) and medications, including antipsychotics. In patients taking antipsychotics, management requires lowering the dosage, switching to another agent, or discontinuing antipsychotics altogether. Benztropine and diphenhydramine are not helpful in relieving antipsychotic-induced dysphagia (Dziewas et al. 2007).

Globus Hystericus

Globus hystericus is the persistent sensation of a lump in the throat. Despite the condition's name, careful ear, nose, and throat evaluation yields some measure of physiological abnormality in most patients (Leelamanit et al. 1996). Although the time course varies, the condition is benign and almost always gradually resolves in response to recommended treatment, reassurance, and, in cases of concomitant panic disorder, anxiolytics.

Gastroesophageal Reflux Disease

Gastroesophageal reflux disease (GERD) is common in North America and Western Europe but rare elsewhere. Studies examining the association of GERD with selective serotonin reuptake inhibitors (SSRIs), anxiety, and depression have not had uniform results, although the larger, population-based studies suggest independent increased risk with each of these variables (Jansson et al. 2007; van Soest et al. 2007). GERD patients who have a history of sexual or physical abuse are more prone to bring their symptoms to medical attention than those with no history of abuse (Mizyed et al. 2009).

Noncardiac Chest Pain

Noncardiac chest pain occurs in up to 25% of the population annually and is often nearly identical to the pain of cardiac ischemia, prompting many emergent assessments. Although panic disorder and other anxiety disorders are more common in patients with noncardiac chest pain than in the general population (Fass and Dickman 2006), other factors, such as esophageal hypersensitivity, are also likely to play a role.

Hyperemesis Gravidarum

Hyperemesis gravidarum requires sufficient nausea and vomiting in pregnancy to provoke ketonuria and weight loss; it affects up to 2% of women. In years past, this diagnosis was often attributed to ambivalence regarding the pregnancy, but evidence does not support this (Kim et al. 2009). Medical interventions include intravenous hydration and pharmacotherapy (Bottomley and Bourne 2009).

Anticipatory Nausea and Vomiting

Anticipatory nausea and vomiting is most commonly associated with chemotherapy but can also occur in association with any other situation or condition that was previously linked in the patient's experience with nausea and vomiting. Behavioral interventions are the most helpful, benzodiazepines are sometimes effective, and conventional antiemetics are not at all useful (Matteson et al. 2002).

Dyspepsia and Peptic Ulcer Disease

Dyspepsia and peptic ulcer disease have prompted psychiatric investigation for more than 80 years; multiple factors have been identified (e.g., *H. pylori,* NSAIDs, alcohol, nicotine) and new treatments introduced (e.g., proton-pump inhibitors). Nonetheless, stress and anxiety continue to be associated with the occurrence of dyspepsia and peptic ulcer disease, underscoring the value of including stress reduction and anxiolytic strategies in any treatment plan (Crone and Dobbelstein 2011).

Irritable Bowel Syndrome

IBS is the presence of abdominal discomfort or pain that has occurred for 12 or more weeks (not necessarily consecutive) in the prior 12 months and is characterized by at least two of the following: 1) onset is associated with a change in the frequency of bowel movements (diarrhea or constipation); 2) onset is associated with a change in the form of the stool (loose, watery, or pellet-like); and 3) the discomfort or pain is relieved with defecation. Patients commonly complain of feelings of abdominal distension or incomplete evacuation, as well as unusual straining or, conversely, urgency (Creed and Olden 2005).

Epidemiology

The prevalence of IBS is uncertain because the spectrum of severity is broad and because existing studies have examined variable age groups with different diagnostic criteria. Also, only a portion of people with IBS seek medical attention. One U.S. householder survey identified a prevalence of about 10% (Drossman et al. 1993). The association of IBS with the following extraintestinal nonpsychiatric disorders is high: temporomandibular joint disorder (65%), chronic fatigue syndrome (50%), chronic pelvic pain (50%), fibromyalgia (50%), and interstitial cystitis (30%) (Riedl et al. 2008; Whitehead et al. 2002).

Psychiatric Issues

Psychiatric issues are both implicit and explicit:

- Patients with IBS make two to three times as many health care visits per year as control subjects. The majority of these visits are for extraintestinal somatic complaints, reflecting significant distress and erosion of quality of life (Whitehead et al. 2002).
- Stress is a common forerunner of IBS and an important predictor of outcome for patients with IBS. Interpersonal stresses are important despite a frequent inclination among these patients to discount the relevance of such tensions (Crone and Dobbelstein 2011).
- Past sexual and physical abuse is associated with up to a threefold increase in incidence of IBS among individuals reporting past sexual abuse (Drossman et al. 1995).

- Panic disorder, anxiety, and depression are reported in 50%–60% of patients with IBS seeking specialty care, with a trend toward anxiety in initial presentations but depression in those who have sought medical attention over time (Creed and Olden 2005).

Management

Methodological complexities prevent clear conclusions about the management of IBS, but the following considerations may serve as a starting point for a clinician's decision making:

- Cognitive-behavioral therapy is more effective than education and may be especially practical when high anxiety is present (Drossman et al. 2003).
- Interpersonal psychotherapy may be particularly apt for individuals who have experienced sexual abuse (Creed et al. 2003).
- Tricyclic antidepressants are more suitable for depressed patients with diarrhea-predominant IBS; adherence must be monitored to assess and ensure efficacy, because side effects often prompt discontinuation (Drossman et al. 2003; Ford et al. 2009).
- SSRIs hold an advantage for depressed patients with constipation-predominant IBS (Creed et al. 2003). Paroxetine may be an exception due to its anticholinergic activity.
- When pain is the primary target symptom for an antidepressant, the clinician should explain this use to the patient to eliminate the risk of discontinuation when the patient is subsequently displeased to discover that the medication prescribed is an antidepressant (Creed and Olden 2005).

Inflammatory Bowel Disease

Inflammatory bowel disease (IBD) is a group of conditions that include Crohn's disease, ulcerative colitis, and the less common collagenous colitis, lymphocytic colitis, and microscopic colitis. The etiologies are cryptic but appear to involve the confluence of genetic and environmental factors that produce a grossly magnified intestinal inflammatory response in at-risk individuals (Kucharzik et al. 2006). The linkage between IBD and psychiatric disorders may have reciprocal elements: not only is IBD associated with increased anxiety and depression, but these conditions are sometimes associated with increased severity of IBD signs and symptoms. Recent attention has addressed whether dysfunctional neuroimmunoregulatory circuits form a common pathway for both IBD and depression (Graff et al. 2009).

Epidemiology

Although subclinical cases of ulcerative colitis are often attributed to infectious colitis, the annual incidence of ulcerative colitis has remained fairly stable in the United States at 10–12 per 100,000. In sharp contrast, the annual incidence of Crohn's disease has increased steadily as society has modernized and is at 6–8 per 100,000. The association between societal development and the increasing prevalence of IBD has been consistently and recurrently observed throughout the world (Shanahan and Bernstein 2009; Thia et al. 2008). Both ulcerative colitis and Crohn's disease have a bimodal distribution, with peak incidences in the second and third decades, and again in the sixth and seventh decades.

Psychiatric Issues

Comorbid Anxiety and Depression

The rigor of studies exploring the prevalence of anxiety and depression in patients with IBD has improved substantially in the past 10 years. Conservatively, depression occurs at least twice as frequently in patients with IBD as in general community samples. Although anxiety occurs less often than depression in patients with IBD, anxiety is still more prevalent in IBD patients than in the general community. Earlier studies suggested that anxiety may occur more often with Crohn's disease and depression with ulcerative colitis, but the majority of more recent studies that evaluated these inflammatory disorders separately found Crohn's disease and ulcerative colitis to be comparable in regard to psychiatric comorbidity. Similarly, the rates of psychiatric disorders in patients with IBD are roughly equivalent to those in patients with several other chronic medical illnesses, such as diabetes mellitus and rheumatoid arthritis (Graff et al. 2009).

Anxiety and Depression as Potential Risk Factors for IBD Onset

No definitive evidence indicates that either anxiety or depression raises the risk of IBD onset, but some studies have noted relationships that warrant continued exploration (Graff et al. 2009). For example, the onset of IBD symptoms occurred earlier in patients with lifetime mood or anxiety disorders, and the majority of these patients experienced the psychiatric disorders 2 years or more before IBD was established (Walker et al. 2008).

Anxiety and Depression as Risk Factors for IBD Exacerbation

Moderate evidence suggests that both anxiety and depression are often intensified during IBD symptom flares. A small body of prospective literature indicates that depression is associated with higher IBD activity, shorter intervals until IBD relapse, and less chance of remission with infliximab treatment (Mardini et al. 2004; Mittermaier et al. 2004; Persoons et al. 2005).

Psychiatric Sequelae of Treatment

Corticosteroids are commonplace among the salicyclates and immunomodulators used to treat IBD. High dosages of corticosteroids may be required, but sustained high dosing is rarely essential. In one study, 50% of patients receiving daily prednisone ≥20 mg experienced psychiatric symptoms, and 10% of those were hospitalized for either mania or depression (Fardet al al. 2007). The incidence of adverse psychiatric events is dose related. Mania is more likely early in treatment, whereas depression more commonly emerges later, including during the tapering phase (Graff et al. 2009).

Management

Screening for Anxiety and Depression

Ongoing active assessment for psychiatric comorbidity in patients with IBD is important because of the association between IBD flares and the occurrence of anxiety and depression, as well as the risk of decreased treatment adherence by patients who are depressed (Nigro et al. 2001).

Pharmacological Versus Psychological Treatment

Pharmacological agents are often prescribed by primary care or gastroenterology specialists, sparing the patient a psychiatric referral. The incidence of relapse is higher, however, when patients discontinue medication than when they stop psychological therapies, and many patients with IBD do not wish to add another medication to their daily regimen. Psychotherapy has the disadvantage of diminished access and potentially higher cost. Because adherence may prove an important determinant of efficacy, the clinician and patient should discuss the treatment options and proceed with the patient's preferred form of care (Fotaki et al. 2008; Graff et al. 2009). The following information may help with the choice:

- SSRIs and serotonin-norepinephrine reuptake inhibitors (SNRIs) offer relative safety and efficacy but have a higher incidence of gastrointestinal side effects, including nausea and diarrhea, that can impact quality of life for patients with IBD. The increase in upper gastrointestinal bleeding with SSRIs and SNRIs can be reduced by concomitant acid-suppressing medications; however, in one study, concomitant NSAIDs increased the risk of gastrointestinal bleeding eightfold (de Abajo and Garcia-Rodriguez 2008).
- Bupropion and mirtazapine have different side-effect profiles than the SSRIs and SNRIs. Bupropion does not interfere with sexual function, an issue that can be of particular importance for some IBD patients for whom treatment has introduced challenges with intimacy (Graff et al. 2009). Weight gain, desired by some but not all patients with IBD, is more likely with mirtazapine.
- Psychological modalities, particularly cognitive-behavioral therapies, have repeatedly been found to reduce anxiety and depression and to improve overall function in patients with IBD. Although unequivocal evidence of reduction in IBD severity has been more elusive, the psychological benefits have persisted in 12-month follow-ups (Graff et al. 2009).

Hepatitis C Virus

Hepatitis C virus (HCV), whose existence was proved in 1989, is the most common blood-borne infection in the United States.

Epidemiology

An estimated 3.2 million persons in the United States and as many as 300 million worldwide have HCV, and no vaccine is available to protect against infection. The incidence declined throughout the 1990s but has plateaued since 2003. HCV is the major cause of chronic liver disease and hepatocellular carcinoma, as well as a leading reason for liver transplantation. Intravenous drug use remains the most common risk factor; transmission requires percutaneous or mucosal exposure.

Psychiatric Issues

Psychiatric issues, including depression, anxiety, fatigue, irritability, and neuro-cognitive complaints, are common among patients with chronic HCV.

- Intravenous drug use is common among individuals with high psychiatric comorbidity, including other substance abuse, mood disorders, and psychotic disorders, who are later infected with HCV (Loftis et al. 2006).
- HCV replication in the central nervous system is associated with changes in frontal white matter neurotransmitter levels, which are correlated with impaired attention and concentration (Foster 2009). HCV also appears to stimulate increased inflammatory cytokines and tumor necrosis factor, which are associated with the "sickness behavior" syndrome (Quelhas and Lopes 2009).
- Medical complications and comorbidities, including cirrhosis, diabetes mellitus, hepatocellular carcinoma, and coinfection with HIV or hepatitis B virus, significantly erode health-related quality of life (Nash et al. 2009).
- Interferon-α is associated with depression, fatigue, anxiety, and irritability in 30%–80% of patients (Schaefer and Mauss 2008).

Management

Management of patients with HCV requires anticipatory vigilance because the incidence of psychiatric problems is high and the consequences of inadequate or absent treatment may include diminished adherence to an antiviral regimen, thereby magnifying the eventual decay in overall health. Most adverse effects of interferon-α occur in the first 3 months of treatment, leading some intravenous drug users to erroneously conclude that they are experiencing withdrawal effects and to return to substance abuse. This negative cascade may warrant preventive initiation of an SSRI alongside or even before interferon-α therapy begins (Schaefer and Mauss 2008).

Other Conditions

Hepatic Encephalopathy

Hepatic encephalopathy may appear much like delirium in the context of known acute or chronic liver disease; it ranges in severity from subtle confusion to coma. Possible contributors are numerous, and the workup is the same as with delirium. The diagnosis requires the exclusion of other causes. Although serum ammonia is often elevated and lactulose is commonly prescribed, some thoroughly encephalopathic patients will have normal ammonia levels. The cornerstone of treatment is the correction of any identifiable causal factor (Sundaram and Shaikh 2009).

Drug-Induced Hepatic Injury

Drug-induced hepatic injury may occur with most psychotropic medications, but the risk is very low. The idiosyncratic reactions range in severity from unnoticed to catastrophic, cannot be predicted, are not dose dependent, occur at variable intervals following drug initiation, and almost always resolve after the offending agent is discontinued. Women are at increased risk, but individuals with comorbid liver disease are not, although the latter have less capacity to tolerate the added compromise of liver function. Potential culprit medications should be discontinued if a patient's serum alanine transferase exceeds three times normal, but routine prophylactic monitoring in otherwise healthy individuals is not recommended (Crone and Dobbelstein 2011).

Drug-Induced Pancreatic Injury

Drug-induced pancreatic injury has been reported, although rarely, in patients taking antipsychotics, anticonvulsants, and antidepressants, irrespective of class. The mechanism of causation is not known and is not dose dependent but usually occurs in the early weeks following drug initiation. Patients with multiple concomitant medications, as well as individuals with cancer, Crohn's disease, and HIV, are at higher risk. Prompt discontinuation of the drug typically leads to resolution; rechallenge with the same drug is not recommended (Crone and Dobbelstein 2011).

References

Bottomley C, Bourne T: Management strategies for hyperemesis. Best Pract Res Clin Obstet Gynaecol 23:549–564, 2009

Creed F, Olden KW: Gastrointestinal disorders, in The American Psychiatric Publishing Textbook of Psychosomatic Medicine. Edited by Levenson JL. Washington, DC, American Psychiatric Publishing, 2005, pp 465–481

Creed F, Fernandes L, Guthrie E, et al: The cost-effectiveness of psychotherapy and paroxetine for severe irritable bowel syndrome. Gastroenterology 124:303–317, 2003

Crone CC, Dobbelstein CR: Gastrointestinal disorders, in The American Psychiatric Publishing Textbook of Psychosomatic Medicine, 2nd Edition. Edited by Levenson JL. Washington, DC, American Psychiatric Publishing, 2011, pp 463–490

de Abajo FJ, Garcia-Rodriguez LA: Risk of upper gastrointestinal tract bleeding associated with selective serotonin reuptake inhibitors and venlafaxine therapy: interaction with nonsteroidal anti-inflammatory drugs and effect of acid-suppressing agents. Arch Gen Psychiatry 65:795–803, 2008

Drossman DA, Li Z, Andruzzi E, et al: U.S. householder survey of functional gastrointestinal disorders: prevalence, sociodemography, and health impacts. Dig Dis Sci 38:1569–1580, 1993

Drossman DA, Talley NJ, Leserman J, et al: Sexual and physical abuse and gastrointestinal illness: review and recommendations. Ann Intern Med 123:782–794, 1995

Drossman DA, Toner BB, Whitehead WE, et al: Cognitive-behavioral therapy versus education and desipramine versus placebo for moderate to severe functional bowel disorders. Gastroenterology 125:19–31, 2003

Dziewas R, Warnecke T, Schnabel M, et al: Neuroleptic-induced dysphagia: case report and literature review. Dysphagia 22:63–67, 2007

Fardet L, Flahault A, Kettaneh A, et al: Corticosteroid-induced clinical adverse events: frequency, risk factors, and patient's opinion. Br J Dermatol 157:142–148, 2007

Fass R, Dickman R: Non-cardiac chest pain: an update. Neurogastroenterol Motil 18:408–417, 2006

Ford AC, Talley NJ, Schoenfeld PS, et al: Efficacy of antidepressants and psychological therapies in irritable bowel syndrome: systematic review and meta-analysis. Gut 58:367–378, 2009

Foster GR: Quality of life considerations for patients with chronic hepatitis C. J Viral Hepat 16:605–611, 2009

Fotaki M, Roland M, Boyd A, et al: What benefits will choice bring to patients? Literature review and assessment of implications. J Health Serv Res Policy 13:178–184, 2008

Graff LA, Walker JR, Bernstein CN, et al: Depression and anxiety in inflammatory bowel disease: a review of comorbidity and management. Inflamm Bowel Dis 15:1105–1118, 2009

Jansson C, Nordenstedt H, Wallander MA, et al: Severe gastroesophageal reflux symptoms in relation to anxiety, depression and coping in a population-based study. Aliment Pharmacol Ther 26:683–691, 2007

Kim DR, Connolly KR, Cristancho P, et al: Psychiatric consultation of patients with hyperemesis gravidarum. Arch Womens Ment Health 12:61–67, 2009

Kucharzik T, Maaser C, Lugering A, et al: Recent understanding of IBD pathogenesis: implications for future therapies. Inflamm Bowel Dis 12:1068–1083, 2006

Leelamanit V, Geater A, Sinkitjaroenchai W: A study of 111 cases of globus hystericus. J Med Assoc Thai 79:460–467, 1996

Loftis JM, Matthews AM, Hauser P: Psychiatric and substance use disorders in individuals with hepatitis C: epidemiology and management. Drugs 66:155–174, 2006

Mardini HE, Kip KE, Wilson JW: Crohn's disease: a two-year prospective study of the association between psychological distress and disease activity. Dig Dis Sci 49:492–497, 2004

Matteson S, Roscoe J, Hickok J, et al: The role of behavioral conditioning in the development of nausea. Am J Obstet Gynecol 186:S239–S243, 2002

Mittermaier C, Dejaco C, Waldhoer T, et al: Impact of depressive mood on relapse in patients with inflammatory bowel disease: a prospective 18-month follow-up study. Psychosom Med 66:79–84, 2004

Mizyed I, Fass SS, Fass R: Review article: gastro-oesophageal reflux disease and psychological comorbidity. Aliment Pharmacol Ther 29:351–358, 2009

Nash KL, Bentley I, Hirschfield GM: Managing hepatitis C virus infection. BMJ 339:37–42, 2009

Nigro G, Angelini G, Bruna Grosso S, et al: Psychiatric predictors of non-compliance in inflammatory bowel disease. J Clin Gastroenterol 32:66–68, 2001

Persoons P, Vermeire S, Demyttenaere K, et al: The impact of major depressive disorder on the short and long-term outcome of Crohn's disease treatment with infliximab. Aliment Pharmacol Ther 22:101–110, 2005

Quelhas R, Lopes A: Psychiatric problems in patients infected with hepatitis C before and during antiviral treatment with interferon-alpha: a review. J Psychiatr Pract 15:262–281, 2009

Riedl A, Schmidtmann M, Stengel A, et al: Somatic comorbidities of irritable bowel syndrome: a systematic analysis. J Psychosom Res 64:573–582, 2008

Schaefer M, Mauss S: Hepatitis C treatment in patients with drug addiction: clinical management of interferon-alpha-associated psychiatric side effects. Curr Drug Abuse Rev 1:177–187, 2008

Shanahan F, Bernstein CN: The evolving epidemiology of inflammatory bowel disease. Curr Opin Gastroenterol 25:301–305, 2009

Sundaram V, Shaikh OS: Hepatic encephalopathy: pathophysiology and emerging therapies. Med Clin North Am 93:819–836, 2009

Thia KT, Loftus EV Jr, Sandborn WJ, et al: An update on the epidemiology of inflammatory bowel disease in Asia. Am J Gastroenterol 103:3167–3182, 2008 van Soest EM, Dieleman JP, Siersema PD, et al: Tricyclic antidepressants and the risk of reflux esophagitis. Am J Gastroenterol 102:1870–1877, 2007

Walker JR, Ediger JP, Graff LA, et al: The Manitoba IBD cohort study: a population-based study of the prevalence of lifetime and 12-month anxiety and mood disorders. Am J Gastroenterol 103:1989–1997, 2008

Whitehead WE, Palsson O, Jones KR, et al: Systematic review of the comorbidity of irritable bowel syndrome with other disorders: what are the causes and implications? Gastroenterology 122:1140–1156, 2002

23

HIV and AIDS

In 1981, the first cases of AIDS (acquired immunodeficiency syndrome) were reported to the CDC (then called the Center for Disease Control; now known as the Centers for Disease Control and Prevention). Since that time, the HIV (human immunodeficiency virus) epidemic has expanded to become one of the greatest public health challenges, both nationally and globally. The millionth case of AIDS in the United States occurred in 2007 (CDC 2008). Despite significant advances in HIV testing, prevention, and treatment in the United States, the human toll has been substantial.

Epidemiology

Cases of HIV/AIDS

From 2004 through 2007, the estimated number of newly diagnosed HIV/AIDS cases in the 34 states that have confidential name-based HIV reporting increased 15% (CDC 2008). In 2007, the estimated rate in the 34 states was 21.1 per 100,000 population.

Age Group

From 2004 through 2007, the estimated number of newly diagnosed HIV/AIDS cases decreased among children (less than 13 years of age) and persons ages 30–39 years. The estimated number of HIV/AIDS cases remained stable among persons ages 13–14 years and increased among persons ages 15–29 and ages 40 and older (CDC 2008).

Race and Ethnicity

From 2004 through 2007, the estimated number of newly diagnosed HIV/AIDS cases increased among all races and ethnic groups (CDC 2008). Blacks accounted for 51% of all HIV/AIDS cases diagnosed in 2007, and rates of cases in the black population were over eight times higher than in the white population and three times higher than in the Hispanic/Latino population.

Sex

From 2004 through 2007, the estimated number of newly diagnosed HIV/AIDS cases increased approximately 18% among males and 8% among females (CDC 2008). Males accounted for 74% of all HIV/AIDS cases among adults and adolescents.

Transmission Category

From 2004 through 2007, the estimated number of newly diagnosed HIV/AIDS cases increased among men who have sex with men and among men and women with high-risk heterosexual contact. Numbers remained stable among injection drug users (CDC 2008). Men who have sex with men and persons exposed through high-risk heterosexual contact accounted for 53% and 32%, respectively, of all HIV/AIDS cases diagnosed.

Progression to AIDS

Of all HIV infections diagnosed in 2006 in the 34 states with confidential name-based HIV reporting, 36% progressed to AIDS within 12 months after HIV infection was diagnosed. AIDS was diagnosed within 12 months after the diagnosis of HIV infection for larger percentages of persons ages 35 years and older, Hispanics/Latinos, male injection drug users, and males with HIV infection attributed to high-risk heterosexual contact (CDC 2008).

Survival After AIDS Diagnosis

Increase in Survival Over the Years

Survival from the year of diagnosis increased each year during the period 1998–2005; year-to-year improvements were smaller during the period 2001–2005. From 2003 through 2007, the estimated number of deaths of persons with AIDS who resided in the 50 states and the District of Columbia decreased 17% (CDC 2008).

Impact of Highly Active Antiretroviral Therapy

Major gains have occurred in treating HIV disease as a result of the effectiveness of highly active antiretroviral therapy (HAART). AIDS is no longer one of the top three causes of death in the United States (Halman et al. 2002). Patients with HIV disease as well as HIV specialists now generally perceive HIV disease as a chronic medical condition rather than a relentlessly progressive infection.

Psychiatric Manifestations

Neuropsychiatric Syndromes

Neuropsychiatric Symptoms

Neuropsychiatric complications in patients with AIDS include memory deficits, concentration impairment, dementia, psychomotor slowing, motor deficits, apathy, withdrawal, depression, and psychosis. In the late stages of the disease, the following are common: disorientation, profound slowing, severe dementia, focal neurological signs, secondary neurological disorders (e.g., tumors, central nervous system [CNS] toxoplasmosis), seizures, and agitation.

Multiple Causes of Neuropsychiatric Syndromes

Patients with AIDS may have neuropsychiatric sequelae that are caused by primary effects of the virus itself; neurotoxic by-products of the immune responses to the virus; indirect consequences of systemic disease (e.g., hypoxia, fatigue, malnutrition), intracranial tumors, or infections that occur as a result of the immunocompromised state; and adverse effects of medications used to treat CNS AIDS disorders.

Changes in Mental Status

HIV-related conditions that may present with changes in mental status include HIV dementia, toxoplasmosis, cytomegalovirus, CNS lymphoma, cryptococcal meningitis, and progressive multifocal leukoencephalopathy (Della Penna and Treisman 2005).

Need for Aggressive Management

Unless the patient is near death from nonneurological causes, aggressive diagnostic workup and management are indicated when new neuropsychiatric symptoms emerge in AIDS patients. Treatment is possible for many AIDS-related CNS disorders, especially toxoplasmosis, herpes simplex infection, and CNS lymphoma.

Adverse Effects of HIV/AIDS Medications

HIV/AIDS medications may have adverse effects that cause neuropsychiatric symptoms. The frequency with which mental status changes are due to medication side effects has increased. In more systemically ill patients, the use of more medications—medications that are more effective at crossing the blood-brain barrier and medications in combination with one another—has resulted in neuropsychiatric syndromes. The most common psychiatric side effects are asthenia, insomnia, depression, delirium, mania, and irritability. The symptoms are often mild and nonspecific, but some may become the focus of psychiatric consultation.

Neuropsychiatric Syndromes in HIV Infection Without AIDS

Neuropsychiatric syndromes may occur in HIV-infected patients without AIDS. Secondary psychiatric syndromes can occur in these patients without AIDS, although less commonly than in patients with AIDS. When neuropsychiatric findings occur shortly after infection, symptoms are those of acute viral encephalitis. Neuropsychiatric findings in early presentations of HIV-related dementing processes tend to involve subcortical, integrative, and executive functions; these include visuospatial integration, visuospatial memory, reaction time, verbal fluency, nonverbal fluency, problem solving, conceptual skills, set shifting, concentration, speed of mental processing, and mental flexibility. Language and related general intellectual skills are usually spared.

Psychiatric Conditions

Delirium

Up to half of AIDS patients who require skilled nursing care have at least one episode of delirium documented (Uldall and Berghuis 1997). Patients with HIV-associated dementia are at increased risk for delirium. Etiologies for delirium that are common in HIV/AIDS patients are hypoxia with pneumocystis pneumonia, malnutrition, CNS infections and neoplasms, systemic infections, HIV nephropathy, and medication toxicity (especially polypharmacy) (Watkins et al. 2011). Acute HIV infection itself may also cause an acute encephalopathy (Bialer et al. 2000).

HIV-Associated Dementia

Risk factors.   In the pre-HAART era, risk factors associated with development of HIV-associated dementia included higher HIV ribonucleic acid (RNA) viral load, lower educational level, older age, illicit drug use, and female sex. However, in the post-HAART era, depression is more predictive of the severity of HIV-associated dementia (Watkins et al. 2011).

Pathophysiology.   Mechanisms of neuronal death in HIV-associated dementia are not clear, but possibilities include glutamate overstimulation, cerebrospinal fluid HIV RNA, and presence of other substances associated with dementia, including quinolinic acid, prostaglandins, and neopterin (Nebuloni et al. 2001).

Clinical characteristics.   The most typical HIV-associated dementia presentation is that of a subcortical dementia, with memory and psychomotor speed impairment, apathy, and movement disorders. Late symptoms may include worsened motor symptoms and accelerated memory impairment. Psychiatric symptoms may occur as part of HIV-associated dementia, including depression, hypomania, impulsivity, and emotional lability.

Diagnosis.   Magnetic resonance imaging (MRI) often shows significant white matter lesions, as well as cortical and subcortical atrophy, in patients with HIV-associated dementia (Watkins et al. 2011). Functional MRI in HIV-positive patients may predate clinical signs or deficits on cognitive tests (Ernst et al. 2002).

Depression

Depressive symptoms and depressive disorders are more common among HIV-infected persons than in the general population. The cause-effect considerations are complex: HIV disease and associated medical complications can cause secondary mood syndromes, and depression is also a risk factor for behavioral disturbances that may increase exposure to HIV infection (Watkins et al. 2011). In addition, fatigue may be confused with depression. In fact, in persons with HIV, fatigue has been found to be more associated with depression than with HIV disease progression.

Mania

Like depression, mania is more frequent in patients with AIDS than in the general population (Halman et al. 1993). Mania or hypomania may be primary or secondary. Secondary mania in AIDS may present differently than primary bipolar mania (Ellen et al. 1999); patients with secondary mania have prominent irritable mood, cognitive changes, and psychomotor slowing, instead of hyperactivity, severe presentation, and malignant course.

Substance Use Disorders

Substance abuse is a vector for the spread of HIV, and it is the psychiatric diagnostic category with the highest prevalence of HIV infection (Beyer et al. 2007). Patients with dual diagnoses (substance use disorders and other psychiatric disorders) who also are infected with HIV are overrepresented in HIV treatment. Neuropsychological tests suggest that substance abuse can contribute to cognitive decline in HIV-associated dementia. Substance use in general, and cocaine use in particular, may augment HIV replication in the CNS and increase HIV encephalopathy risk by rendering the blood-brain barrier more permeable to HIV (Watkins et al. 2011). Substance use is also associated with significantly diminished adherence to treatment regimens such as HAART (Chander et al. 2006).

Anxiety Disorders

Substantial and consistent evidence indicates that anxiety, trauma, and stressful events may negatively affect HIV disease progression by decreasing CD4 T lymphocytes, increasing viral load, and accelerating clinical decline and mortality (Leserman 2008; Strachan et al. 2007). Posttraumatic stress disorder (PTSD) may occur at increased rates in HIV-infected persons (Martinez et al.

2002). PTSD symptoms are associated with frequency of high-risk behaviors, including prostitution, injection drug use, and unsafe sexual practices. PTSD patients are at elevated risk for other anxiety disorders, depression, and substance abuse.

Personality Disorders

Prevalence rates of personality disorders among HIV-infected patients (20%–35%) exceed rates found in the general population (10%) (Johnson et al. 1995). Personality disorders in this population are associated with higher rates of substance abuse, sharing needles, risky sexual behaviors, frequent sex with multiple partners, and treatment nonadherence.

Psychiatric Treatment

For the treatment and management of patients with HIV disease, the psychiatrist must take into consideration a wide range of etiological factors, including premorbid primary psychiatric disorders, disorders secondary to HIV-related CNS infections, advanced systemic disease, and neuropsychiatric side effects of commonly used HIV/AIDS medications (Halman et al. 2002). Advanced systemic disease and HIV-1 CNS infection can constrain the pharmacotherapeutic options available to the psychiatric consultant (Ferrando et al. 2010). Psychotherapeutic interventions must take into account the perspectives of patients who come from communities that often have been marginalized, socially disenfranchised, and impoverished. Management plans frequently require liaison with community-based HIV/AIDS service organizations and highly diverse social and family support groups.

Delirium

Management of HIV-associated delirium, which is similar to that for delirium in general, involves searching for etiologies and correcting them when possible, behavioral and environmental interventions, and judicious pharmacotherapy (see Chapter 7, "Delirium"). Low dosages of high-potency, or atypical, antipsychotics are used with some success, although this off-label use is based on case reports and case series. Anticholinergic medications may worsen delirium; patients with HIV-associated dementia should be assumed to be vulnerable to extrapyramidal symptoms. Benzodiazepines may exacerbate delirium and should be used with caution in patients who abuse drugs; however, benzodiazepines may be necessary when a patient has a withdrawal delirium from alcohol or sedative-hypnotics.

HIV-Associated Dementia

The impact of HAART on cognitive outcomes has not been as robust as its impact on other AIDS-related conditions (Watkins et al. 2011). When combination antiretroviral therapy is administered, cognitive improvement appears to be related to a medication's CNS penetration index, which may vary by individual patient for a given dosage (Cysique et al. 2009). Improvement may occur within weeks after initiating therapy and may be persistent over at least a year. Benefit may be maximized by choosing antiretroviral medications that reach therapeutic concentrations in the CNS.

Depression

Antidepressants

Antidepressants have good response rates. Antidepressant nonadherence is the most common reason for ineffective medication response, and adverse effects are the most common reason for nonadherence. Fortunately, selective serotonin reuptake inhibitors (SSRIs) are generally well tolerated and effective in HIV-related major depressive disorder, with a 60%–80% response rate and no deleterious effects on immune status (Halman et al. 2002). Studies of antidepressant efficacy among HIV-infected patients, however, are notable for substantial placebo response and attrition (Rabkin et al. 1999), suggesting that other factors are important, for example, the status of the doctor-patient relationship.

Caution is required when SSRIs are used to treat depression in HIV/AIDS patients. The dosing principle of starting low and increasing slowly applies. Drug interactions can occur between SSRIs and some antiretroviral therapies because of competition for cytochrome P450 3A3/3A4 metabolism. Because citalopram and sertraline have little interaction with these enzymes, they are preferred over other SSRIs in treating depression in HIV-positive patients receiving antiretroviral treatment. If used, fluoxetine or paroxetine should be started at 10 mg/day and increased to the standard dosage after 7–10 days (Halman et al. 2002).

Psychostimulants

Psychostimulants may have a role in the treatment of some patients. At low dosages, both dextroamphetamine and methylphenidate have been reported in case series to be effective for HIV-related major depression, as primary agents (Fernandez and Levy 1992) or as adjuvant agents, with response rates up to 80%. They are especially effective for anergia, apathy, and anorexia. Some patients also report improved mood, attention, and concentration. Although stimulants are not usually first-line treatments for major depression, they should be considered as an adjunct or a substitute for conventional antidepressants in patients with a predominance of apathy compared with sadness, and in patients who are unable to tolerate the side effects of conventional antidepressants. Stimulants should also be considered for depression in the terminally ill patient with HIV who may not live long enough for a traditional antidepressant to take effect. Psychostimulants should be used with caution in patients who have motor problems.

Mania

Although mood stabilizers have not been systematically studied in patients with HIV/AIDS, case reports suggest that traditional mood stabilizers, especially lithium, are not tolerated by patients with HIV/AIDS as well as they are by physically healthy bipolar patients. Patients with HIV/AIDS have less tolerance for lithium's adverse effects, including nausea, vomiting, diarrhea, tremor, and cognitive changes. Antipsychotics, especially low-potency agents, may also be poorly tolerated. Late-stage patients may be especially prone to side effects of mood stabilizers and antipsychotics. Low initial dosages of any psychiatric medications should be used, and titration should be slow. Valproic acid and carbamazepine have been used successfully, but liver enzymes and hematopoietic markers should be monitored closely. Because of medication sensitivities, many manic AIDS patients end up being treated with low-dosage, high-potency antipsychotic monotherapy.

Substance Use Disorders

Substance use disorders must be aggressively treated because of their morbidity and because of their associations with HIV-associated risk behaviors and nonadherence to treatment (Disney et al. 2006). An example of effective prevention is the enrollment of opiate-dependent patients at risk for HIV infection into methadone maintenance programs, resulting in sustained reductions in HIV risk and lower incidence of HIV infection (Della Penna and Treisman 2005).

Posttraumatic Stress Disorder

Persons at risk for HIV infection and HIV-infected individuals should be routinely screened for PTSD and treated as needed (see Chapter 6, "Anxiety"). Ignoring PTSD has serious consequences for this population's welfare and for public health (Watkins et al. 2011) because of the association of PTSD with poor health behaviors, psychiatric comorbidity, and high-risk sexual behaviors.

Personality Disorder

Treatment principles for patients with HIV/AIDS who present with personality complications include a number of techniques from cognitive-behavioral therapy and dialectical behavior therapy traditions (Watkins et al. 2011):

- Focus on the patient's thoughts, not feelings.
- Use a behavioral contract for patient to improve adherence.
- Emphasize constructive rewards (e.g., money saved from not buying drugs can be used for clothes or food).
- Use relapse prevention techniques to change habitual ways of behaving.
- Develop a coordinated treatment plan in concert with medical providers.

References

Beyer JL, Taylor L, Gersing KR, et al: Prevalence of HIV infection in a general psychiatric outpatient population. Psychosomatics 48:31–37, 2007

Bialer PA, Wallack JJ, McDaniel S: Human immunodeficiency virus and AIDS, in Psychiatric Care of the Medical Patient, 2nd Edition. Edited by Stoudemire A, Fogel BS, Greenberg D. New York, Oxford University Press, 2000, pp 871–887

Centers for Disease Control and Prevention: HIV/AIDS Surveillance Report, 2008. Available at: www.cdc.gov/hiv/surveillance/resources/reports/2008report/webaddress.htm. Accessed January 1, 2011.

Chander G, Himelhoch S, Moore RD: Substance abuse and psychiatric disorders in HIV-positive patients: epidemiology and impact on antiretroviral therapy. Drugs 66:769–789, 2006

Cysique LA, Vaida F, Letendre S, et al: Dynamics of cognitive change in HIV-positive patients initiating antiretroviral therapy. Neurology 73:342–348, 2009

Della Penna ND, Treisman GJ: HIV/AIDS, in The American Psychiatric Publishing Textbook of Psychosomatic Medicine. Edited by Levenson JL. Washington, DC, American Psychiatric Publishing, 2005, pp 599–627

Disney E, Kidorf M, Koldner K, et al: Psychiatric comorbidity is associated with drug use and HIV risk in syringe exchange participants. J Nerv Ment Dis 194:577–583, 2006

Ellen SR, Judd FK, Mijch AM, et al: Secondary mania in patients with HIV infection. Aust NZ J Psychiatry 33:353–360, 1999

Ernst T, Change L, Jovicich J, et al: Abnormal brain activation on functional MRI in cognitively asymptomatic HIV patients. Neurology 59:1343–1349, 2002

Fernandez F, Levy JK: Psychopharmacotherapy of psychiatric syndromes in asymptomatic and symptomatic HIV infection. Psychiatr Med 9:377–394, 1992

Ferrando SJ, Levenson JL, Owen JA: Infectious diseases, in Manual of Psychopharmacology in the Medically Ill. Edited by Ferrando SJ, Levenson JL, Owen JA. Washington, DC, American Psychiatric Publishing, 2010, pp 371–404

Halman MH, Worth JL, Sanders KM, et al: Anticonvulsant use in the treatment of manic syndromes in patients with HIV-1 infection. J Neuropsychiatry Clin Neurosci 5:430–434, 1993

Halman MH, Bialer P, Worth JL, et al: HIV Disease/AIDS, in The American Psychiatric Publishing Textbook of Consultation-Liaison Psychiatry: Psychiatry in the Medically Ill, 2nd Edition. Edited by Wise MG, Rundell JR. Washington, DC, American Psychiatric Publishing, 2002, pp 807–851

Johnson JG, Williams JBW, Rabkin JG, et al: Axis I psychiatric symptomatology associated with HIV infection and personality disorder. Am J Psychiatry 152:551–554, 1995

Leserman J: Role of depression, stress, and trauma in HIV disease progression. Psychosom Med 70:539–545, 2008

Martinez A, Israelski D, Walker C, et al: Posttraumatic stress disorder in women attending human immunodeficiency virus outpatient clinics. AIDS Patient Care STDS 16:283–291, 2002

Metzger et al. 1998

Nebuloni M, Pellegrinelli A, Ferri A, et al: Beta amyloid precursor protein and patterns of HIV p24 immunohistochemistry in different brain areas of AIDS patients. AIDS 15:571–575, 2001

Rabkin JG, Wagner GJ, Rabkin R: Fluoxetine treatment for depression in patients with HIV and AIDS: a randomized, placebo-controlled trial. Am J Psychiatry 156:101–107, 1999

Strachan ED, Bennet WR, Russo J, et al: Disclosure of HIV status and sexual orientation independently predicts increased absolute CD4 cell counts over time for psychiatric patients. Psychosom Med 69:74–80, 2007

Uldall KK, Berghuis JP: Delirium in AIDS patients: recognition and medication factors. AIDS Patient Care STDS 11:435–441, 1997

Watkins CC, Della Penna ND, Angelino AA, et al: HIV/AIDS, in The American Psychiatric Publishing Textbook of Psychosomatic Medicine, 2nd Edition. Edited by Levenson JL. Washington, DC, American Psychiatric Publishing, 2011, pp 637–665

24

Obstetrics

Untreated maternal psychiatric illness has consequences not only for the mother, but also for the developing fetus, the infant, and the child. The peak incidence of affective disorders in women, at ages 25–44 years, coincides with childbearing years. Most women with psychiatric disorders do not receive mental health care regardless of pregnancy status (Vesga-Lopez et al. 2008). Those women who do receive psychiatric treatment often discontinue taking psychotropic medication while they are attempting to conceive, are pregnant, or are breast-feeding. A careful risk-benefit analysis is needed as women and their physicians consider the negative effects of untreated mental illness versus the risk of exposure to psychotropics for the fetus and infant.

Epidemiology

Pregnancy and Childbirth

Pregnancy per se is not associated with an increased risk of most psychiatric disorders. In pregnant and postpartum women, younger age, singleness, exposure to traumatic or stressful life events, pregnancy complications, and overall poor health increase the risk of psychiatric disorders (Vesga-Lopez et al. 2008). Childbirth is associated with an increased risk of inpatient psychiatric readmission for mothers during the first postpartum month, but thereafter, the rates decrease and nonmothers have a higher risk for readmission. A diagnosis of bipolar disorder is the strongest predictor of readmission during the first postpartum month (Munk-Olsen et al. 2009).

Mood Disorders

An estimated 10%–15% of women experience depression during pregnancy, the postpartum period, or both (Bennett et al. 2004; Gavin et al. 2005). Studies have suggested that the rate of mood disorders is similar in pregnant and nonpregnant women, although a large national survey found that pregnant women are significantly less likely than nonpregnant women to have a mood disorder (Vesga-Lopez et al. 2008). Postpartum blues, characterized by labile mood, irritability, and tearfulness, is a transient state that typically peaks at 3–5 days postpartum and occurs in 50% of women (Miller 2002). The risk of major depressive disorder appears to be increased in the postpartum period (Vesga-Lopez et al. 2008).

Anxiety Disorders

Anxiety disorders are common during the perinatal period. Some studies report higher rates of obsessive-compulsive disorder and generalized anxiety disorder in postpartum women (Ross and McLean 2006), but other data suggest similar rates (Vesga-Lopez et al. 2008). Situational anxiety warrants consideration, and inquiring about a history of negative obstetrical or other medical experiences may help identify the source of anxiety or even of posttraumatic stress disorder (PTSD) symptoms.

Substance Abuse

Alcohol use is less frequent among pregnant and postpartum women than nonpregnant women, but illicit drug use is the same. Methamphetamine use is rising among pregnant women and has become the primary substance for which pregnant women enter inpatient substance abuse treatment, accounting for 25% of all admissions in 2006 (Terplan et al. 2009).

Postpartum Psychosis

Postpartum psychosis is a psychiatric emergency requiring hospitalization. This diagnosis has garnered considerable attention because 1 in 25 mothers with postpartum psychosis commits infanticide (Spinelli 2009). The majority of women with postpartum psychosis have bipolar disorder. Clinically, the presentation can be similar to delirium with cognitive dysfunction and disorganization, including waxing and waning, bizarre behavior, delusions, and impaired sensorium (Wisner et al. 1994). New-onset psychosis necessitates a differential diagnostic evaluation comparable to that performed with a nongravid patient.

The following are major risk factors for postpartum psychosis (Jones and Craddock 2001):

- History of psychosis following prior childbirth (relapse rates approach 70%)
- History of bipolar disorder
- Family history of postpartum psychosis

Schizophrenia

A variety of pregnancy, birth, and neonatal complications have been reported for women with schizophrenia. Adverse outcomes include a higher incidence of placental abruption, low-birth-weight infants, and increased risk of cardiovascular congenital anomalies (Jablensky et al. 2005).

Maternal Depression, Adverse Reproductive Outcomes, and Comorbid Medical Problems

Preterm Delivery

The data are mixed regarding the association between depression during pregnancy and preterm delivery (Yonkers et al. 2009). One prospective study found that infants exposed to either depression or selective serotonin reuptake inhibitors (SSRIs) continuously across gestation were more likely to be born preterm, with preterm birth rates of more than 20% (Wisner et al. 2009).

Comorbid Medical Illness

Comorbid medical illness may increase risk of depression. Postpartum depression rates are higher among women with epilepsy, especially those who are multiparous or receiving multiple antiepileptic drugs, than in the general population (Galanti et al. 2009). Women with diabetes, even without a prior history of depression, had twice the risk of developing postpartum depression during the year following delivery than women without diabetes (Kozhimannil et al. 2009).

Screening for Depression

Multiple depression screening instruments are easy to administer and require less than 10 minutes to complete. The Edinburgh Depression Scale was designed specifically for screening for depression in pregnancy and the postpartum period. It has good sensitivity and specificity, and it is a reliable instrument for repeated evaluations of depressive symptoms during pregnancy (Bunevicius et al. 2009). Other instruments with high sensitivity are the Patient Health Questionnaire–9 and the Postpartum Depression Screening Scale (American College of Obstetricians and Gynecologists Committee on Obstetric Practice 2010).

Treatment of Depression and Anxiety During Pregnancy

High Risk of Relapse With Antidepressant Discontinuation

Women with depression, including those who have a history of recurrent depressive illness, are likely to discontinue antidepressant use during attempts to conceive or after conception. Physicians must assist women in making an informed choice not only about the risks of prenatal exposure to medication, but also about the risk of relapse if treatment is discontinued. In a study of women receiving antidepressant treatment for major depression prior to pregnancy, 45% of women relapsed during pregnancy, and among those who relapsed, 70% had discontinued antidepressant treatment and 25% had continued treatment (Cohen et al. 2006). In the group who relapsed, 50% relapsed within the first trimester and 90% by the end of the second trimester.

General Approach

For the drug-naïve patient with mild depressive symptoms, psychotherapy is considered first-line treatment. Evidence supports the use of interpersonal therapy to address grief, interpersonal role disputes, role transitions, and interpersonal deficits (Spinelli and Endicott 2003). Minimal data exist on the use of cognitive-behavioral therapy (CBT) for pregnant women, although its efficacy has been established for other populations. The decision to use medication is based on the severity of depression, the number and frequency of depressive episodes, and the history of response to medication. Table 24–1 provides general guidelines for choosing an antidepressant medication for women during pregnancy.

Pharmacological Management

The potential risks of in utero exposure to antidepressant medications depend on numerous factors, including gestational age, duration of exposure, and comorbid factors. All psychotropic medications cross the placenta, although umbilical cord concentrations of antidepressants and their metabolites are lower than maternal concentrations (Hendrick et al. 2003).

Selective Serotonin Reuptake Inhibitors

Overall, limited evidence exists of teratogenic effects from SSRI use in pregnancy. Increased risks of congenital cardiac malformations (reported with paroxetine), craniosynostosis, and omphalocele have been found, but the data are mixed and absolute risk is low (Alwan et al. 2007; Louik et al. 2007). The risk of pregnancy complications, such as miscarriage, preterm birth, and low birth weight appears to be low, but these findings are controversial. Two prospective studies have found an association between antidepressant use and preterm birth (Suri et al. 2007; Wisner et al. 2009). Exposure to SSRIs late in pregnancy has been associated with transient neonatal complications, including jitteriness, mild respiratory distress, weak cry, and poor muscle tone. Limited data suggest a possible association between maternal use of SSRIs in the latter half of pregnancy and persistent pulmonary hypertension of the newborn, although the absolute risk is small (6–12 affected infants per 1,000 exposed fetuses) (Chambers et al. 1996, 2006). Gestational hypertension and preeclampsia have been reported to occur more frequently in women exposed to SSRIs dur-

Table 24–1.   Guidelines for medication use during pregnancy or breast-feeding

1. Perform a risk-benefit analysis.

2. Document the mother's problems in daily living and her ability to care for the fetus/infant, target symptoms, and the rationale for medication use.

3. Record all drug exposures (prescribed, over-the-counter, herbal, and illicit) during pregnancy and the postpartum period, if the patient is breast-feeding. Ask about and document alcohol consumption during pregnancy.

4. Obtain informed consent. Discuss with the mother the risks and unknown aspects of taking psychotropic medication while pregnant or breast-feeding, to include the remote possibility of long-term effects on the child. Document this discussion, and have the patient sign the informed consent, especially if the patient insists on taking medications despite recommendations to the contrary (e.g., patient has a severe, chronic psychotic illness that responds only to clozapine and insists on breast-feeding despite recommendations against breast-feeding while taking clozapine). If the patient's capacity to make an informed decision is influenced by the illness, have the spouse participate in the decision-making process and have him also sign the informed consent.

5. Use a medication that has worked in the past, unless contraindicated.

6. Choose a medication that has some data rather than a novel compound with no data.

7. Attempt monotherapy. Data on combination pharmacotherapy do not exist. Do not forget that electroconvulsive therapy is the treatment of choice when a woman has a psychotic depression.

8. While the patient is breast-feeding, try to avoid prescribing medications that require invasive monitoring (e.g., clozapine).

9. Use the minimum effective dosage.

10. Urge the mother who is breast-feeding to take doses so that the medication level in breast milk is minimized at the time the infant nurses (i.e., take medication immediately after the infant nurses, or take dose immediately prior to infant's long afternoon nap).

Source. Reprinted from Llewellyn A, Stowe ZN: "Psychotropic Medications in Lactation." *Journal of Clinical Psychiatry* 59 (suppl 2):41–52, 1998. Used with permission.

ing late pregnancy, but a causal relationship has not been determined (Toh et al. 2009).

Fluoxetine. Fluoxetine is the best studied drug in pregnant women and the SSRI with the largest amount of long-term follow-up of exposed infants. Its long half-life predisposes to accumulation in the neonate, and the rate of transfer to the baby through breast-feeding is higher than for other SSRIs.

Sertraline. Sertraline has very low serum levels in breast-fed infants and thus can be a good option for mothers who plan to breast-feed. Sertraline may also be associated with less fetal medication exposure near delivery (Hendrick et al. 2003).

Paroxetine. Paroxetine is not considered first-line treatment for pregnant women because of contradictory data regarding cardiac malformations in exposed infants; however, it is generally not recommended that a woman who is taking paroxetine should switch to an alternative agent (American College of Obstetricians and Gynecologists Committee on Practice Bulletins—Obstetrics 2008).

Citalopram and escitalopram. Studies have generally been positive regarding the safety of citalopram for pregnant women, although one study reported an increased risk of septal defects (Pedersen et al. 2009), and another found increased risk of the pooled group of defects consisting of anencephaly, omphalocele, and craniosynostosis (Alwan et al. 2007). Minimal data are available for escitalopram.

Serotonin-Norepinephrine Reuptake Inhibitors

One prospective cohort study found no increased risk of congenital anomalies following gestational exposure to the serotonin-norepinephrine reuptake inhibitor (SNRI) venlafaxine (Einarson et al. 2001).

Mirtazapine

Data on pregnancy outcomes after exposure to mirtazapine are limited. However, case reports suggest that mirtazapine is effective for treatment-resistant hyperemesis gravidarum (Guclu et al. 2005; Rohde et al. 2003).

Bupropion

Bupropion is classified by the U.S. Food and Drug Administration as Category B, which indicates no evidence of risk in humans (American College of Obstetricians and Gynecologists Committee on Practice Bulletins—Obstetrics 2008). Bupropion may be especially useful for patients who have not responded to other medications, who have attentional disorders, or who need help with smoking cessation.

Tricyclic Antidepressants

Most studies have found that tricyclic antidepressants (TCAs) are not associated with congenital abnormalities (Simon et al. 2002), and long-term studies have shown no differences in IQ, language, or temperament between children exposed to TCAs in utero and nonexposed children (Nulman et al. 2002). Withdrawal syndromes during the perinatal period have been noted (Altshuler et al. 1996).

Benzodiazepines

A possible association exists between first-trimester exposure to benzodiazepines and the development of cleft lip, cleft palate, and other congenital anomalies, although the data have been conflicting, and if an increased risk exists, the absolute risk is low (Altshuler et al. 1996; Dolovich et al. 1998). Exposure to benzodiazepines close to the time of labor and delivery has been associated with transient neonatal intoxication characterized by hypotonia (floppy infant syndrome), poor respiratory effort, hypothermia, and feeding difficulties, in addition to neonatal withdrawal syndromes including restlessness, hypertonia, hyperreflexia, tremulousness, diarrhea, and vomiting (Altshuler et al. 1996; McElhatton 1994).

Electroconvulsive Therapy

No randomized controlled trial of electroconvulsive therapy (ECT) during pregnancy has been conducted. A review of 339 cases found comparable response rates between pregnant and nonpregnant women, and the risk of adverse events appears to be low (Anderson and Reti 2009). ECT should be considered for women with psychotic symptoms, catatonia, or suicidal ideation (with intent) requiring immediate intervention.

Treatment of Postpartum Depression

Psychotherapy

Compared with usual postpartum care, psychosocial and psychological interventions have been shown to reduce depressive symptoms. Interpersonal, psychodynamic, CBT, and group psychotherapy may be effective (Dennis 2005). The most evidence exists for interpersonal therapy, which has been found to improve depressive symptoms and social adjustment (O'Hara et al. 2000), as well as to reduce the likelihood of the development of postpartum depression (Zlotnick et al. 2006).

Pharmacotherapy

Only a few randomized placebo-controlled treatment studies have been conducted in women with postpartum depression (Appleby et al. 1997; Yonkers et al. 2008); therefore, antidepressants are used in this population based on extrapolation of results from studies in the general population. A randomized trial comparing nortriptyline and sertraline for postpartum depression found similar efficacy and side-effect burden for these agents (Wisner et al. 2006).

Breast-Feeding and Drugs

Antidepressants and Breast-Feeding

All psychotropic medications are transferred into breast milk and passed on to the nursing infant. In a pooled analysis of antidepressant drug levels in lactating mothers, breast milk, and nursing infants, Weissman et al. (2004) found that nortriptyline, paroxetine, and sertraline usually produce undetectable infant levels and, therefore, are the preferred choices for breast-feeding women. Fluoxetine produced the highest proportion of infant levels. Possible adverse effects of antidepressants in the infant include irritability, sedation, poor weight gain, and change in feeding patterns. The benefits of breast-feeding generally outweigh the relatively low risk of antidepressant medication, but each patient deserves a careful risk-benefit analysis.

Benzodiazepines and Breast-Feeding

Benzodiazepines should be used cautiously for treating women who are breast-feeding. Low dosages and careful monitoring are necessary because sedation and withdrawal can occur in infants.

Treatment of Bipolar Disorder During Pregnancy and the Postpartum Period

High Risk for Recurrence

During the immediate postpartum period, women with bipolar disorder have nearly a sevenfold higher risk of admission for a first episode and a twofold higher risk for a recurrent episode, compared with nonpregnant and nonpostpartum women (Yonkers et al. 2004). In a prospective study, the overall risk of at least one recurrence was 71%. Compared with subjects who continued mood stabilizer treatment, those who discontinued mood stabilizer treatment had a twofold higher risk of recurrence, and the time to recurrence was fourfold shorter (Viguera et al. 2007b).

Mood Stabilizers

Lithium

In a study of women with bipolar disorder treated with lithium, rates of recurrence during the first 40 weeks after lithium discontinuation were similar for pregnant and nonpregnant women but then substantially increased postpartum, although the risk was lower if lithium discontinuation was gradual (Viguera et al. 2000). Lithium exposure during the first trimester has been associated with a 20-fold increased risk of developing Ebstein's anomaly, but the absolute rate is still low (1/1,000). The most common toxicity effect during labor is the floppy infant syndrome. During pregnancy, the dosage generally needs to be titrated upward due to increased renal excretion as pregnancy progresses. Some researchers recommend decreasing the dosage prior to labor, due to the rapid reduction in vascular volume during delivery. For mothers who breast-feed, lithium use has been discouraged, although some evidence suggests that lithium use in nursing mothers is well tolerated by the infant (Viguera et al. 2007a).

Valproate

Valproate is considered a human teratogen because of its association with neural tube defects, fetal valproate syndrome, and possible long-term adverse neurocognitive effects. The neural tube defect rate in babies whose mothers take valproate is about 5%–9%, an effect related to use of the medication 17–30 days postconception. Folate supplementation has been found to reduce the risk of neural tube defects. In contrast to the risk to infants exposed to valproate during pregnancy, the risk to infants who are breast-fed by mothers treated with valproate is low (Yonkers et al. 2004).

Carbamazepine

Carbamazepine should generally be avoided during pregnancy due to its association with minor and major malformations, including craniofacial defects and fingernail hypoplasia. Studies have not yet definitively shown whether carbamazepine is associated with an increased risk of developmental delay or neural tube defects. Teratogenicity is enhanced when it is coadministered with another anticonvulsant, particularly valproate. The American Academy of Pediatrics Committee on Drugs (2000) considers carbamazepine to be compatible with breast-feeding.

Lamotrigine

Newport et al. (2008b) reported decreased risk of bipolar disorder recurrence in pregnant women who took lamotrigine compared with those who discontinued mood stabilizer treatment. Also, lamotrigine's fetal safety seems to compare favorably with that of other agents used to manage bipolar disorder, although more data are needed. The rate of lamotrigine excretion into human breast milk is similar to that observed with other antiepileptic drugs (Newport et al. 2008a).

Use of Antipsychotics During Pregnancy and the Postpartum Period

First-Generation Antipsychotics

Exposure of pregnant women to low-potency antipsychotics for hyperemesis gravidarum resulted in a 0.4% relative increased risk for congenital anomalies associated with first-trimester exposure, but no specific malformation was identified (Altshuler et al. 1996). A prospective study of haloperidol found no difference in rates of major malformations between the haloperidol group and the control group (Diav-Citrin et al. 2005). Infants should be monitored, because an extrapyramidal syndrome has been observed in babies exposed in utero to first-generation antipsychotics. Some experts consider the risk associated with first-generation antipsychotics to be less than with mood stabilizers. Limited data on the use of first-generation antipsychotics in women who breast-feed do not suggest adverse effects (Yonkers et al. 2004).

Second-Generation Antipsychotics

Limited evidence is available to suggest that second-generation antipsychotics are associated with teratogenesis or neonatal toxicity, although further studies are needed. One prospective study found no increased risk of birth defects but a small increased risk for low birth weight (McKenna et al. 2005); in contrast, another study showed an elevated risk for infants being large for gestational age (Newham et al. 2008). Very few studies are available regarding the use of antipsychotics during breast-feeding. Because psychosis and bipolar disorder usually require long-term treatment and the data on safety of antipsychotics during lactation are limited, the benefits of breast-feeding must be weighed against the potential risks of medication (Fortinguerra et al. 2009; Gentile 2008).

References

Altshuler LL, Cohen L, Szuba MP, et al: Pharmacologic management of psychiatric illness during pregnancy: dilemmas and guidelines [see comment]. Am J Psychiatry 153:592–606, 1996

Alwan S, Reefhuis J, Rasmussen SA, et al: Use of selective serotonin-reuptake inhibitors in pregnancy and the risk of birth defects. N Engl J Med 356:2684–2692, 2007

American Academy of Pediatrics Committee on Drugs: Use of psychoactive medication during pregnancy and possible effects on the fetus and newborn. Pediatrics 105:880–887, 2000

American College of Obstetricians and Gynecologists Committee on Obstetric Practice: Committee opinion no. 453: screening for depression during and after pregnancy. Obstet Gynecol 115:394–395, 2010

American College of Obstetricians and Gynecologists Committee on Practice Bulletins—Obstetrics: ACOG practice bulletin: clinical management guidelines for obstetrician-gynecologists number 92, April 2008 (replaces practice bulletin number 87, November 2007). Use of psychiatric medications during pregnancy and lactation. Obstet Gynecol 111:1001–1020, 2008

Anderson EL, Reti IM: ECT in pregnancy: a review of the literature from 1941 to 2007. Psychosom Med 71:235–242, 2009

Appleby L, Warner R, Whitton A, et al: A controlled study of fluoxetine and cognitive-behavioural counselling in the treatment of postnatal depression. BMJ 314:932–936, 1997

Bennett HA, Einarson A, Taddio A, et al: Prevalence of depression during pregnancy: systematic review. (Erratum in Obstet Gynecol 103:1344, 2004.) Obstet Gynecol 103:698–709, 2004

Bunevicius A, Kusminskas L, Pop VJ, et al: Screening for antenatal depression with the Edinburgh Depression Scale. J Psychosom Obstet Gynaecol 30:238–243, 2009

Chambers CD, Johnson KA, Dick LM, et al: Birth outcomes in pregnant women taking fluoxetine. N Engl J Med 335:1010–1015, 1996

Chambers CD, Hernandez-Diaz S, Van Marter LJ, et al: Selective serotonin-reuptake inhibitors and risk of persistent pulmonary hypertension of the newborn. N Engl J Med 354:579–587, 2006

Cohen LS, Altshuler LL, Harlow BL, et al: Relapse of major depression during pregnancy in women who maintain or discontinue antidepressant treatment. (Erratum in JAMA 296:170, 2006.) JAMA 295:499–507, 2006

Dennis CL: Psychosocial and psychological interventions for prevention of postnatal depression: systematic review [see comment in BMJ 331:5–6, 2005]. BMJ 331:15, 2005

Diav-Citrin O, Shechtman S, Ornoy S, et al: Safety of haloperidol and penfluridol in pregnancy: a multicenter, prospective, controlled study. J Clin Psychiatry 66:317–322, 2005

Dolovich LR, Addis A, Vaillancourt JM, et al: Benzodiazepine use in pregnancy and major malformations or oral cleft: meta-analysis of cohort and case-control studies. BMJ 317:839–843, 1998

Einarson A, Fatoye B, Sarkar M, et al: Pregnancy outcome following gestational exposure to venlafaxine: a multicenter prospective controlled study. Am J Psychiatry 158:1728–1730, 2001

Fortinguerra F, Clavenna A, Bonati M: Psychotropic drug use during breastfeeding: a review of the evidence. Pediatrics 124:e547–e556, 2009

Galanti M, Newport DJ, Pennell PB, et al: Postpartum depression in women with epilepsy: influence of antiepileptic drugs in a prospective study. Epilepsy Behav 16:426–430, 2009

Gavin NI, Gaynes BN, Lohr KN, et al: Perinatal depression: a systematic review of prevalence and incidence. Obstet Gynecol 106:1071–1083, 2005

Gentile S: Infant safety with antipsychotic therapy in breast-feeding: a systematic review. J Clin Psychiatry 69:666–673, 2008

Guclu S, Gol M, Dogan E, et al: Mirtazapine use in resistant hyperemesis gravidarum: report of three cases and review of the literature. Arch Gynecol Obstet 272:298–300, 2005

Hendrick V, Stowe ZN, Altshuler LL, et al: Placental passage of antidepressant medications. Am J Psychiatry 160:993–996, 2003

Jablensky AV, Morgan V, Zubrick SR, et al: Pregnancy, delivery, and neonatal complications in a population cohort of women with schizophrenia and major affective disorders. Am J Psychiatry 162:79–91, 2005

Jones I, Craddock N: Familiality of the puerperal trigger in bipolar disorder: results of a family study. Am J Psychiatry 158:913–917, 2001

Kozhimannil KB, Pereira MA, Harlow BL: Association between diabetes and perinatal depression among low-income mothers. JAMA 301:842–847, 2009

Llewellyn A, Stowe ZN: Psychotropic medications in lactation. J Clin Psychiatry 59 (suppl 2):41–52, 1998

Louik C, Lin AE, Werler MM, et al: First-trimester use of selective serotonin-reuptake inhibitors and the risk of birth defects. N Engl J Med 356:2675–2683, 2007

McElhatton PR: The effects of benzodiazepine use during pregnancy and lactation. Reprod Toxicol 8:461–475, 1994

McKenna K, Koren G, Tetelbaum M, et al: Pregnancy outcome of women using atypical antipsychotic drugs: a prospective comparative study. J Clin Psychiatry 66:444–449; quiz 546, 2005

Miller LJ: Postpartum depression. JAMA 287:762–765, 2002

Munk-Olsen T, Laursen TM, Mendelson T, et al: Risks and predictors of readmission for a mental disorder during the postpartum period. Arch Gen Psychiatry 66:189–195, 2009

Newham JJ, Thomas SH, MacRitchie K, et al: Birth weight of infants after maternal exposure to typical and atypical antipsychotics: prospective comparison study. (Erratum in Br J Psychiatry 192:477, 2008.) Br J Psychiatry 192:333–337, 2008

Newport DJ, Pennell PB, Calamaras MR, et al: Lamotrigine in breast milk and nursing infants: determination of exposure. Pediatrics 122:e223–e231, 2008a

Newport DJ, Stowe ZN, Viguera AC, et al: Lamotrigine in bipolar disorder: efficacy during pregnancy. Bipolar Disord 10:432–436, 2008b

Nulman I, Rovet J, Stewart DE, et al: Child development following exposure to tricyclic antidepressants or fluoxetine throughout fetal life: a prospective, controlled study. Am J Psychiatry 159:1889–1895, 2002

O'Hara MW, Stuart S, Gorman LL, et al: Efficacy of interpersonal psychotherapy for postpartum depression. Arch Gen Psychiatry 57:1039–1045, 2000

Pedersen LH, Henriksen TB, Vestergaard M, et al: Selective serotonin reuptake inhibitors in pregnancy and congenital malformations: population based cohort study. BMJ 339:b3569, 2009

Rohde A, Dembinski J, Dorn C: Mirtazapine (Remergil) for treatment resistant hyperemesis gravidarum: rescue of a twin pregnancy. Arch Gynecol Obstet 268:219–221, 2003

Ross LE, McLean LM: Anxiety disorders during pregnancy and the postpartum period: a systematic review. J Clin Psychiatry 67:1285–1298, 2006

Simon GE, Cunningham ML, Davis RL: Outcomes of prenatal antidepressant exposure. Am J Psychiatry 159:2055–2061, 2002

Spinelli MG: Postpartum psychosis: detection of risk and management. Am J Psychiatry 166:405–408, 2009

Spinelli MG, Endicott J: Controlled clinical trial of interpersonal psychotherapy versus parenting education program for depressed pregnant women. Am J Psychiatry 160:555–562, 2003

Suri R, Altshuler L, Hellemann G, et al: Effects of antenatal depression and antidepressant treatment on gestational age at birth and risk of preterm birth. Am J Psychiatry 164:1206–1213, 2007

Terplan M, Smith EJ, Kozloski MJ, et al: Methamphetamine use among pregnant women. Obstet Gynecol 113:1285–1291, 2009

Toh S, Mitchell AA, Louik C, et al: Selective serotonin reuptake inhibitor use and risk of gestational hypertension [see comment]. Am J Psychiatry 166:320–328, 2009

Vesga-Lopez O, Blanco C, Keyes K, et al: Psychiatric disorders in pregnant and postpartum women in the United States. Arch Gen Psychiatry 65:805–815, 2008

Viguera AC, Nonacs R, Cohen LS, et al: Risk of recurrence of bipolar disorder in pregnant and nonpregnant women after discontinuing lithium maintenance. Am J Psychiatry 157:179–184, 2000

Viguera AC, Newport DJ, Ritchie J, et al: Lithium in breast milk and nursing infants: clinical implications. Am J Psychiatry 164:342–345, 2007a

Viguera AC, Whitfield T, Baldessarini RJ, et al: Risk of recurrence in women with bipolar disorder during pregnancy: prospective study of mood stabilizer discontinuation. Am J Psychiatry 164:1817–1824; quiz 1923, 2007b

Weissman AM, Levy BT, Hartz AJ, et al: Pooled analysis of antidepressant levels in lactating mothers, breast milk, and nursing infants. Am J Psychiatry 161:1066–1078, 2004

Wisner KL, Peindl K, Hanusa BH: Symptomatology of affective and psychotic illnesses related to childbearing. J Affect Disord 30:77–87, 1994

Wisner KL, Hanusa BH, Perel JM, et al: Postpartum depression: a randomized trial of sertraline versus nortriptyline. J Clin Psychopharmacol 26:353–360, 2006

Wisner KL, Sit DKY, Hanusa BH, et al: Major depression and antidepressant treatment: impact on pregnancy and neonatal outcomes. Am J Psychiatry 166:557–566, 2009

Yonkers KA, Wisner KL, Stowe Z, et al: Management of bipolar disorder during pregnancy and the postpartum period. Am J Psychiatry 161:608–620, 2004

Yonkers KA, Lin H, Howell HB, et al: Pharmacologic treatment of postpartum women with new-onset major depressive disorder: a randomized controlled trial with paroxetine. J Clin Psychiatry 69:659–665, 2008

Yonkers KA, Wisner KL, Stewart DE, et al: The management of depression during pregnancy: a report from the American Psychiatric Association and the American College of Obstetricians and Gynecologists. Obstet Gynecol 114:703–713, 2009

Zlotnick C, Miller IW, Pearlstein T, et al: A preventive intervention for pregnant women on public assistance at risk for postpartum depression. Am J Psychiatry 163:1443–1445, 2006

25

Oncology

Depression and Anxiety

A frequent misconception is that depression and anxiety are normal and expected for patients with cancer; this attitude minimizes the significance of the patients' suffering from these psychiatric disorders. Depression and anxiety are more common in cancer patients than in the general population, and are at least as prevalent as in other medically ill patients. Depression influences treatment compliance and efficacy, quality of life, functional status, hospital length of stay, and possibly prognosis and mortality (Miller and Massie 2006; Reich 2008). Effective treatment includes both psychosocial and psychopharmacological interventions.

Depression

Prevalence

Limitations in research methodology and lack of standardization in diagnostic criteria contribute to wide variations in prevalence rates of depression in patients with cancer. Age, gender, type of cancer, treatment, and severity of illness also influence depression rates. A review of the literature found a mean prevalence rate of 25%, with rates ranging from 2%–50% (McDaniel et al. 1995).

Risk Factors for Depression

The following are risk factors for depression in patients with cancer (McDaniel et al. 1995; Miller and Massie 2006):

- Poorly controlled pain
- Advanced cancer stage
- Previous history of depression
- Pancreatic, oropharyngeal, and breast cancers
- Poor functional status
- Family history of depression/suicide
- Treatment with medications known to be associated with depression

Diagnostic Considerations

Many symptoms that occur in the context of cancer overlap with the DSM-IV-TR criteria for major depressive episode (American Psychiatric Association 2000), prompting debate as to whether these shared symptoms should be included or excluded when criteria are considered in making a psychiatric diagnosis. Anorexia, weight loss, fatigue, sleep disturbance, cognitive impairment, and psychomotor slowing can each be caused by pathophysiological processes related to the cancer itself or treatment. An inclusive approach that includes all symptoms of depression regardless of the possible contributory etiologies is most often used clinically. For research purposes, the exclusive approach improves specificity by removing fatigue and anorexia from the criteria necessary for depression, and instead emphasizing depressed mood, anhedonia, and hopelessness (von Ammon Cavanaugh et al. 2001) (see also Chapter 10, "Mood Disorders").

Suicide

Estimates of suicide risk vary, but compared with the general population, cancer patients have at least a slightly higher risk for suicide (Hem et al. 2004). Male patients with cancer of the respiratory tract or prostate cancer have been shown to have a fourfold increased risk (Hem et al. 2004; Llorente et al. 2005). Risk factors include uncontrolled pain, advanced disease, fatigue, male gender, delirium, and hopelessness. Hopelessness is a stronger predictor of suicide than is depression in patients with advanced terminal cancer (Chochinov et al. 1998).

Medical Consequences of Depression

Substantial data have been published regarding the role of psychological factors or stress in cancer onset, progression, or survival. Due to methodological limitations, publication bias, and confounding factors, the findings are contradictory and inconclusive (Massie and Miller 2011). Studies that support an association between psychological factors and cancer outcomes generally are unable to demonstrate a clear causal relationship. The data are mixed, but evidence is available to suggest that depression may be associated with elevated cancer risk, and stronger evidence suggests that depression affects cancer progression (Spiegel and Giese-Davis 2003). Depression may affect the course of the illness due to the impact on treatment adherence and desire for life-sustaining therapy. Musselman et al. (2001) reported that 35% of patients with malignant melanoma who developed depression during treatment with interferon-α discontinued treatment, compared with 5% who were not depressed.

Pharmacological Treatments for Depression

Few studies have been reported on randomized placebo-controlled trials of antidepressants in patients with cancer. Selection of an antidepressant often depends on the side-effect profile and drug-drug interactions.

Selective serotonin reuptake inhibitors. Because of their tolerability, selective serotonin reuptake inhibitors (SSRIs) are first-line treatment for depression. SSRIs can cause initial suppression of appetite, but this effect usually subsides within a few weeks. Serotonin-mediated nausea can occur, especially at the onset of treatment, but can be reduced with ondansetron. Inhibitors of cytochrome P450 2D6, such as fluoxetine, paroxetine, bupropion, and duloxetine, may prevent conversion of tamoxifen, which is a prodrug, into its active metabolite, thereby reducing its effectiveness, and therefore these drugs should be avoided in patients taking tamoxifen (Henry et al. 2008). Fluoxetine has the longest half-life, which can be advantageous for patients who have periods of inability to take anything by mouth. Citalopram, sertraline, fluoxetine, and mirtazapine (a mixed-action antidepressant; see below) have been found effective for depression induced by interferon-α in patients with cancer or hepatitis C (Miller and Massie 2006).

Novel and mixed-action antidepressants. Patients with insomnia, anorexia-cachexia, or nausea may benefit from mirtazapine because of its sedative properties, appetite stimulation, and antiemetic effect. Venlafaxine and duloxetine have been demonstrated to improve neuropathic pain. Bupropion can be stimulating and decrease fatigue, but it usually should be avoided in patients who are at risk of seizures (Miller and Massie 2006).

Tricyclic antidepressants.   The side-effect profile of the tricyclic antidepressants (TCAs) limits their use in patients with cancer, and therefore TCAs should be considered primarily for patients who have comorbid neuropathic pain.

Psychostimulants and wakefulness-promoting agents.   The rapid onset of action of the psychostimulants (methylphenidate and dextroamphetamine) and modafinil can be a significant advantage over antidepressants in some circumstances, especially for patients with very short life expectancies. Psychostimulants can promote a sense of well-being, increase energy and appetite, and improve concentration. In patients treated with opioids, psychostimulants may counteract sedation and potentiate the analgesic effects. Side effects include insomnia, anxiety and agitation, tachycardia, and rarely psychosis.

Psychosocial Interventions for Depression

Various psychotherapeutic interventions are used for cancer patients, including psychoeducational, supportive, cognitive-behavioral, existential, psychodynamic, life narrative, dignity-conserving, and meaning-centered therapies. Psychotherapy may be done individually, in a group setting, or with the patient's caregiver (Miller and Massie 2006). The evidence for efficacy of different psychosocial interventions has varied widely. The goals of treatment are to reduce emotional distress, provide education, provide social support, improve coping, and facilitate resolution of problems. Earlier studies suggested that group therapy might extend survival in patients with breast cancer (Spiegel et al. 1989) and malignant melanoma (Fawzy et al. 1993), but subsequent studies have not substantiated this finding (Ross et al. 2002).

Anxiety

Prevalence

Mixed anxiety and depressive symptoms are generally more prevalent than anxiety alone in cancer patients. One study showed that nearly one-half of cancer patients self-reported significant anxiety, but the rate of anxiety disorders was 18%, which is similar to the rate in the general population (Stark et al. 2002).

Diagnostic Considerations

Anxiety is a normal reaction to unpredictability, loss of control, and the threat of death. Fears related to pain, dependency, disfigurement, and disability may arise in patients with cancer. Anxiety increases prior to surgical interventions, during chemotherapy and radiotherapy, and with progression of the illness, but anxiety may also occur before routine visits even without evidence of cancer recurrence. Somatic symptoms, including tachycardia, shortness of breath, abdominal discomfort, diaphoresis, and feelings of hyperarousal, are common with anxiety. Patients may experience irritability, insomnia, and poor concentration due to intrusive thoughts related to their prognosis (Miller and Massie 2006). Anxiety disorders need to be recognized not only because of the associated psychological distress, but also because anxiety may contribute to noncompliance with treatment or abrupt discontinuation of treatment.

Phobias.   Patients may experience phobias triggered by the medical environment, such as fear of needles, blood, or hospitals. Patients who are confined to the hospital may experience agoraphobia, and claustrophobia often occurs in patients who require magnetic resonance imaging or radiotherapy.

Posttraumatic stress disorder.   Patients may develop posttraumatic stress disorder (PTSD) after completion of cancer treatment. Younger age, lower income, less education, advanced disease, and longer hospitalizations are associated with increased PTSD symptoms (Cordova et al. 1995; Jacobsen et al. 1998).

Misdiagnosis of anxiety as primary psychiatric disorder.   Anxiety can be misdiagnosed as a primary psychiatric disorder when it is a side effect of medication or is secondary to medical causes such as dyspnea or uncontrolled pain. Restlessness may be caused by corticosteroids, stimulants, or antiemetic dopamine-blocking agents (due to akathisia) (Massie and Miller 2011). Medical causes of anxiety in cancer patients are listed in Table 25–1.

Treatment of Anxiety

Psychological interventions, including cognitive-behavioral therapy, relaxation techniques, psychoeducation, and supportive therapy, have demonstrated effi-

Table 25–1.   Medical causes of anxiety in cancer patients

Uncontrolled pain

Corticosteroids

Dopamine-blocking antiemetics (e.g., metoclopramide, prochlorperazine)

Opioid or benzodiazepine withdrawal

Chemotherapy and radiotherapy

Dyspnea

Metabolic abnormalities

Hypoglycemia

Encephalopathy

cacy in the short-term treatment of mild to moderate anxiety (Jacobsen and Jim 2008). Pharmacological treatment may be necessary to alleviate severe anxiety, and benzodiazepines are often the first-line treatment. Alprazolam and lorazepam reduce anticipatory nausea and vomiting, as well as postchemotherapy nausea and vomiting (Greenberg et al. 1987). Elderly patients in particular need to be monitored for somnolence and mental status changes when treated with a benzodiazepine. Low-dose antipsychotics should be considered for patients who are both confused and anxious. For patients who have significant respiratory compromise, a low-dose antihistamine (e.g., hydroxyzine) or an antipsychotic may be effective. If anxiety develops in the setting of a preexisting anxiety disorder or panic disorder, treatment with an SSRI is indicated.

Mania

Corticosteroids are the most frequent cause of mania in cancer patients. If high-dose corticosteroids are planned as part of a chemotherapy regimen, subsequent cycles may be preceded by initiation of valproate or lithium (in the absence of contraindications) to avert recurrent episodes of mania. Mania with psychotic features may be confused with delirium. Interferon-α-2b has also been reported to induce mania or mixed states (Greenberg et al. 2000).

Pain

Pain is most often caused by direct effects of the tumor or complications of treatment, but unrelated sources of pain also need to be considered. Compared to cancer patients without pain, cancer patients with pain have lower levels of functioning, increased depressive symptoms, and decreased quality of life (Tavoli et al. 2008). Uncontrolled pain, adverse effects of opioids, and fear of pain contribute to depressive symptoms. Depressive symptoms that develop in the setting of poorly controlled pain should not be assumed to represent an autonomous depression unless the symptoms persist despite adequate pain relief. One review found a prevalence of both pain and depression of 35%, and pain intensity was shown to positively correlate with depression. Although the evidence suggests an association between pain and depression, insufficient data are available to support a causal relationship (Laird et al. 2009).

Management

Effective treatment frequently involves a multidisciplinary approach, which may include oncology, anesthesia, psychiatry, psychology, physical therapy, pharmacy, and nursing. Pharmacotherapy is the mainstay of treatment and should be individualized to the patient. The risk of addiction in patients who receive opioids for cancer pain is minimal and should rarely limit treatment.

Cancer-Related Fatigue

Cancer-related fatigue is reported as the most frequent and disabling symptom in 60%–90% of patients with advanced cancer. The prevalence of fatigue among patients receiving chemotherapy is greater than 60%. Factors identified as contributing to cancer fatigue include pain, emotional distress, insomnia, anemia, and hypothyroidism (Mock et al. 2000), as well as chemotherapy, radiation therapy, and other medications (e.g., opioids, sedatives) (Table 25–2). Much cancer fatigue, however, does not have an apparent cause; the underlying mechanism has not been clearly identified but may include abnormal inflammatory response and cytokine release or disruption of the hypothalamic-pituitary-adrenal axis (Minton et al. 2008).

Table 25–2.   Causes of cancer-related fatigue

Cancer treatment
  Interferon
  Chemotherapy
  Irradiation
Pain
Anemia
Nutritional deficits
Hormone imbalance
  Thyroid
  Estrogen
  Androgens
Immune response
Cytokine release
Drug effects
  Opioids
  Sedatives
Psychiatric disorders
  Sleep disruption
  Depression

Source.   Reprinted from Massie MJ, Miller K: "Oncology," in *The American Psychiatric Publishing Textbook of Psychosomatic Medicine,* 2nd Edition. Edited by Levenson JL. Washington, DC, American Psychiatric Publishing, 2011, p. 532. Used with permission.

Management

Some evidence suggests that methylphenidate improves fatigue (Bruera et al. 2003). Stronger support exists for treatment with hematopoietic agents to relieve fatigue associated with chemotherapy-induced anemia. Antidepressants are not indicated because cancer-related fatigue and depression are different entities (Minton et al. 2008).

Delirium

Delirium occurs in 15%–40% of hospitalized cancer patients and is associated with a 30-day mortality rate of 25%. In a study of patients with non–central nervous system cancers, 35% had a single cause of delirium identified and 65% had multiple etiologies. The most common causes were medications (usually opioids) and metabolic abnormalities. Delirium improved in 65% of the patients, although it was a poor overall prognostic factor (Tuma and DeAngelis 2000). Antineoplastic and immunotherapeutic agents can cause altered mental status and delirium (Massie and Miller 2011) (Table 25–3).

Cancer-Related Anorexia-Cachexia Syndrome

Cancer-related anorexia-cachexia syndrome (CACS) is a hypercatabolic state associated with poor appetite and reduced body weight due to loss of muscle mass and adipose tissue. Many agents have been evaluated for the treatment of CACS, but only corticosteroids and progestational agents (e.g., megestrol acetate) have proven benefit (Yavuzsen et al. 2005).

Treatment of Hot Flashes

Vasomotor symptoms can be caused by surgically induced menopause, premature cessation of ovarian function caused by chemotherapy, or the use of adjuvant hormone therapy (e.g., tamoxifen, anastrozole). Hot flashes in women with breast cancer are difficult to treat because estrogen therapy is contraindicated and because some SSRIs (e.g., paroxetine and fluoxetine) interfere with tamoxifen metabolism. SSRIs, serotonin-norepinephrine reuptake inhibitors (SNRIs), clonidine, gabapentin, and megestrol effectively reduce hot flashes (Loprinzi et al. 2007; Nelson et al. 2006).

End-of-Life Care

The dying patient is often comfortable talking about death, but family members and sometimes the hospital staff may be reluctant to engage in such conversations. A minority of patients with advanced cancer have end-of-life

Table 25–3.   Neuropsychiatric side effects of common chemotherapeutic agents

Agent	Side effects
Hormones	
Corticosteroids	Mild to severe insomnia, hyperactivity, anxiety, depression, psychosis with prominent manic features
Tamoxifen	Sleep disorder, irritability
Biologicals	
Cytokines	Encephalopathy
Interferon	Depression, suicidality, mania, psychosis, delirium, akathisia, seizures
Interleukin-2	Dysphoria, delirium, psychosis, seizures
Chemotherapy agents	
L-Asparaginase	Somnolence, lethargy, delirium, depression
Chlorambucil	Hallucinations, lethargy, seizures, stupor, coma
Capecitabine	Multifocal leukoencephalopathy, cerebellar ataxia, reversible neuromuscular syndrome: trismus, slurred speech, confusion, ocular abnormalities
Cisplatin	Encephalopathy (rare), sensory neuropathy
Cytarabine	Delirium, seizures, leukoencephalopathy
5-Fluorouracil	Fatigue, rare seizures or confusion, cerebellar syndrome
Gemcitabine	Fatigue
Ifosfamide	Lethargy, seizures, drunkenness, cerebellar signs, delirium, hallucinations
Methotrexate	Intrathecal regimens: possible leukoencephalopathy (acute and delayed forms) High dose: possible transient delirium
Procarbazine	Somnolence, depression, delirium, psychosis, cerebellar disorder
Taxanes	Sensory neuropathy, fatigue, depression
Thalidomide	Fatigue, reversible dementia
Vincristine, vinblastine, vinorelbine	Depression, fatigue, encephalopathy

Table 25–3. Neuropsychiatric side effects of common chemotherapeutic agents *(continued)*

Agent	Side effects
Multikinase inhibitors	
Sorafenib, sunitinib, bevacizumab	Posterior leukoencephalopathy syndrome

Source. Reprinted from Massie MJ, Miller K: "Oncology," in *The American Psychiatric Publishing Textbook of Psychosomatic Medicine,* 2nd Edition. Edited by Levenson JL. Washington DC, American Psychiatric Publishing, 2011, p. 531. Copyright 2011, American Psychiatric Association. Used with permission.

discussions with their physicians. Such exchanges are associated with less aggressive medical care near death; more aggressive care is associated with decreased quality of life and a higher risk of major depressive disorder in bereaved caregivers (Wright et al. 2008).

References

American Psychiatric Association: Diagnostic and Statistical Manual of Mental Disorders, 4th Edition, Text Revision. Washington, DC, American Psychiatric Association, 2000

Bruera E, Driver L, Barnes EA, et al: Patient-controlled methylphenidate for the management of fatigue in patients with advanced cancer: a preliminary report. J Clin Oncol 21:4439–4443, 2003

Chochinov HM, Wilson KG, Enns M, et al: Depression, hopelessness, and suicidal ideation in the terminally ill. Psychosomatics 39:366–370, 1998

Cordova MJ, Andrykowski MA, Kenady DE, et al: Frequency and correlates of post-traumatic-stress-disorder–like symptoms after treatment for breast cancer. J Consult Clin Psychol 63:981–986, 1995

Fawzy FI, Fawzy NW, Hyun CS, et al: Malignant melanoma: effects of an early structured psychiatric intervention, coping, and affective state on recurrence and survival 6 years later. Arch Gen Psychiatry 50:681–689, 1993

Greenberg DB, Surman OS, Clarke J, et al: Alprazolam for phobic nausea and vomiting related to cancer chemotherapy. Cancer Treat Rep 71:549–550, 1987

Greenberg DB, Jonasch E, Gadd MA, et al: Adjuvant therapy of melanoma with interferon-alpha-2b is associated with mania and bipolar syndromes. Cancer 89:356–362, 2000

Hem E, Loge JH, Haldorsen T, et al: Suicide risk in cancer patients from 1960 to 1999. J Clin Oncol 22:4209–4216, 2004

Henry NL, Stearns V, Flockhart DA, et al: Drug interactions and pharmacogenomics in the treatment of breast cancer and depression. Am J Psychiatry 165:1251–1255, 2008

Jacobsen PB, Jim HS: Psychosocial interventions for anxiety and depression in adult cancer patients: achievements and challenges. CA Cancer J Clin 58:214–230, 2008

Jacobsen PB, Widows MR, Hann DM, et al: Posttraumatic stress disorder symptoms after bone marrow transplantation for breast cancer. Psychosom Med 60:366–371, 1998

Laird BJ, Boyd AC, Colvin LA, et al: Are cancer pain and depression interdependent? A systematic review. Psychooncology 18:459–464, 2009

Llorente MD, Burke M, Gregory GR, et al: Prostate cancer: a significant risk factor for late-life suicide. Am J Geriatr Psychiatry 13:195–201, 2005

Loprinzi CL, Kugler JW, Barton DL, et al: Phase III trial of gabapentin alone or in conjunction with an antidepressant in the management of hot flashes in women who have inadequate control with an antidepressant alone: NCCTG N03C5. J Clin Oncol 25:308–312, 2007

Massie MJ, Miller K: Oncology, in The American Psychiatric Publishing Textbook of Psychosomatic Medicine, 2nd Edition. Edited by Levenson JL. Washington, DC, American Psychiatric Publishing, 2011, pp 525–550

McDaniel JS, Musselman DL, Porter MR, et al: Depression in patients with cancer: diagnosis, biology, and treatment. Arch Gen Psychiatry 52:89–99, 1995

Miller K, Massie MJ: Depression and anxiety. Cancer J 12:388–397, 2006

Minton O, Richardson A, Sharpe M, et al: A systematic review and meta-analysis of the pharmacological treatment of cancer-related fatigue. J Natl Cancer Inst 100:1155–1166, 2008

Mock V, Atkinson A, Barsevick A, et al: NCCN practice guidelines for cancer-related fatigue. Oncology 14:151–161, 2000

Musselman DL, Lawson DH, Gumnick JF, et al: Paroxetine for the prevention of depression induced by high-dose interferon alfa. N Engl J Med 344:961–966, 2001

Nelson HD, Vesco KK, Haney E, et al: Nonhormonal therapies for menopausal hot flashes: systematic review and meta-analysis. JAMA 295:2057–2071, 2006

Reich M: Depression and cancer: recent data on clinical issues, research challenges and treatment approaches. Curr Opin Oncol 20:353–359, 2008

Ross L, Boesen EH, Dalton SO, et al: Mind and cancer: does psychosocial intervention improve survival and psychological well-being? Eur J Cancer 38:1447–1457, 2002

Spiegel D, Giese-Davis J: Depression and cancer: mechanisms and disease progression [see comment]. Biol Psychiatry 54:269–282, 2003

Spiegel D, Bloom JR, Kraemer HC, et al: Effect of psychosocial treatment on survival of patients with metastatic breast cancer. Lancet 2:888–891, 1989

Stark D, Kiely M, Smith A, et al: Anxiety disorders in cancer patients: their nature, associations, and relation to quality of life. J Clin Oncol 20:3137–3148, 2002

Tavoli A, Montazeri A, Roshan R, et al: Depression and quality of life in cancer patients with and without pain: the role of pain beliefs. BMC Cancer 8:177, 2008

Tuma R, DeAngelis LM: Altered mental status in patients with cancer [see comment]. Arch Neurol 57:1727–1731, 2000

von Ammon Cavanaugh S, Furlanetto LM, Creech SD, et al: Medical illness, past depression, and present depression: a predictive triad for in-hospital mortality. Am J Psychiatry 158:43–48, 2001

Wright AA, Zhang B, Ray A, et al: Associations between end-of-life discussions, patient mental health, medical care near death, and caregiver bereavement adjustment. JAMA 300:1665–1673, 2008

Yavuzsen T, Davis MP, Walsh D, et al: Systematic review of the treatment of cancer-associated anorexia and weight loss. J Clin Oncol 23:8500–8511, 2005

26

Pulmonary Disease

Very few experiences command the personal attention demanded by hunger for air. Whether diminished oxygenation occurs suddenly as with an asthmatic attack or insidiously as with chronic obstructive pulmonary disease (COPD), it may compromise cognition, kindle anxiety, threaten contentment, and intrude upon an individual's life with suffocating insistence. Lung disease is common. Psychiatric morbidity may aggravate or be exacerbated by pulmonary problems and the management strategies designed to relieve those problems, whether pharmacological or procedural. In turn, psychiatric medication may ease suffering but impede recovery if not used wisely.

Common Pulmonary Conditions

Chronic Obstructive Pulmonary Disease

COPD is widespread, costly, and deadly. The worldwide prevalence ranges from 10% to 23% in men, and half that in women. The direct and indirect costs in the United States for each person with COPD exceed $3,000 annually. COPD is presently the fourth leading cause of death in the world but is projected to be the third by 2020 (Putman-Casdorph and McCrone 2009).

Anxiety Disorders

Anxiety disorders, particularly generalized anxiety disorder and panic disorder, not only are much more prevalent in patients with COPD than in the general population, but also are associated with increased mortality and decreased functional status and quality of life (Brenes 2003; Putman-Casdorph and McCrone 2009). Posttraumatic stress disorder was identified in 25%–45% of patients who required mechanical ventilation in the course of critical illness, including acute lung injury and acute respiratory distress syndrome (Davydow et al. 2008; Shanmugam et al. 2007). Other sources of anxiety symptoms include nicotine withdrawal and some bronchodilators.

Pharmacological management.   Low dosages of a short-acting benzodiazepine, such as lorazepam, may be judiciously used if carefully monitored, especially in patients prone to carbon dioxide (CO_2) retention. Large, sufficiently powered trials of selective serotonin reuptake inhibitors, tricyclic antidepressants, and buspirone in patients with COPD have not been reported, but small studies suggest that these agents are effective and reasonably tolerated, although onset to benefit may require weeks (Jain and Lolak 2009; Shapiro et al. 2011). Short-term relief for individuals who cannot safely tolerate benzodiazepines may be achieved with off-label use of gabapentin, hydroxyzine, pregabalin, or some antipsychotics. Nicotine replacement will relieve the acute withdrawal anxiety that these patients experience when hospitalized.

Psychotherapy and other strategies.   Biofeedback, cognitive-behavioral therapy (CBT), progressive relaxation, and pulmonary rehabilitation are sometimes helpful for anxiety disorders in patients with COPD, although results vary. These approaches have the advantage of not requiring patient adherence to a psychotropic medication regimen in a population that often already feels burdened by pharmacology and is prone to poor medication compliance (Maurer et al. 2008).

Depression

Depression is common among patients with COPD. Although prevalence rates vary from 20% to 70% in various studies (Maurer et al. 2008; Solano et al. 2006), patients with stable COPD have the lowest rates, followed by those who recently recovered from an acute exacerbation, followed by those with ongoing severe disease (Jain and Lolak 2009).

Management.   Management strategies, including antidepressants, CBT, pulmonary rehabilitation, and electroconvulsive therapy have all been used safely and effectively for depression in patients with COPD, although outcome data are less plentiful for depression than for anxiety disorders (Putman-Casdorph and McCrone 2009; Schak et al. 2008). Patients who smoke and hope to stop may benefit from selection of bupropion as an antidepressant.

Asthma

Asthma afflicted about 24.5 million Americans in 2009 (American Lung Association 2011). Age-adjusted mortality rates rise in socioeconomically disadvantaged groups. Although asthma was once construed as a truly psychosomatic illness with psychological causation, current research focuses instead on the complex interrelationship between asthma and psychological factors because this web can complicate both accurate diagnosis and effective management.

Anxiety Disorders

Anxiety disorders, particularly panic disorder and posttraumatic stress disorder, are nearly twice as common in patients with asthma as in those without (Jain and Lolak 2009; Roy-Byrne et al. 2008). Cause and effect may be interdependent: evidence suggests that poor mental health and increased stress can contribute to airway instability, whereas some asthma medications increase anxiety (Jain and Lolak 2009).

Psychopharmacological management.   Psychopharmacological management of anxiety disorders in patients with asthma is the same as for other patients with anxiety disorders, although benzodiazepines should be used cautiously in individuals with a known propensity for CO_2 retention.

Psychotherapy and other strategies.   Although results are encouraging, psychological interventions such as biofeedback, relaxation therapy, and CBT have not been sufficiently studied in patients with asthma to affirm definitive effectiveness (Yorke et al. 2007).

Depression

In older adults with asthma, depression occurs more commonly than anxiety disorders and is associated with increased use of health care resources and increased likelihood of medical hospitalization within the subsequent year (Jain and Lolak 2009).

Management.   Management strategies, whether pharmacological or psychological, should be chosen with particular attention to the patient's investment in treatment, because depressed mood contributes to less commitment to self-care and adherence to the treatment plan.

Ventilator Dependence

As the population has aged, the medical comorbidity in patients undergoing major surgical interventions has increased; infections and other postoperative complications increase the duration of ventilator dependence. The psychiatrist is often consulted when the patient does not make the desired progress toward ventilator independence. Delirium, anxiety, and depression may all compromise or delay successful ventilator weaning (Shapiro et al. 2011). Anger, frustration, loneliness, and discouragement are commonly experienced by individuals obliged to remain on a ventilator (Castillo and Egan 1974; Pattison and Watson 2009).

Delirium

Delirium in ventilator-dependent patients may be particularly aggravated by hypoxia, pain, analgesics, sedatives, and sleep deprivation; other common precipitants of delirium, such as infection and metabolic derangements, are also frequent.

Management.   Management may sometimes require thorough sedation with propofol or dexmedetomidine until other physiological and metabolic aberrations are addressed. However, continuous sedation by infusion is associated with increased duration of mechanical ventilation, longer hospital lengths of stay, and increased rates of organ failure (Brush and Kress 2009). Reversing the delirium, when possible, is imperative to clear the path for an accurate assessment of anxiety or depression and to enable the patient to collaborate constructively in the ventilator weaning process.

Anxiety

Anxiety may be fueled in ventilator-dependent patients by inability to talk; loss of independence; immersion in a tangle of tubes and insistent alarms; excessively rapid taper of sedatives; inability to move, cough, or use the toilet; fear of the uncertain future; and the presence of gowned and masked staff and visitors.

Management.   Management of anxiety in ventilator-dependent patients may include judicious use of benzodiazepines. Other agents with less potential for a direct effect on respiratory function include antipsychotics, such as haloperidol (with the added advantage of its ability to be given intravenously); the anxiolytic hydroxyzine (except when anticholinergic effects may outweigh the benefit); and possibly the anticonvulsant gabapentin. Equally important, by encouraging the patient to make persistent attempts at communication (e.g., lip articulation or writing), explaining to the patient the surroundings and meaning of the various alarms and functions of the different teams, and consistently coaching the patient in weaning strategies, health care providers better enable the patient to recapture some sense of understanding and participation, if not control.

Depression

A ventilator-dependent patient may develop depression or demoralization when faced with an unexpectedly prolonged intensive care stay, feelings that one's family is being unduly burdened, loss of autonomy and independent identity, ambivalence about consenting for the procedure, uncertain prognosis, and lack of connection with and trust of a staff that changes with each shift.

Management.   Management of depression in a ventilator-dependent patient requires consideration of the typically long latency of response to conventional antidepressant agents. A small case report literature exists on the use of stimulants such as methylphenidate to alleviate depression more quickly and thereby allow the patient to engage in weaning and pulmonary rehabilitation sooner than would otherwise have been possible (Rothenhausler et al. 2000).

Restrictive Lung Diseases

Idiopathic Pulmonary Fibrosis

Idiopathic pulmonary fibrosis is the most common of the interstitial lung diseases. It primarily affects adults older than 40 years. No cure is available; immunosuppressive medications are used to suppress disease activity. Progressive dyspnea increases anxiety, and depression is estimated to occur in 25% of patients (Shanmugam et al. 2007).

Sarcoidosis

Sarcoidosis can affect multiple organ systems, but the lungs are a primary target. Of these patients, 5%–10% will have central nervous system involvement and may present with depression, psychosis, or cognitive decline. Depression occurs twice as frequently in patients with pulmonary sarcoidosis as in the general population; women experience a higher likelihood than men (Shanmugam et al. 2007). Stress has been associated with increased disease activity and progression; quality of life deteriorates with the diagnosis of sarcoidosis (Jain and Lolak 2009).

Pulmonary Hypertension

Pulmonary hypertension is a chronic disease of progressively increasing pulmonary arterial pressure that develops insidiously, often escaping detection for years after the first symptoms occur. Over the past 10 years, inhaled and oral prostacyclins (e.g., iloprost and sildenafil, respectively) and endothelin-antagonist drugs (e.g., bosentan) have improved mean survival from 2 years to 6–7 years. However, these agents are expensive ($18,000–$36,000 annually), and the improved exercise capacity has not yet been shown to translate into improved quality of life or other dimensions of mental health (Wryobeck et al. 2007).

Psychiatric Issues

Psychiatric issues for patients with pulmonary hypertension include panic disorder, present in 20% of patients, and depression, diagnosed in 10% (Shafazand et al. 2004). Additionally, patients with pulmonary hypertension experience significant reductions in their functional capacity but do not appear ill to family and friends, a fact that increases their social isolation and further impairs their ability to adapt to a foreshortened future and constricted role in life.

End-of-Life Issues

Palliative care deserves discussion among patients with pulmonary hypertension, but timing is difficult. In one study of 132 patients who received attempted cardiopulmonary resuscitation, it was unsuccessful in 80%, and only 8% survived beyond 1 week (Hoeper et al. 2002). Cessation of prostacyclins, particularly when administered intravenously, can precipitate death within hours or less; this has been likened to a decision to remove a conscious patient from ventilator support (Wryobeck et al. 2007), imposing a weighty decision on the patient and family.

Hyperventilation Syndrome

Hyperventilation syndrome (HVS) may occur in 10% of the population, although females in their 30s and 40s are at highest risk. An increased rate of breathing is easy to spot, but respiratory alkalosis and its sequelae of dizziness and paresthesias may also result from a less obvious increase in the depth of breathing. Although benign and usually self-limited to minutes (but occasionally hours), HVS needs to be distinguished from medical causes of hyperventilation (e.g., pulmonary embolus, coronary insufficiency, diabetic ketoacidosis, salicylate ingestion, asthma, carbon monoxide poisoning) to ensure appropriate intervention. The majority of patients with HVS episodes recover spontaneously; others find beta-blockers, sedatives, or the bag rebreathing method helpful (Coffman and Levenson 2011; Shanmugam et al. 2007).

Tuberculosis

Tuberculosis had been steadily waning in the latter half of the twentieth century following the discovery in 1951 that isoniazid was an effective antitubercular agent. However, with the advent of AIDS, increasing substance abuse, and the emergence of drug-resistant strains, the incidence of tuberculosis is now increasing once again. Individuals who abuse alcohol and other substances are at increased risk of acquiring tuberculosis. Alcohol dependence and a history of mental illness also increase the risk of mania or psychosis with isoniazid therapy (Coffman and Levenson 2011).

Psychiatric Symptoms Associated With Pulmonary Medications

Systemic Corticosteroids

Systemic corticosteroids, especially when administered in higher dosages (e.g., prednisone 80 mg/day or more), are well known to induce emotional lability, acute dysphoria, mania, cognitive dysfunction, and even psychosis.

Management

Management by steroid dosage reduction or by addition of antipsychotics, benzodiazepines, anticonvulsants, or lithium has been effective, although anticonvulsant or lithium augmentation requires more time and is therefore more practical when sustained use of steroids is anticipated (Shanmugam et al. 2007).

Theophylline

Theophylline, although not commonly used in the hospital, may increase restlessness and anxiety, lower the seizure threshold, and increase lithium clearance by 20%–30% (Coffman and Levenson 2011).

Inhaled Bronchodilators and Anticholinergics

Inhaled bronchodilators and anticholinergics do not appear to have significant psychiatric side effects (Shanmugam et al. 2007).

Rifampin

Rifampin, used in tuberculosis treatment, affects multiple cytochrome P450 isoenzymes; through 3A4 induction, rifampin can decrease effective levels of diazepam, valproic acid, and tricyclic antidepressants (Coffman and Levenson 2011).

References

American Lung Association: Trends in Asthma Morbidity and Mortality. July 2011. Available at: http://www.lungusa.org/finding-cures/our-research/epidemiology-and-statistics-rpts.html. Accessed July 29, 2011.

Brenes GA: Anxiety and chronic obstructive pulmonary disease: prevalence, impact, and treatment. Psychosom Med 65:963–970, 2003

Brush DR, Kress JP: Sedation and analgesia for the mechanically ventilated patient. Clin Chest Med 30:131–141, 2009

Castillo A, Egan H: How it feels to be a ventilator patient. Respir Care 19:289–293, 1974

Coffman K, Levenson JL: Lung disease, in The American Psychiatric Publishing Textbook of Psychosomatic Medicine, 2nd Edition. Edited by Levenson JL. Washington, DC, American Psychiatric Publishing, 2011, pp 441–462

Davydow DS, Desai SV, Needham DM, et al: Psychiatric morbidity in survivors of the acute respiratory distress syndrome: a systematic review. Psychosom Med 70:512–519, 2008

Hoeper MM, Galié N, Murali S, et al: Outcome after cardiopulmonary resuscitation in patients with pulmonary arterial hypertension. Am J Respir Crit Care Med 165:341–344, 2002

Jain A, Lolak S: Psychiatric aspects of chronic lung disease. Curr Psychiatry Rep 11:219–225, 2009

Maurer J, Rebbapragada V, Borson S, et al: Anxiety and depression in COPD: current understanding, unanswered questions, and research needs. Chest 134 (suppl):43S–56S, 2008

Pattison N, Watson J: Ventilatory weaning: a case study of protracted weaning. Nurs Crit Care 14:75–85, 2009

Putman-Casdorph H, McCrone S: Chronic obstructive pulmonary disease, anxiety, and depression: state of the science. Heart Lung 38:34–47, 2009

Rothenhausler HB, Ehrentraut S, von Degenfeld G, et al: Treatment of depression with methylphenidate in patients difficult to wean from mechanical ventilation in the intensive care unit. J Clin Psychiatry 61:750–755, 2000

Roy-Byrne PP, Davidson KW, Kessler RC, et al: Anxiety disorders and comorbid medical illness. Gen Hosp Psychiatry 30:208–225, 2008

Schak KM, Mueller PS, Barnes R, et al: The safety of ECT in patients with chronic obstructive pulmonary disease. Psychosomatics 49:208–211, 2008

Shafazand S, Goldstein MK, Doyle RL, et al: Health-related quality of life in patients with pulmonary arterial hypertension. Chest 126:1452–1459, 2004

Shanmugam G, Bhutani S, Khan DA, et al: Psychiatric considerations in pulmonary disease. Psychiatr Clin North Am 30:761–780, 2007

Shapiro PA, Fedoronko DA, Epstein LA, et al: Psychiatric aspects of heart and lung disease in critical care. Heart Fail Clin 7:109–125, 2011

Solano JP, Gomes B, Higginson IJ: A comparison of symptom prevalence in far advanced cancer, AIDS, heart disease, chronic obstructive pulmonary disease and renal disease. J Pain Symptom Manage 31:58–69, 2006

Wryobeck JM, Lippo G, McLaughlin V, et al: Psychosocial aspects of pulmonary hypertension: a review. Psychosomatics 48:467–475, 2007

Yorke J, Fleming SL, Shuldham C: Psychological interventions for adults with asthma: a systematic review. Respir Med 101:1–14, 2007

27

Rehabilitation Medicine

Rehabilitation medicine is a diverse specialty: patients are young and old, abruptly deprived of health or debilitated by inexorable senescence, whole in body but not mind, or perhaps fully cognizant but unable to move. Regardless of whether the issue at hand is acute or chronic, restoration of function to whatever degree possible invariably requires the attention and effort of a multidisciplinary team. Such teams are often well integrated and frequently include a psychologist who provides a wide range of vital services to the patient and family. Consequently, a request for psychiatric consultation often arises well into the course of the patient's rehabilitative work, after other strategies have fallen short. The prudent psychiatrist remembers that he or she is joining an existing team and, in developing an understanding of the patient, will harvest history and observations from the full spectrum of caregivers, some of whom spend extended daily time with the patient. Although the range of problems encountered in rehabilitation medicine is broad, only three of the more common difficulties that prompt psychiatric evaluation are discussed in this chapter: traumatic brain injury (TBI), stroke, and spinal cord injury.

Traumatic Brain Injury

TBI is common, costly, and consequential (Fann et al. 2011; Rao and Lyketsos 2002). Of the 2 million Americans who incur a TBI each year, 25% are hospitalized. Although improved acute care has dramatically reduced mortality, it has thereby increased morbidity and long-term disability. The incidence of TBI is bimodal: vehicular accidents, violence, sports, and workplace injury cause a peak incidence in young adults ages 15–24 years, and falls account for a second peak in the over-60 population. Alcohol is associated with half of all cases. The sequelae of TBI are substantial: 25% of those who sustain an injury are unable to return to work in the year following the event, and many of these individuals require occupational, speech, and physical therapy to recapture a measure of independent function. Cognitive and behavioral difficulties range from mild to severe and frequently do not correlate with overt signs of injury, adding complexity to the individual's efforts to reengage society.

Primary Brain Injury

Primary brain injury includes both focal and diffuse damage due to mechanical forces at the time of the trauma.

Focal Injury

Focal injury is typically caused by a direct blow to the head. The internal architecture of the skull, with bony ridges cradling the inferior aspect of the frontal and temporal lobes, renders these locations especially susceptible to coup-contrecoup injuries.

Cerebral contusion.   Cerebral contusion commonly results in a loss of consciousness. Although recovery is the rule, focal neurological signs and symptoms such as headache, altered coordination and balance, disorientation, confusion, and seizures may persist for several weeks. Generally, structural damage is not evident on imaging studies, although postinjury edema may occur (Simon et al. 1999).

Subdural hematoma.   Subdural hematoma is caused by venous shearing in the space between the dura mater lining the interior of the skull and the arachnoid mater that wraps the cortex. Acute subdural hematomas often result from extreme acceleration or deceleration injuries and, without rapid surgical decompression, result in a mortality rate approaching 75%. In contrast, chronic subdural hematomas may develop over weeks and remain largely asymptomatic (Marik et al. 2002).

Epidural hematoma. Epidural hematoma is usually associated with a lateral skull fracture, rupture of the middle meningeal artery or vein, and temporal or temporoparietal injury. Initial loss of consciousness may be followed by a deceptive return of lucidity before neurological decline begins to accelerate; urgent surgical evacuation of the clot is imperative (Marik et al. 2002).

Diffuse Axonal Injury

Diffuse axonal injury is more commonly the result of rotational forces or rapid changes in velocity rather than direct trauma. Computed tomography is commonly unrevealing; diffusion-weighted magnetic resonance imaging may disclose axonal edema, but this edema is not typically immediately evident. Normal results from head imaging followed by changes in cognition and consciousness should alert the physician to diffuse injury (Lezak 1995).

Secondary Brain Injury

Secondary brain injury is the result of a cascade of physiological changes that develop in the wake of trauma and often in concert with the more gradual development of swelling that introduces increased pressure and structural challenge within the fixed boundaries of the skull.

Prognostic Factors

The following premorbid factors are associated with less favorable outcomes for patients with TBI (Silver et al. 2002):

- Comorbid substance abuse disorder
- Older age
- Lower IQ
- History of prior brain injury

The following posttraumatic factors are associated with less favorable outcomes:

- Loss of consciousness greater than 5 minutes
- Amnesia greater than 12 hours
- New onset or exacerbation of preexisting seizures

Clinical Disorders and Syndromes

Personality Patterns and Associated Behaviors

Personality patterns and associated behaviors change in 25% of individuals with TBI; changes may include aggression, apathy, disinhibition, labile affect, and poor social manners. These patients may be uncharacteristically careless, irritable, oblivious, suspicious, and unkempt (Koponen et al. 2002).

Cognitive Dysfunction

After TBI, patients may experience memory, language, and executive function disorders. Retraining can, over time, ease but not erase the net debilitation. Neuropsychological testing is essential to adequately assess executive deficits and design a focused rehabilitation program.

Chronic Pain

Chronic pain is an underdiagnosed result of TBI; the incidence is independent of posttraumatic stress disorder (PTSD) and depression (Nampiaparampil 2008).

Mood Disorders

Mood disorders occur in 25% of individuals following a mild TBI, and higher rates occur in those with more severe injuries. Prior substance abuse or mood disorder, less education, and erratic employment history presage a higher incidence of depression (Dikman et al. 2004). In one study of more than 500 adults with TBI, less than half who met criteria for major depression received antidepressants or counseling; the occurrence of major depression was an independent predictor of poorer quality of life 1 year after injury (Bombardier et al. 2010). Pseudobulbar affect is discussed later in this chapter in the section on stroke.

Anxiety Disorders

Anxiety disorders, most commonly generalized anxiety disorder and PTSD, may also develop after TBI.

Substance Abuse or Dependence

Substance abuse or dependence is a substantial risk factor for patients with TBI. In multiple studies, "at-risk" alcohol drinking patterns were present in more than 50% of patients, and toxicology evidence of illicit substance use was present in more than one-third of patients. Although substance abuse rates decline following TBI, problematic use persists and complicates the multiple challenges faced by patients with TBI (Graham and Cardon 2008).

War-Related Traumatic Brain Injury

War-related TBI has become an increasing medical concern. In one survey of 2,525 U.S. Army infantry soldiers approximately 3 months after a year-long deployment in Iraq, 5% reported injuries resulting in loss of consciousness, and 10% reported injuries with altered mental status. Of those who lost consciousness, 45% met criteria for PTSD, compared with 25% of those who experienced altered mental status, 15% of the soldiers with non-TBI injuries, and 10% of those who were uninjured (Hoge et al. 2008). The contextual factors of combat-related injury (e.g., less likely role of substance use as a causative factor, injury's occurrence during service to country, occupational consequences of injury) may influence the psychiatric aftermath in comparison with civilian injury, but data are not yet available.

Neuropsychiatric sequelae of war-related TBIs have been grouped as follows (Halbauer et al. 2009):

- Cognitive dysfunctions, including difficulties in memory, attention, and language
- Neurobehavioral disorders, such as depression, PTSD, and sleep problems
- Somatosensory disruptions, frequently caused by trauma to sensory organs
- Somatic symptoms, primarily headache and chronic pain
- Substance dependence

Treatment and Management

Treatment and management of the consequences of TBI are best addressed by an integrated and multidisciplinary effort. The disruptions experienced by patients with TBI are often complex, crossing multiple domains and extending beyond the injured person.

Coordinated Rehabilitation

When possible, coordinated rehabilitation, with contributions from social work, occupational therapy, psychology, and psychiatry, will enable the patient to maximize his or her potential. The following components may be helpful:

- Cognitive rehabilitation
- Stress management
- Creating structure and developing routine
- Family education

Pharmacotherapy

Pharmacotherapy is an important adjunct for patients with Axis I disorders, severe behavioral disturbances, or both. The injured brain is often more sensitive and may require longer to respond fully, underscoring the importance of beginning with a low dose, advancing slowly, and coaching patience and persistence to individuals who often find such qualities in short supply.

Antidepressants. Selective serotonin reuptake inhibitors (SSRIs) improve mood and diminish aggression (Perino et al. 2001). Careful consideration should be given before using bupropion, which lowers seizure threshold, or tricyclic antidepressants (TCAs), which increase sensitivity to side effects, including orthostasis and anticholinergic aggravation of cognitive dysfunction.

Stimulants. Dopamine agonists have been used to target post-TBI apathy and fatigue. Methylphenidate has demonstrated improved mental processing speed and reduced intensive care unit and hospital length of stay after acute TBI, but neither of these benefits was correlated with methylphenidate's effect on depression (Moein et al. 2006; Whyte et al. 1997). Amantadine has also demonstrated improved cognition and executive function in patients with TBI (Kraus et al. 2005; Sawyer et al. 2008).

Anticonvulsants. Anticonvulsants stabilize mania. Lithium use is not recommended due to increased adverse effects and possible neurotoxicity.

Antipsychotics. Antipsychotics may calm agitation (Kim and Bijlani 2006), but psychiatrists should consider avoiding high-potency, strongly anticholinergic, and seizure threshold–lowering antipsychotics. Patients with TBI are more sensitive to extrapyramidal side effects.

Benzodiazepines. Benzodiazepines may calm and relieve anxiety, but in TBI patients, they have narrower therapeutic index free of cognitive and motor compromise compared with their use in non-TBI patients.

Stroke

About 800,000 Americans annually have strokes, and about half of these individuals develop neuropsychiatric aftereffects (Carson et al. 2011). Eight-five percent of strokes are ischemic, and three-quarters of individuals survive the first year following ischemic strokes. The remaining 15% of strokes are hemorrhagic, and only one-third of individuals with hemorrhagic strokes survive the first year. The prevalence of stroke survivors in America is about 3 million. Stroke is the most common cause of disability and the third most common cause of death in the United States.

Stroke Sequelae

Stroke sequelae may include alterations in mental status, cognition, and behavior.

Delirium

Delirium affects one-third of patients in the days immediately following a stroke and is associated with a longer length of hospitalization and increased risk of subsequent dementia (Henon et al. 1999).

Depression

Depression occurs in one-third of stroke patients, with a peak incidence 6–24 months poststroke (Hackett et al. 2005). Probability is increased for patients with a prior history of depression, poor premorbid function, and isolation, but probability is not related to severity of the stroke itself (Ouimet et al. 2001). If untreated, poststroke depression contributes to diminished long-term social and motor function, as well as increased mortality, with odds ratios of 3.1 at 12 months and 2.2 at 24 months (House et al. 2001).

Anxiety

Anxiety occurs in about 25% of poststroke patients and more often than not is accompanied by comorbid depression (Carson et al. 2011).

Cognitive Impairment

Cognitive impairment, including dementia, occurs in 25% of poststroke patients (Carson et al. 2011).

Behavioral Changes

Some behavioral changes correlate approximately to the location of the stroke lesion and may overlap with the symptoms of specific psychiatric disorders (Huffman et al. 2010):

- Orbitofrontal region—disinhibition and irritability
- Dorsolateral frontal lobe—executive dysfunction
- Medial frontal lobe—apathy and abulia
- Left frontal lobe—nonfluent (Broca's) aphasia
- Left temporal lobe—fluent (Wernicke's) aphasia and short-term memory impairment to verbal and written stimuli
- Left parietal lobe—acalculia, agraphia, and right/left disorientation
- Right frontal lobe—motor dysprosody
- Right temporal lobe—sensory dysprosody and short-term memory impairment to nonverbal stimuli (e.g., music)
- Right parietal lobe—anosognosia, constructional apraxia, and hemineglect
- Occipital lobes—cortical blindness with unawareness of the visual disturbance

Other Behavioral Phenomena

Pseudobulbar affect. Pseudobulbar affect, also described as emotional incontinence, occurs in multiple neurological conditions that affect the central nervous system and is characterized by incongruent episodes of laughter or crying that erupt without the control of the patient, often in inappropriate settings that prompt frustration and embarrassment, and that do not correspond to any experience of relief at having expressed felt emotion on the part of the patient (Chriki et al. 2006).

Catastrophic reaction. Catastrophic reaction typically includes an outburst of anger, frustration, desperation, and acute dysphoria in the poststroke period when the individual is confronted with either a change or a challenge, such as moving from one's home to a skilled nursing facility. The incidence may be higher in individuals with a history of psychiatric illness and left-hemispheric involvement; catastrophic reaction overlaps considerably but not completely with poststroke depression (Huffman et al. 2010).

Poststroke fatigue.   Poststroke fatigue, which is distinct from depression and characterized by early exhaustion after physical or mental activity and consequent aversion to activity, occurs in 25%–50% of poststroke patients and may significantly inhibit rehabilitation effort; basal ganglia and brain stem strokes are associated with greater risk (Annoni et al. 2008; Tang et al. 2010).

Treatment

Depression and Anxiety

Antidepressants.   SSRIs and TCAs are effective for poststroke depression, as demonstrated in several placebo-controlled trials. SSRIs may be better tolerated and have the potential advantage of contributing to reduced platelet aggregation (Bhogal et al. 2005; Hackett et al. 2005; Ramasubbu and Patten 2003; Starkstein et al. 2008). Although less well studied, venlafaxine proved effective in a small series, and only two of 30 patients experienced an increase in blood pressure (Kucukalic et al. 2007); mirtazapine has also been shown to be effective (Niedermaier et al. 2004). A meta-analysis from 16 randomized placebo-controlled trials suggested that the duration of antidepressant use beyond the initial month was associated with incremental further improvement (Chen et al. 2006).

Stimulants.   Uncontrolled prospective and retrospective studies support the efficacy and tolerability of stimulants in patients with poststroke depression (Grade et al. 1998; Masand and Tesar 1996). Stimulants have the advantage of more rapid onset of benefit, thereby facilitating patient motivation and collaboration with physical therapy and other rehabilitative efforts.

Benzodiazepines.   Benzodiazepines can relieve anxiety but are not effective for comorbid depression and may impede rehabilitation by blunting cognition and contributing to gait instability.

Cognitive-behavioral therapy.   Uncontrolled studies of cognitive-behavioral therapy for poststroke depression have been inconclusive (Lincoln and Flannaghan 2003; Starkstein et al. 2008), but a randomized controlled trial of problem-solving therapy suggested probable benefit in preventing depression over the first year after a stroke (Robinson et al. 2008).

Cognitive Impairment

Although many studies have been designed to clarify whether pharmacotherapy can enhance natural neuroplasticity and recovery, definitive data are lacking. Low-dose levodopa may improve recovery from aphasia (Seniow et al. 2009), and noradrenergic and dopaminergic agents appear to hold the most promise among other options (Czlonkowska and Lesniak 2009). Conversely, use of dopamine antagonists and benzodiazepines ought to be avoided (Czlonkowska and Lesniak 2009) unless clearly necessary. In poststroke patients, escitalopram improved motor and cognitive outcome at 12 months, independent of its effect on depression (Jorge et al. 2010). Other studies have shown that both SSRIs and TCAs improve cognitive function when comorbid depression is present (Kimura et al. 2000).

Pseudobulbar Affect

In small trials of patients, TCAs and SSRIs have proved helpful for treating pseudobulbar affect, even in the absence of depression. Dextromethorphan/quinidine combinations (the latter serves only as an inhibitor of dextromethorphan metabolism) have also demonstrated efficacy (Rosen and Cummings 2007).

Poststroke Fatigue

Poststroke fatigue was not alleviated by fluoxetine, but modafinil may prove helpful in patients with brain stem and diencephalic stroke (Brioschi et al. 2009).

Spinal Cord Injury

Although devastating, spinal cord injury (SCI) is relatively uncommon (about 1.25 million Americans are currently affected). Each of the following categories accounts for about 25% of all SCIs: motor vehicular accidents, occupational accidents, sporting and recreational injury, and falls (Carson et al. 2011; "One degree of separation" 2009). Males are twice as likely to be affected as females, and more than half of SCI patients are less than age 30 years at the time of injury. Half of all SCIs result in paraplegia and the other half in quadriplegia. Improved life expectancy translates into prolonged financial and caregiver burdens.

Psychiatric Comorbidities

Prompt psychiatric consultation is recommended when patients with SCI have any of the following comorbidities: alcohol abuse and dependence, depression, PTSD, or sexual dysfunction.

Alcohol Abuse and Dependence

Problematic drinking prior to injury (up to 50%) and intoxication at the time of injury (up to 40%) identify patients with SCI whose long-term outcome may be improved by initiating discussion of the role of alcohol use and the benefits of moderation, if not abstinence (Bombardier 2000; Turner et al. 2003).

Depression

Depression in patients with SCI presents a paradoxical challenge: although depression is prevalent in 25% of patients with SCI and is associated with increased morbidity and mortality, multiple studies have shown that caregivers expect depression to occur much more frequently and therefore both overestimate its occurrence and conclude that its absence betrays denial. Perversely, this expectation or normalization of depression may also lead to undertreatment in patients who do meet diagnostic criteria for major depression (Fann et al. 2011).

Posttraumatic Stress Disorder

PTSD is rare in individuals with quadriplegia but occurs in 20% of those with paraplegia; this disparity may reflect decreased awareness of physiological arousal in those with higher-level lesions. PTSD may be more likely to occur in those whose SCI was sustained in combat or who had prior exposure to violence (Kennedy and Duff 2001).

Sexual Dysfunction

Sexual dysfunction is commonly addressed by occupational therapists working with patients with SCI. The level and completeness of injury determine the degree of difficulty with lubrication in women, and of erectile and ejaculatory function in men. The capacity to experience orgasm may approach 50% in men and women, independent of injury characteristics (Fann et al. 2011). Substantive assessment and treatment strategies exist (Basson and Rees 2011).

Treatment

Treatment studies for psychiatric disorders in patients with SCI are uncommon. Psychiatrists must treat patients based on thoughtful integration of the known physiological sequelae of SCI and knowledge about the mechanism of action and likely side effects of various medications.

Pharmacological Agents

Patients with SCI are liable to gain weight and develop glucose intolerance and decreased gastrointestinal motility; they are also at increased risk of orthostasis and venous thrombosis (Fann et al. 2011). These are reasons to prefer SSRIs over TCAs, and perhaps bupropion over mirtazapine. Antispasticity agents are often sedating, emphasizing the potential merit of activating rather than soporific antidepressants.

Psychological Assistance

The preponderance of young, active patients and the circumstances under which SCIs occur may imbue the disability with particular meaning for patients; for example, feelings of self-recrimination and guilt are possible. These feelings deserve attention and may provide an opportunity for illustrating the practical value of developing cognitive-behavioral skills. For individuals whose premorbid routine included high activity levels, effective intervention and collaboration with the rehabilitation team may benefit from deliberate use of cognitive-behavioral therapy to reinforce participation in physical and occupational therapies.

References

Annoni JM, Staub F, Bogousslavsky J, et al: Frequency, characterization and therapies of fatigue after stroke. Neurol Sci 29:S244–S246, 2008

Basson R, Rees PM: Sexual dysfunction, in The American Psychiatric Publishing Textbook of Psychosomatic Medicine, 2nd Edition. Edited by Levenson JL. Washington, DC, American Psychiatric Publishing, 2011, pp 361–380

Bhogal SK, Teasell R, Foley N, et al: Heterocyclics and selective serotonin reuptake inhibitors in the treatment and prevention of poststroke depression. J Am Geriatr Soc 53:1051–1057, 2005

Bombardier CH: Alcohol and traumatic disability, in The Handbook of Rehabilitation Psychology. Edited by Frank R, Elliott T. Washington, DC, American Psychological Association Press, pp 399–416, 2000

Bombardier CH, Fann JR, Temkin NR, et al: Rates of major depressive disorder and clinical outcomes following traumatic brain injury. JAMA 303:1938–1945, 2010

Brioschi A, Gramigna S, Werth E, et al: Effect of modafinil on subjective fatigue in multiple sclerosis and stroke patients. Eur Neurol 62:243–249, 2009

Carson AJ, Zeman A, Stone J, et al: Neurology and neurosurgery, in The American Psychiatric Publishing Textbook of Psychosomatic Medicine, 2nd Edition. Edited by Levenson JL. Washington, DC, American Psychiatric Publishing, 2011, pp 759–795

Chen Y, Guo JJ, Zhan S, et al: Treatment effects of antidepressants in patients with post-stroke depression: a meta-analysis. Ann Pharmacother 40:2115–2122, 2006

Chriki LS, Bullain SS, Stern TA: The recognition and management of psychological reactions to stroke: a case discussion. Prim Care Companion J Clin Psychiatry 8:234–240, 2006

Czlonkowska A, Lesniak M: Pharmacotherapy in stroke rehabilitation. Expert Opin Pharmacother 10:1249–1259, 2009

Dikman SS, Bombardier CH, Machamer JE, et al: Natural history of depression in traumatic brain injury. Arch Phys Med Rehabil 85:1457–1464, 2004

Fann JR, Kennedy R, Bombardier CH: Physical medicine and rehabilitation, in The American Psychiatric Publishing Textbook of Psychosomatic Medicine, 2nd Edition. Edited by Levenson JL. Washington, DC, American Psychiatric Publishing, 2011, pp 855–899

Grade C, Redford B, Chrostowski J, et al: Methylphenidate in early poststroke recovery: a double-blind, placebo-controlled study. Arch Phys Med Rehabil 79:1047–1050, 1998

Graham DP, Cardon AL: An update on substance use and treatment following traumatic brain injury. Ann NY Acad Sci 1141:148–162, 2008

Hackett ML, Anderson CS, House AO: Management of depression after stroke: a systematic review of pharmacological therapies (review). Stroke 36:1098–1103, 2005

Halbauer JD, Ashford JW, Zeitzer JM, et al: Neuropsychiatric diagnosis and management of chronic sequelae of war-related mild to moderate traumatic brain injury. J Rehabil Res Dev 46:757–796, 2009

Henon H, Lebert F, Durieu I, et al: Confusional state in stroke: relation to pre-existing dementia, patient characteristics and outcome. Stroke 30:773–779, 1999

Hoge CW, McGurk D, Thomas JL, et al: Mild traumatic brain injury in U.S. soldiers returning from Iraq. N Engl J Med 358:453–463, 2008

House A, Knapp P, Bamford J, et al: Mortality at 12 and 24 months after stroke may be associated with depressive symptoms at 1 month. Stroke 32:696–701, 2001

Huffman JC, Brennan MM, Smith FA, et al: Patients with neurologic conditions. I: seizure disorders (including nonepileptic seizures), cerebrovascular disease, and traumatic brain injury, in Massachusetts General Hospital Handbook of General Hospital Psychiatry, 6th Edition. Edited by Stern TA, Fricchione GL, Cassem NH, et al. Philadelphia, PA, Saunders Elsevier, 2010, pp 237–253

Jorge RE, Acion L, Moser D, et al: Escitalopram and enhancement of cognitive recovery following stroke. Arch Gen Psychiatry 67:187–196, 2010

Kennedy P, Duff J: Post traumatic stress disorder and spinal cord injuries. Spinal Cord 39:1–10, 2001

Kim E, Bijlani M: A pilot study of quetiapine treatment of aggression due to traumatic brain injury. J Neuropsychiatry Clin Neurosci 18:547–549, 2006

Kimura M, Robinson RG, Kosier JT: Treatment of cognitive impairment after poststroke depression: a double-blind treatment trial. Stroke 31:1482–1486, 2000

Koponen S, Taiminem T, Portin R, et al: Axis I and II psychiatric disorders after traumatic brain injury: a 30-year follow-up study. Am J Psychiatry 159:1315–1321, 2002

Kraus MF, Smith GS, Butters M, et al: Effects of the dopaminergic agent and NMDA receptor antagonist amantadine on cognitive function, cerebral glucose metabolism and D2 receptor availability in chronic traumatic brain injury: a study using positron emission tomography (PET). Brain Inj 19:471–479, 2005

Kucukalic A, Bravo-Mehmedbasic A, Kulenovic AD, et al: Venlafaxine efficacy and tolerability in the treatment of post-stroke depression. Psychiatr Danub 19:56–60, 2007

Lezak MD: Neuropsychological Assessment, 3rd Edition. New York, Oxford University Press, 1995

Lincoln NB, Flannaghan T: Cognitive behavioral psychotherapy for depression following strokes: a randomized controlled trial. Stroke 34:111–115, 2003

Marik PE, Varon J, Trask T: Management of head trauma. Chest 122:699–711, 2002

Masand PS, Tesar GE: Use of stimulants in the medically ill. Psychiatr Clin North Am 19:515–547, 1996

Moein H, Khalili HA, Keramatian K: Effect of methylphenidate on ICU and hospital length of stay in patients with severe and moderate traumatic brain injury. Clin Neurol Neurosurg 108:539–542, 2006

Nampiaparampil DE: Prevalence of chronic pain after traumatic brain injury: a systematic review. JAMA 300:711–719, 2008

Niedermaier N, Bohrer E, Schulte K, et al: Prevention and treatment of poststroke depression with mirtazapine in patients with acute stroke. J Clin Psychiatry 65:1619–1623, 2004

One degree of separation: paralysis and spinal cord injury in the United States. Christopher and Dana Reeve Foundation. March 30, 2009. Available at: www.christopherreeve.org. Accessed January 1, 2011.

Ouimet MA, Primeau F, Cole MG: Psychosocial risk factors in poststroke depression: a systematic review. Can J Psychiatry 46:819–828, 2001

Perino C, Rago R, Cicolin A, et al: Mood and behavioral disorders following traumatic brain injury: clinical evaluation and pharmacological management. Brain Inj 15:139–148, 2001

Ramasubbu R, Patten SB: Effect of depression on stroke morbidity and mortality (review). Can J Psychiatry 48:250–257, 2003

Rao V, Lyketsos CG: Psychiatric aspects of traumatic brain injury. Psychiatr Clin North Am 25:43–69, 2002

Robinson RG, Jorge RE, Moser DJ, et al: Escitalopram and problem-solving therapy for prevention of poststroke depression. JAMA 299:2391–2400, 2008

Rosen HF, Cummings J: A real reason for patients with pseudobulbar affect to smile. Ann Neurol 34:717–719, 2007

Sawyer E, Mauro LS, Ohlinger MJ: Amantadine enhancement of arousal and cognition after traumatic brain injury. Ann Pharmacother 42:247–252, 2008

Seniow J, Litwin M, Litwin T, et al: New approach to the rehabilitation of post-stroke focal cognitive syndrome: effect of levodopa combined with speech and language therapy on functional recovery from aphasia. J Neurol Sci 283:214–218, 2009

Silver JM, Hales RE, Yudofsky SC: Neuropsychiatric aspects of traumatic brain injury, in The American Psychiatric Publishing Textbook of Neuropsychiatry and Clinical Neurosciences, 4th Edition. Edited by Yudofsky SC, Hales RE. Washington, DC, American Psychiatric Publishing, 2002, pp 625–672

Simon RP, Aminoff MJ, Greenberg DA: Clinical Neurology, 4th Edition. Stamford, CT, Appleton and Lange, 1999, pp 1–49

Starkstein SE, Mizrahi R, Power BD: Antidepressant therapy in post-stroke depression. Expert Opin Pharmacother 9:1291–1298, 2008

Tang WK, Chen YK, Mok V, et al: Acute basal ganglia infarcts in poststroke fatigue: an MRI study. J Neurol 257:178–182, 2010

Turner AP, Bombardier CH, Rimmele CT: A typology of alcohol use patterns among persons with recent traumatic brain injury or spinal cord injury: implications for treatment matching. Arch Phys Med Rehabil 84:358–364, 2003

Whyte J, Hart T, Schuster K, et al: Effects of methylphenidate on attentional function after traumatic brain injury: a randomized, placebo-controlled trial. Am J Phys Med Rehabil 76:440–450, 1997

28

Transplantation

More than 20,000 transplantations occur in the United States each year, and well over 100,000 individuals are on waiting lists. Psychosomatic medicine psychiatrists commonly participate in consultations during pretransplant, perioperative, recovery, and posttransplant periods. The degree to which the psychiatrist is accepted as a member of the transplant team depends on several factors (Skotzko and Strouse 2002): the ability to communicate effectively and succinctly with other team members; the extent to which his or her clinical judgment is trusted; the ability to effectively defuse adverse transplant team member reactions to patients; and the ability to work collaboratively and effectively with other transplant team members.

General Issues

Psychiatric Symptoms

Long waits for transplants and graft survival rates (e.g., 10-year graft survival rates of 35% for kidneys and 45% for livers) create stresses for transplantation candidates, recipients, and families (DiMartini et al. 2011). The biological manifestations of organ failure and the treatments administered as part of organ failure and transplantation care cause significant neuropsychiatric morbidity during all phases of care of transplantation candidates and patients.

Health Systems

Psychiatric factors such as psychotic symptoms, personality disorders, social support, and substance use patterns are related to transplantation outcome measures in positive and negative directions (Kotlyar et al. 2008). Psychiatric consultation findings are associated with medical outcomes, including length of stay, readmission duration, adherence with medications, and even mortality (Foster et al. 2009). Psychosomatic medicine psychiatrists have important roles in helping the transplant team manage psychiatric symptoms and disorders that impact outcomes.

Patient Categories

Research related to psychiatric factors that are important in transplantation outcomes has focused mostly on kidney, liver, and heart transplantations, which account for almost 90% of all solid organ transplants performed in the United States (DiMartini et al. 2011). Over 11,000 kidney transplants are performed annually, compared with about 4,000 liver transplants, 3,600 bone marrow transplants, 2,000 heart transplants, 1,800 pancreas transplants, and 900 lung transplants (DiMartini et al. 2011). Most transplantation psychiatry programs in the United States conceptualize their consultative practices around pretransplantation, perioperative and postsurgical recovery, and posttransplantation periods.

Pretransplantation Issues

End-Organ Failure

Neuropsychiatric differential diagnosis and psychopharmacological management can be quite complicated in patients being evaluated for transplantation with organ failure, and in patients with organ failure who do not qualify for or who do not receive transplants. The medications usually recommended by psychosomatic medicine psychiatrists to treat psychiatric symptoms may require significant caution and alteration in the setting of end-organ failure.

Renal Disease

Reduced renal clearance requires avoidance (or careful monitoring when use is necessary) of medications predominantly excreted by the kidneys; these medications include lithium, gabapentin, topiramate, and methylphenidate (DiMartini et al. 2011). In addition, some psychotropic medications, including venlafaxine, have active metabolites that are excreted largely by the kidneys. Hypoalbuminemia associated with renal disease can increase free drug concentrations.

Liver Disease

Pharmacological issues.   Loss of liver tissue and decreased hepatic perfusion decrease metabolism of medications, effectively raising drug levels. This elevation in drug levels, in turn, heightens risks of increased liver toxicity and drug adverse effects and interactions. Therefore, doses of psychiatric medications, when used, are reduced 25%–75% from usual levels, depending on the degree of liver disease (DiMartini et al. 2011).

Hepatic encephalopathy.   Hepatic encephalopathy is characterized by altered consciousness, cognitive impairment, and disorientation, and may include affective lability, perceptual disturbances, and asterixis. A fluctuating course is the pattern. Treatment focuses on reducing the production and absorption of ammonia. Lactulose is an osmotic laxative that is usually an effective treatment.

Heart Disease

Diminished cardiac capacity may lead to "third spacing" and increased volume of distribution of drugs into interstitial tissues, resulting in decreased drug metabolism and clearance (Shammas and Dickstein 1988). Hepatically cleared drugs are more affected in heart failure than are renally cleared drugs.

Lung Disease

Acute hypoxia may reduce splanchnic blood flow to the liver, decreasing drug metabolism and increasing drug levels. Hypoxia may also lead to reduced renal blood flow.

Psychiatric Pretransplantation Evaluation

Donor Evaluations

Heart transplants involve brain-dead donors; other types of transplants frequently involve living family donors. The consulting psychiatrist should evaluate potential interpersonal, marital, or family problems encountered by donor families. For example, the psychiatrist should consider whether a family's "black sheep" is donating out of a conscious or an unconscious desire to improve his or her standing in the family system.

Kidney donors. Living donors now outnumber cadaver donors for kidney transplants (DiMartini et al. 2011). The mortality rate for kidney donors is very low, calculated to be 0.03% (Surman and Prager 2004). Although preoperative donor anxiety may occur, it is generally self-limited when donors are psychiatrically screened beforehand (Surman and Prager 2004).

Liver donors. For right hepatic lobe liver donation by a living donor, morbidity is only about 1%, although medical complications occur in 36% and serious complications in 15%, reinforcing the need for careful psychiatric consultation (DiMartini et al. 2011) to assure appropriateness of candidacy for donation. Although psychiatric complications following liver donation are uncommon (4%) when donors are psychiatrically screened (Trotter et al. 2007), they may be serious and include suicidal behaviors. Postdonation mental health and quality of life outcomes are poorer for patients with predonation psychiatric diagnoses (DuBay et al. 2009). Although predonation psychiatric diagnoses do not exclude a patient from being a donor, psychiatrists should remain available for support to donors following transplantation procedures, especially when there are preexisting psychiatric issues.

Transplantation Recipient Evaluation

The psychiatric consultant on the transplant team conducts a wide-ranging evaluation of potential transplantation recipients. The presence or absence of a psychiatric disorder is only one factor in the overall assessment. Successful transplantation outcomes have been reported in patients who have mental retardation, anxiety disorders, mood disorders, substance use disorders, and personality disorders (Surman and Prager 2004). Factors such as allograft success, strength of social supports, and history of medical treatment adherence are also important considerations in behavioral evaluation of potential organ recipients.

Absolute contraindications.

- Active substance abuse
- Psychosis that limits capacity for informed consent or adherence
- Active suicidal ideation
- Factitious disorder with physical symptoms

- Consistent nonadherence to medical treatment
- Unwillingness to participate in necessary psychiatric treatment
- Unstable current mania

Relative contraindications.

- Dementia or other persistent cognitive dysfunction
- Inadequate psychosocial resources to support adherence
- Treatment-resistant mood disorder
- Schizophrenia
- Personality disorder with consequences for adherence
- Eating disorder
- Prominent and unmanageable behavioral dyscontrol
- Treatment-refractory psychiatric illness

Rating scales. Two scales are available for the clinical categorization of readiness for organ transplantation from a psychiatric perspective: the Psychosocial Assessment of Candidates for Transplantation (PACT; Olbrisch et al. 1989) and the Transplant Evaluation Rating Scale (TERS; Twillman et al. 1993). Both scales weight or consider psychiatric diagnoses, substance abuse, health behaviors, adherence, social support, and coping mechanisms. Both the PACT and TERS have good interrater reliability and predictive power (Skotzko and Strouse 2002).

Perioperative and Postsurgical Recovery Period Issues

Delirium and Other Secondary Psychiatric Disorders

Transplantation recipients are at risk for postoperative delirium and other secondary psychiatric disorders due to any of the following: existing central nervous system consequences of organ failure; the residua of general anesthesia; sometimes lengthy transplant surgery; volume and electrolyte shifts associated with surgery and perfusion of the new organ; postoperative opiate analgesia; effects of transplantation-specific medications, such as cyclosporine; and the potential complications of coagulopathy, fever, and infections.

Neuropsychiatric Effects of Immunosuppressive Medications

Cyclosporine

Tremor, restlessness, and headaches are common in patients taking cyclosporine. Up to one-third of patients may experience more severe side effects, such as seizures, delirium, or psychosis (DiMartini et al. 2011). Rare but potentially life-threatening side effects include central pontine myelinolysis and brain abscess.

Tacrolimus

Although the neuropsychiatric adverse effects of tacrolimus are similar to those of cyclosporine, they occur less frequently (Emiroglu et al. 2009). Intravenous administration may increase the relative risk, and the effects are dose related.

Mycophenolate Mofetil

Although considered better tolerated than its predecessor azathioprine, mycophenolate is nevertheless associated with neuropsychiatric symptoms in 3%–20% of transplant recipients who receive it. Effects include anxiety, depression, delirium, seizures, paresthesias, neuropathy, psychosis, and somnolence (DiMartini et al. 2011). The precise contribution of this medication to neuropsychiatric syndromes is hard to define because it is often given in combination with tacrolimus or cyclosporine.

Corticosteroids

High-dose steroids may be used in the acute postoperative period to treat acute rejection. Psychiatric side effects of corticosteroids may include dose-related delirium, psychosis, and mood changes.

Drug Interactions

Tacrolimus, mycophenolate, and cyclosporine are each largely metabolized by cytochrome P450 (CYP) 3A4. Psychotropic medications that inhibit this enzyme should be avoided; these include fluvoxamine, nefazodone, fluoxetine, sertraline, most tricyclic antidepressants, escitalopram, desvenlafaxine, and venlafaxine. In particular, fluvoxamine and nefazodone should be avoided due to the potential for potent enzyme inhibition. As of now, because CYP3A4 cannot be reliably tested pharmacogenomically, clinical knowledge and judgment are necessary to avoid potentially life-threatening drug interactions.

Posttransplantation Issues

Transplantation and Quality of Life

The physical benefits of transplantation have a markedly positive impact on posttransplantation psychological functioning and quality of life (Bravata et al. 1999; Vermuelen et al. 2009). Quality of life is an important outcome cited by patients in terms of reasons for pursuing transplantation to start with. Particularly for transplantations with relatively limited long-term survival (i.e., lung and heart transplants), quality of life and psychosocial functioning are important elements to weigh in the decision to have a transplant (Barbour et al. 2006).

Psychiatric Disorders and Posttransplantation Outcomes

Effect on Survival

Psychiatric disorders affect survival. Posttransplantation survival can be shortened by the presence of psychiatric illness, especially depression (Havik et al. 2007; Owen et al. 2006). Neurotoxic effects of immunosuppressive medications are more frequent in patients with excessive alcohol use prior to transplantation (DiMartini et al. 2008).

Risk of Resuming Risky Health Behaviors

The risk of postoperative resumption of risky health behaviors that were associated with the original end organ disease is significant. For example, 5%–20% of liver transplant recipients who had alcoholic liver disease may relapse to alcohol the first year after transplantation (Dew et al. 2008; DiMartini et al. 2006), and 15% or more of smokers who receive heart transplants may start smoking again (Nagele et al. 1997). Risk of alcohol use after liver transplant must be continually monitored.

Immunosuppressive Drug–Related Neuropsychiatric Syndromes

Immunosuppressive drugs can cause chronic neuropsychiatric syndromes. The use of chronic immunosuppressive drugs may be responsible for psychopathology that will need to be managed in ongoing psychiatric care that occurs in concert with posttransplantation medical care. The same precautions about neuropsychiatric adverse effects of medication and about drug interactions apply throughout the posttransplantation period, even when chronic immunosuppressant medication doses have equilibrated.

References

Barbour KA, Blumenthal JA, Palmer SM: Psychosocial issues in the assessment and management of patients undergoing lung transplantation. Chest 129:1367–1374, 2006

Bravata DM, Olkin I, Barnato AE, et al: Health-related quality of life after liver transplantation: a meta-analysis. Liver Transpl Surg 5:318–331, 1999

Dew MA, DiMartini AF, Steel J, et al: Meta-analysis of risk for relapse to substance use after transplantation of the liver or other solid organs. Liver Transpl 14:159–172, 2008

DiMartini A, Day N, Dew MA, et al: Alcohol consumption patterns and predictors of use following liver transplantation for alcoholic liver disease. Liver Transpl 12:813–820, 2006

DiMartini A, Fontes P, Dew MA, et al: Age, model for end-stage liver disease score, and organ functioning predict posttransplant tacrolimus neurotoxicity. Liver Transpl 14:815–822, 2008

DiMartini AF, Sotelo JL, Dew MA: Organ transplantation, in The American Psychiatric Publishing Textbook of Psychosomatic Medicine, 2nd Edition. Edited by Levenson JL. Washington, DC, American Psychiatric Publishing, 2011, pp 725–758

DuBay DA, Holtzman S, Adcock L, et al: Adult right-lobe living liver donors: quality of life, attitudes, and predictors of donor outcomes. Am J Transplant 9:1169–1178, 2009

Emiroglu R, Ayvaz I, Moray G, et al: Tacrolimus-related neurologic and renal complications in liver transplantation: a single-center experience. Transplant Proc 38:619–621, 2009

Foster LW, McLellan L, Rybicki L, et al: Utility of the Psychosocial Assessment of Candidates for Transplantation (PACT) scale in allogeneic BMT. Bone Marrow Transplant 44:375–380, 2009

Havik OE, Sivertsen B, Relbo A, et al: Depressive symptoms and all-cause mortality after heart transplantation. Transplantation 84:97–103, 2007

Kotlyar DS, Burke A, Campbell MS, et al: A critical review of candidacy for orthotopic liver transplantation in alcoholic liver disease. Am J Gastroenterol 103:734–743, 2008

Nagele H, Kalmar P, Rodiger W: Smoking after heart transplantation: an underestimated hazard? Eur J Cardiothorac Surg 12:70–74, 1997

Olbrisch ME, Levenson J, Hamer R: The PACT: a rating scale for the study of clinical decision making in psychosocial screening criteria for organ transplant candidates. Clin Transplant 3:164–169, 1989

Owen JE, Bonds CL, Wellisch DK: Psychiatric evaluations of heart transplant candidates: predicting post-transplant hospitalizations, rejection episodes, and survival. Psychosomatics 47:213–222, 2006

Shammas FV, Dickstein K: Clinical pharmacokinetics in heart failure: an updated review. Clin Pharmacokinet 15:94–113, 1988

Skotzko CE, Strouse TB: Solid organ transplantation, in The American Psychiatric Publishing Textbook of Consultation-Liaison Psychiatry: Psychiatry in the Medically Ill, 2nd Edition. Edited by Wise MG, Rundell JR. Washington, DC, American Psychiatric Publishing, 2002, pp 623–655

Surman OS, Prager LM: Organ failure and transplantation, in Massachusetts General Hospital Handbook of General Hospital Psychiatry, 5th Edition. Edited by Stern TL, Fricchione GL, Cassem NH, et al. St. Louis, MO, Mosby, 2004, pp 641–670

Trotter JF, Hill-Callahan MM, Gillespie BW: Severe psychiatric problems in right hepatic lobe donors for living donor liver transplantation. Transplantation 83:1506–1508, 2007

Twillman RK, Manetto C, Wolcott DL: The Transplant Evaluation Rating Scale: a revision of the psychosocial levels system for evaluating organ transplant candidates. Psychosomatics 34:144–153, 1993

Vermuelen KM, van der Bij W, Erasmus ME, et al: Long-term health-related quality of life after lung transplantation: different predictors for different dimensions. J Heart Lung Transplant 26:188–193, 2009

Index

CPSIA information can be obtained
at www.ICGtesting.com
Printed in the USA
FSHW021922040519
57826FS